Therapeutic Strategies

LIPID DISORDERS

Edited by

Andrew M. Tonkin
Professor of Medicine; Consultant Cardiologist;
Head, Cardiovascular Research Unit, Department of Epidemiology
and Preventive Medicine, School of Public Health and
Preventive Medicine, Monash University, Melbourne, Australia

Foreword by

Eugene Braunwald, MD
Distinguished Hersey Professor of Medicine, Harvard Medical School;
Chairman, TIMI Study Group, Brigham and Women's Hospital, Boston,
Massachusetts, USA

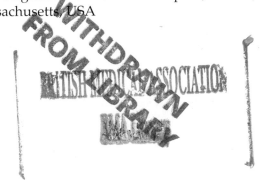

CLINICAL PUBLISHING

OXFORD

Clinical Publishing
an imprint of Atlas Medical Publishing Ltd

Oxford Centre for Innovation
Mill Street, Oxford OX2 0JX, UK
Tel: +44 1865 811116
Fax: +44 1865 251550
Email: info@clinicalpublishing.co.uk
Web: www.clinicalpublishing.co.uk

Distributed in USA and Canada by:
Clinical Publishing
30 Amberwood Parkway
Ashland OH 44805 USA
Tel: 800-247-6553 (toll free within USA and Canada)
Fax: 419-281-6883
Email: order@bookmasters.com

Distributed in UK and Rest of World by:
Marston Book Services Ltd
PO Box 269
Abingdon
Oxon OX14 4YN, UK
Tel: +44 1235 465500
Fax: +44 1235 465555
Email: trade.orders@marston.co.uk

A catalogue record for this book is available from the British Library.

ISBN 13   978 1 84692 034 9
ISBN e-book 978 1 84692 601 3

The publisher makes no representation, express or implied, that the dosages in this book are correct. Readers must therefore always check the product information and clinical procedures with the most up-to-date published product information and data sheets provided by the manufacturers and the most recent codes of conduct and safety regulations. The authors and the publisher do not accept any liability for any errors in the text or for the misuse or misapplication of material in this work.

Project manager: Gavin Smith, GPS Publishing Solutions, Hertfordshire, UK
Typeset by Mizpah Publishing Services Private Limited, Chennai, India
Printed by the MPG Books Group in the UK

Therapeutic Strategies

LIPID DISORDERS

Contents

Editor and Contributors   vii

Foreword   xi

1   A global view of cardiovascular risk factors   1
    C. K. Chow, A. A. Patel

2   Low-density lipoprotein cholesterol as a therapeutic target   15
    J. Armitage, L. Bowman

3   High-density lipoprotein as a therapeutic target   29
    P. Barter, K.-A. Rye

4   Apolipoprotein B in the therapy of atherogenic dyslipoproteinaemias   43
    A. D. Sniderman

5   Management of coronary heart disease patients   59
    K. K. Ray, C. P. Cannon

6   Stroke and transient ischaemic attack prevention   77
    P. Amarenco, P. Lavallée, M. Mazighi, J. Labreuche

7   Diabetes and the metabolic syndrome   87
    A. J. Cameron, J. Shaw, P. Zimmet

8   Hypertension   107
    R. H. Grimm, Jr

9   Treatment of familial hypercholesterolaemia   117
    R. Huijgen, H. J. Avis, B. A. Hutten, M. N. Vissers, J. J. P. Kastelein

10 Lipid lowering in chronic kidney disease   135
    V. Perkovic, M. J. Jardine, M. Gallagher, A. Cass

11 Statins and heart failure   143
    J. Kjekshus

12 Absolute risk assessment in the general population   155
    L. Chen, A. M. Tonkin

13 Pleiotropic effects of statins and potential new indications   177
    J. Davignon, H. Wassef

14 The role of imaging endpoints in clinical trials   195
    S. J. Nicholls

15 Biomarkers in cardiovascular disease   211
    S. Blankenberg, R. B. Schnabel

16 Novel lipid-modifying agents   227
    E. A. Stein, K. M. Kostner, D. R. Sullivan

17 The enhanced evidence base and translation into improved outcomes   245
    A. M. Tonkin

List of abbreviations   263

Index   271

Editor

Andrew M. Tonkin, MBBS, MD, FRACP, FCSANZ, Professor of Medicine; Consultant Cardiologist; Head, Cardiovascular Research Unit, Department of Epidemiology and Preventive Medicine, School of Public Health and Preventive Medicine, Monash University, Melbourne, Australia

Contributors

Pierre Amarenco, MD, Professor of Neurology, INSERM U-698 and Paris-Diderot University, Department of Neurology and Stroke Center, Bichat University Hospital, Paris, France

Jane Armitage, FRCP, FFPH, Professor of Clinical Trials and Epidemiology, University of Oxford; Honorary Consultant in Public Health Medicine, Oxford Radcliffe Trust, Oxford, UK

Hans J. Avis, MD, Department of Vascular Medicine, Academic Medical Center, Amsterdam, The Netherlands

Philip Barter, MBBS, PhD, FRACP, Director and Chief Executive Officer, The Heart Research Institute, Camperdown, New South Wales, Australia

Stefan Blankenberg, MD, Professor of Medicine, Deputy Director, Department of Medicine II, Johannes Gutenberg-University, Mainz, Germany

Louise Bowman, MBBS, MRCP, Clinical Research Fellow, University of Oxford, Oxford, UK

Adrian J. Cameron, BSc(Hons), MPH, Grad Dip Int Hlth, Epidemiologist, Baker IDI Heart and Diabetes Institute, Department of Clinical Diabetes and Epidemiology, Melbourne, Australia

Christopher P. Cannon, MD, Senior Investigator, TIMI Study Group, Cardiovascular Division, Brigham and Women's Hospital; Associate Professor of Medicine, Harvard Medical School, Boston, Massuchsetts, USA

Alan Cass, MBBS, PhD, FRACP, Co-director, Renal Division, The George Institute for International Health, University of Sydney, Sydney, Australia

LEI CHEN, MD, MMed, Endocrinologist, Department of Epidemiology and Preventive Medicine, School of Public Health and Preventive Medicine, Monash University, Melbourne, Australia

CLARA K. CHOW, MBBS, FRACP, PhD, Cardiologist, Population Health Research Institute, McMaster University and Hamilton Health Sciences, Hamilton, Ontario, Canada; The George Institute for International Health, University of Sydney, Sydney, New South Wales, Australia

JEAN DAVIGNON, OC, GOQ, MD, MSc, FRCP(C), FACP, FACN, FAHA, FRSC, Professor of Medicine, University of Montreal; Director, Hyperlipidemia and Atherosclerosis Group, Clinical Research Institute of Montreal, Montreal, Quebec, Canada

MARTIN GALLAGHER, MBBS, FRACP, MPH, Nephrologist and Senior Research Fellow, The George Institute for International Health, University of Sydney, Sydney, Australia

RICHARD H. GRIMM, Jr, MD, MPH, PhD, Professor of Cardiology and Epidemiology, Department of Medicine, Division of Cardiology, University of Minnesota, Minneapolis, Minnesota, USA

ROELAND HUIJGEN, MD, MSc, Department of Vascular Medicine, Academic Medical Center, Amsterdam, The Netherlands

BARBARA A. HUTTEN, PhD, Clinical Epidemiologist, Department of Clinical Epidemiology, Biostatistics and Bioinformatics, Academic Medical Center, Amsterdam, The Netherlands

MEG J. JARDINE, MBBS, PhD, FRACP, Nephrologist and Senior Research Fellow, The George Institute for International Health, University of Sydney, Sydney, Australia

JOHN J. P. KASTELEIN, MD, PhD, Professor of Medicine; Chairman, Department of Vascular Medicine, Academic Medical Center, Amsterdam, The Netherlands

JOHN KJEKSHUS, MD, PhD, Professor, Department of Cardiology, University of Oslo, Rikshospitalet University Clinic, Oslo, Norway

KARAM M. KOSTNER, MD, FRACP, Consultant Cardiologist, Department of Cardiology, Mater Adult Hospital and University of Queensland, Brisbane, Queensland, Australia

JULIEN LABREUCHE, BS, Biostatistician, INSERM U-698 and Paris-Diderot University, Department of Neurology and Stroke Center, Bichat University Hospital, Paris, France

PHILIPPA LAVALLÉE, MD, Associate Professor of Neurology, INSERM U-698 and Paris-Diderot University, Department of Neurology and Stroke Center, Bichat University Hospital, Paris, France

MIKAEL MAZIGHI, MD, PhD, Assistant Professor of Neurology, INSERM U-698 and Paris-Diderot University, Department of Neurology and Stroke Center, Bichat University Hospital, Paris, France

STEPHEN J. NICHOLLS, MBBS, PhD, Cardiologist, Department of Cardiovascular Medicine and Cell Biology, Cleveland Clinic, Cleveland, USA

ANUSHKA A. PATEL, MBBS, SM, PhD, FRACP, Director, Cardiovascular Division, The George Institute for International Health, The University of Sydney, Sydney, NSW; Consultant Cardiologist, Department of Cardiology, Royal Prince Alfred Hospital, Camperdown, New South Wales, Australia

VLADO PERKOVIC, MBBS, PhD, FRACP, Co-director, Renal Division, The George Institute for International Health, University of Sydney, Sydney, Australia

KAUSIK K. RAY, BSc, MBChB, MRCP, MD, MPhil, FACC, FESC, Honorary Consultant Cardiologist, Department of Public Health and Primary Care, University of Cambridge; Department of Cardiology, Addenbrooke's Hospital, Cambridge, UK

KERRY-ANNE RYE, BSc(Hons), PhD, Head, Lipid Research Group, The Heart Research Institute, Camperdown, New South Wales, Australia

RENATE B. SCHNABEL, MD, MSc, Physician and Epidemiologist, Department of Medicine II, Johannes Gutenberg-University, Mainz, Germany

JONATHAN SHAW, MD, MRCP(UK), FRACP, Associate Director / Consultant Physician, Baker IDI Heart and Diabetes Institute, Department of Clinical Diabetes and Epidemiology, Melbourne, Australia

ALLAN D. SNIDERMAN, MD, Edwards Professor of Cardiology, McGill University, Montreal, Quebec, Canada

EVAN A. STEIN, MD, PhD, FRCP(C), FCAP, Voluntary Professor of Pathology and Laboratory Medicine, University of Cincinnati; Director, Metabolic and Atherosclerosis Research Center, Cincinnati, Ohio, USA

DAVID R. SULLIVAN, MBBS, FRACP, FRCPA, Senior Staff Specialist, Department of Clinical Biochemistry, Royal Prince Alfred Hospital, Camperdown, New South Wales, Australia

ANDREW M. TONKIN, MBBS, MD, FRACP, FCSANZ, Professor of Medicine; Consultant Cardiologist; Head, Cardiovascular Research Unit, Department of Epidemiology and Preventive Medicine, School of Public Health and Preventive Medicine, Monash University, Melbourne, Australia

MAUD N. VISSERS, PhD, Scientific Researcher / Nutritionist, Department of Vascular Medicine, Academic Medical Center, Amsterdam, The Netherlands

HANNY WASSEF, MSc, PhD Candidate, McGill University, Hyperlipidemia and Atherosclerosis Group, Clinical Research Institute of Montreal, Montreal, Quebec, Canada

PAUL ZIMMET, MD, PhD, FRACP, FRCN, FTSE, Hon Causa Doctoris (Complutense, Spain), Director Emeritus and Director, International Research, Baker IDI Heart and Diabetes Institute, Department of Clinical Diabetes and Epidemiology, Melbourne, Australia

Foreword

Atherosclerotic vascular disease is by far the most common cause of cardiovascular disease, and therefore among the leading causes of death worldwide. It was in 1910 that the Nobel Prize-winning organic chemist, Professor Adolf Windaus, first identified cholesterol in atherosclerotic plaques in human aortas. This was soon followed by the famous experiments of Anichkov and Chalatow, two young Russian physicians who fed rabbits large quantities of cholesterol and showed that they developed lipid-laden lesions in the aorta. A century has passed since then: numerous observational studies, registries and clinical trials have documented the importance of circulating cholesterol in the development of atherosclerotic lesions of the arterial bed, leading to ischemic heart disease, cerebrovascular disease, peripheral arterial disease, renovascular and aortic disease. Although there are a number of other important atherosclerotic risk factors (such as diabetes mellitus, hypertension, chronic kidney disease, cigarette smoking and abnormally low levels of circulating high-density cholesterol), the elevation of plasma low-density lipoprotein cholesterol concentration is a necessary – albeit not always sufficient – condition for atherogenesis. Therefore, it is imperative that physicians possess a clear understanding of the genesis of dyslipidemias, how the latter lead to atherothrombosis and finally the measures that are now available to treat and/or prevent atherothrombosis.

Andrew Tonkin, a world-renowned epidemiologist and clinical trialist in the field of lipid disorders, has gathered an outstanding group of authors to produce *Therapeutic Strategies in Lipid Disorders*. Although the central focus of this book is on the critical analyses of interventions designed to optimize plasma lipid concentrations, it also pays appropriate attention to diabetes, hypertension and chronic kidney disease, all of which interact with lipids in atherogenesis. The book ends with a truly excellent 'wrap up' chapter by the editor on the translation of scientific evidence into improved clinical outcomes.

This is a very important, well-written book on a crucial subject. It will be useful to and appreciated by scholarly cardiologists, lipidologists, epidemiologists and clinical trialists, especially those who are joining forces to control the pandemic of atherosclerosis.

Eugene Braunwald, MD
Harvard Medical School
Boston, MA

1

A global view of cardiovascular risk factors

C. K. Chow, A. A. Patel

THE GLOBAL IMPACT OF CARDIOVASCULAR DISEASES

Cardiovascular diseases are now the leading causes of morbidity and mortality globally. Previously characterised as conditions largely affecting rich countries, age-specific rates of cardiovascular diseases are declining in most high-income countries, while rapidly increasing in many middle- and low-income countries. In 1990, it was estimated that there were 14 million deaths from cardiovascular diseases worldwide – 5 million of these occurred in populations from high-income countries and 9 million occurred in populations from middle- and low-income countries [1]. By 2020, it is projected that there will be 25 million deaths from cardiovascular diseases worldwide – 6 million in populations from high-income countries and 19 million in populations from middle- and low-income countries [1]. These projections suggest that cardiovascular diseases will continue to be leading causes of morbidity and premature mortality worldwide, but increasingly so in developing regions of the world.

The current and projected burden of cardiovascular diseases in developing countries likely reflects what is often termed an 'epidemiological transition' (Figure 1.1) [2]. This describes how the burden of disease transfers from predominantly maternal and communicable illnesses to chronic non-communicable diseases, broadly reflecting several major changes in society. First, decreasing mortality rates from perinatal conditions and acute infectious diseases result in increased life expectancy, which in turn leads to a higher proportion of individuals reaching middle and old age, during which they are at greater risk of experiencing cardiovascular events. This transition is reflected by observed global increases in life expectancy over the last several decades, with most recent gains occurring in less developed countries. For example, in India, the average life expectancy at birth for men has increased from 41.2 years in the decade 1951–1961 to 61.4 years for the period between 1991 and 1996 [3]. Second, economic development and increasing urbanisation of populations due to greater migration from rural to urban centres, as well as industrialisation of traditionally rural areas, have resulted in marked societal and environmental changes. These, in turn, have been linked to major lifestyle changes such as reduced levels of physical activity and altered dietary patterns, which directly influence the proximate risk factors

Clara K. Chow, MBBS, FRACP, PhD, Cardiologist, Population Health Research Institute, McMaster University and Hamilton Health Sciences, Hamilton, Ontario, Canada; The George Institute for International Health, University of Sydney, Sydney, New South Wales, Australia

Anushka A. Patel, MBBS, SM, PhD, FRACP, Director, Cardiovascular Division, The George Institute for International Health, The University of Sydney, Sydney, NSW; Consultant Cardiologist, Department of Cardiology, Royal Prince Alfred Hospital, Camperdown, New South Wales, Australia

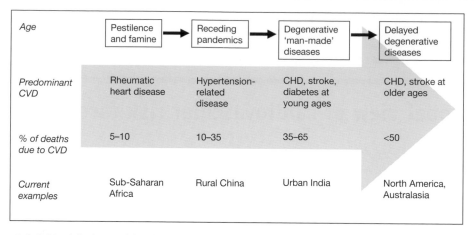

Figure 1.1 Epidemiologic transition (modified with permission from [2]). CHD = coronary heart disease; CVD = cardiovascular diseases.

for the development of cardiovascular diseases. The effects of this epidemiological transition on population levels of cardiovascular risk factors are rapid. Conceptually, such changes are analogous to the development of more adverse risk factor profiles in ethnic groups from countries with lower levels of cardiovascular risk factors migrating to industrialised countries such as the United States [4] or the United Kingdom [5, 6].

Another important feature of the epidemiological transition is a shift from cardiovascular conditions predominantly related to blood pressure, such as haemorrhagic stroke, towards atherothrombotic vascular diseases where other risk factors, including blood lipids and tobacco use, play a greater role. In many East Asian countries, stroke is a relatively more common cause of cardiovascular death, compared to populations in North America, Western Europe and Australasia [7]. Furthermore, in a number of these countries, strokes historically have been represented by a relatively high proportion of the haemorrhagic subtype, likely reflecting the influence of blood pressure-related disorders during this stage of the epidemiological transition [8–11]. By contrast, in high-income countries with predominantly Caucasian populations, most data from studies with reliable stroke subtype verification indicate that approximately three-quarters of all strokes are due to cerebral infarction [12, 13]. However, in many populations in developing countries, there is already substantial evidence of a shift towards increasing predominance of atherothrombotic conditions such as coronary heart disease and ischaemic stroke. For example, in Beijing, China, age-adjusted coronary heart disease mortality rates increased by about 50% in men and 27% in women between 1984 and 1999 [14]. Importantly, with the widespread availability of computed tomography scanning in many parts of China over recent years, there are now reliable data to indicate that at least two-thirds of first-ever strokes in this country are currently due to cerebral infarction [15]. In Korea, national mortality data indicate a large decline in age-adjusted stroke mortality between 1984 and 1999. However, the proportion of ischaemic strokes increased by a factor of about five over this same period, while coronary heart disease mortality increased by over 300% [16]. Surveillance of male industrial workers in Osaka, Japan, between 1963 and 1994 also showed a sharp decline in the incidence of stroke over this period, accompanied by an initial rise and then plateau of coronary disease incidence [17]. A meta-analysis of cross-sectional studies from India indicates that the reported prevalence of coronary heart disease had increased within urban centres in that country from ~1% in 1960 to 8–10% in 1995 [18].

For both developed and developing regions of the world, the socioeconomic consequences of cardiovascular diseases are substantial. In high-income countries, socioeconomically deprived communities suffer the brunt of the burden of cardiovascular diseases [19, 20]. Such groups have both higher rates of and poorer outcomes from cardiovascular diseases, with these observations incompletely explained by different levels of known major cardiovascular risk factors [19]. Other factors likely to contribute to these differences include poor access to healthcare [21, 22], a more toxic physical environment (e.g. less access to good food choices [23], more fast food [24], less opportunities for physical activity [25], more pollution [26]), and less social support for those with known disease [27].

In less developed economies, the peak prevalence of cardiovascular disease is currently in populations of working and child-rearing age, as it was in the Organisation for Economic Cooperation and Development (OECD) countries during the 1950s and 1960s [28, 29]. In low-income countries, more than half of all cardiovascular deaths occur among people aged between 30–69 years of age, compared to about a quarter in high-income countries such as Australia and New Zealand [30]. The younger age at which cardiovascular events occur in developing countries has major socioeconomic consequences for these communities. An example of a region where the working-age population has been devastated by cardiovascular disease is the Russian Federation [31]. In 1984, the cardiovascular disease mortality rate among people aged 55–59 was 600 per 100 000; this had increased by 55% to 929 per 100 000 in 2002 [28]. In the United States, the rate in 1980 for people aged 55–64 was 494 per 100 000; this fell 46% to 247 per 100 000 in 2001 [28, 32]. Life expectancy for Russian males is now less than 60 years. The principal cause of this shortened life expectancy has been attributed to cardiovascular diseases.

Within many middle- and low-income countries, the reversal in socioeconomic gradient for cardiovascular disease incidence that has been observed in higher-income nations is not yet apparent. Higher rates of cardiovascular diseases are currently still seen in richer, urban centres as compared with poorer (usually rural) communities [33]. However, as a consequence of the population distribution in many developing countries (e.g. >70% of the populations of China and India live in rural areas) the absolute burden of cardiovascular diseases is greatest among poorer communities [34]. Rural areas of developing countries generally have a grossly insufficient health infrastructure to provide adequate services for the evaluation and management of cardiovascular risk factors and diseases.

This current and increasing global impact of cardiovascular diseases is an urgent problem that requires examination of a number of important questions relating to the determinants of these conditions. What are the current trends for cardiovascular risk factors across different regions of the world? Are the relationships between established risk factors and cardiovascular diseases similar in different populations? To what extent can cardiovascular diseases be attributed to the major established risk factors globally, and does this vary by region or by risk factor? An understanding of these issues underpins efforts to develop and implement effective preventative and therapeutic strategies to reduce the burden of cardiovascular diseases in different settings worldwide.

GLOBAL TRENDS IN CARDIOVASCULAR RISK FACTORS

Analysis of data from a number of high-income countries suggests that a substantial proportion of the decline in coronary heart disease rates over the past few decades in these regions can be explained by favourable shifts in population-wide risk factor levels [35–39]. For example, recent data from the United States attribute almost half the decline in deaths from coronary disease between 1980 and 2000 to relative declines of ~30% in smoking prevalence, ~4% in mean blood pressure levels, ~6% in mean total cholesterol levels, as well as an ~8% relative increase in levels of physical activity [39]. However, the benefits from these improvements in risk factor levels were partially offset by relative increases in average body mass index (~10%) and the prevalence of diabetes (~40%) over the same period [39]. Furthermore, these overall trends appear to mask more unfavourable shifts in risk factor levels among younger adults, with some evidence that the decline in coronary heart disease mortality rates is levelling off in this subgroup of the US population [40].

Conversely, development of increasingly adverse risk factor levels is being consistently observed across developing regions of the world. For example, the prevalence of high blood pressure in China increased from a crude rate of 7.7% in people aged ≥15 years in 1979/1980 to 11.4% in 1991 [41]. Similar increases in the prevalence of hypertension have been reported in India [42]. The prevalence of cigarette smoking continues to increase in many developing countries, especially in those with few regulatory controls and newly-liberalised economies, and particularly among women [43, 44]. As a result of increasing incomes in many developing countries, cigarettes are becoming more rather than less affordable [45]. Globally, but particularly in middle- and low-income countries, rates of overweight and obesity are rising rapidly. This reflects falling levels of physical activity and increased consumption of high-calorie diets [46]. For example, in Indonesia between 1983 and 1999, major dietary changes included increases in the average consumption of meat, eggs and processed foods, accompanied by a fall in the consumption of cereals [47]. In Brazil, rapid decreases in the rates of childhood malnutrition have been accompanied by an even more rapid increase in adult overweight and obesity, with serial surveys conducted between the 1970s and 1990s indicating that obesity rates doubled or tripled in adult men and women at the extremes of the time series analysed [48]. Changes in lifestyle, particularly in low- and middle-income countries are secondary to a combination of increasing economic prosperity; increasing access to energy-dense low-fibre diets through falling food prices (e.g. of beef) and increased availability of fast foods, snacks and soft drinks; and reduced energy expenditure at home and during work and leisure times [49]. In a cohort study from China, 84% of adults did not own motorised transportation in 1997; however, 14% of households acquired a motorised vehicle between 1989 and 1997. Compared with those whose vehicle ownership did not change, men who acquired a vehicle experienced significantly greater weight gain and were two-thirds more likely to become obese [50].

An alarming rise in the incidence of diabetes is accompanying these increasing rates of overweight and obesity. Global estimates suggest the prevalence of diabetes will increase by ~9% between 2000 and 2030 in established market economies, but will also rise by ~40% in India and Latin America, ~60% in the Middle East and over 90% in sub-Saharan Africa [51]. These projections may be an underestimate of the future prevalence of diabetes; in India, the prevalence of type 2 diabetes has already nearly doubled in some urban areas [52, 53] and has increased three-fold in some rural regions over the past 20 years [54].

Historically, many developing regions of the world have documented highly favourable population distributions of blood lipid levels. Data from the 1960s–1970s from the Western Pacific region indicated very low levels of blood cholesterol (mean levels <3.5 mmol/l) among certain populations from the Papua New Guinean highlands, the Solomon Islands and Western Samoa [55–57]. Similarly low levels of cholesterol have been reported more recently in certain rural Chinese and Indian communities in the early and mid 1990s [58–60]. However, there are now many data indicating large shifts in population-wide levels of blood lipids within these communities over recent decades. In Guangzhou, China, it has been estimated that total cholesterol levels increased by an average of 0.25–0.52 mmol/l (10–20 mg/dl) in the decade between 1983–1984 and 1993–1994 [61]. World Health Organization Monitoring of Trends and Determinants in Cardiovascular Disease (WHO Monica) data from Beijing indicate a much greater 24% increase in total cholesterol levels between 1984 and 1999, from a mean of 4.3–5.3 mmol/l [14]. These data are consistent with a large population-based survey of both rural and urban areas of China in 2000–2001; the age-adjusted mean total cholesterol levels in this study were 4.8 mmol/l and 5.1 mmol/l, respectively [62]. Adverse shifts in the distribution of lipids tend to occur first in urban areas of developing countries [63]. In India, data from selected states show marked urban–rural differences in the prevalence of high cholesterol and other cardiovascular risk factors [60, 64]. For example, one urban study found the prevalence of hypercholesterolaemia (defined as total cholesterol ≥200 mg/dl) increased from 25% to 37% among men in large serial surveys of an urban population between 1995 and 2002 [65], with similar changes observed among women. However, such trends are also now being increasingly seen in rural areas of developing countries. A recent population-based study conducted in a rural South Indian population found that the prevalence among adults of high cholesterol (again defined as total cholesterol ≥200 mg/dl) was 30%, with a similar prevalence of low high-density lipoprotein cholesterol (HDL-C) levels (defined as HDL-C <40 mg/dl) [66]. Adverse shifts in the population distributions of blood lipids have also been described in other developing regions of the world, including Eastern Europe [67], South America [68] and the Middle East [69].

GLOBAL DIFFERENCES IN THE ASSOCIATIONS BETWEEN RISK FACTORS AND CARDIOVASCULAR DISEASES

Much is now known about the nature and magnitude of the associations between major risk factors (such as blood pressure, blood cholesterol, tobacco use, blood glucose and body adiposity) and cardiovascular diseases. Almost universally, these associations are continuous and log-linear, with no obvious threshold values to define clearly abnormal risk factor levels. The Prospective Studies Collaboration (PSC), a meta-analysis of cohort studies predominantly among largely Caucasian populations from developed countries, provides the most reliable information about many of these relationships. This study indicated that each 20 mmHg lower level of systolic blood pressure was associated with a lower risk of coronary heart disease ranging between 30% (at older ages) and over 60% (at younger ages), regardless of the initial systolic blood pressure level [70]. Similarly, for each 1 mmol/l (39 mg/dl) lower level in cholesterol, the risk of ischaemic heart disease was also lower by between 15% (at older ages) and 55% (at younger ages) (Figure 1.2) [71]. While blood pressure is also a strong, continuous determinant of stroke risk, the association between blood cholesterol and stroke is more complex. PSC data indicated a weak positive relationship between total cholesterol and ischaemic stroke, which was substantially confounded by blood pressure levels. Among older individuals, and particularly for those with higher blood pressure levels, total cholesterol was inversely associated with haemorrhagic stroke risk. In the PSC, HDL-C was inversely related to ischaemic heart disease risk, with each 0.3 mmol/l (12 mg/dl) higher level of HDL-C being associated with an approximate one-third lower risk of a coronary event. There was no evidence of any association between HDL-C and stroke risk.

The importance of blood triglycerides as a risk factor for cardiovascular diseases remains controversial. Many epidemiological studies have demonstrated a univariate association between triglycerides and cardiovascular events, particularly in relation to coronary disease. However, this relationship is attenuated and often becomes non-significant after adjusting for major cardiovascular risk factors, particularly HDL-C levels. More recently, the results of separate analyses in European and North American cohorts showing an independent association of either fasting or non-fasting triglyceride levels with cardiovascular risk support the suggestion that at least some triglyceride-rich lipoproteins may have a role in atherogenesis [72–74].

While comparatively fewer long-term observational data are available from populations in developing regions of the world, there is now compelling evidence indicating that the associations between the major established risk factors and cardiovascular diseases are broadly similar across diverse populations. The Asia Pacific Cohort Studies Collaboration (APCSC) is an individual-participant data meta-analysis of prospective cohort studies that includes more than half a million participants from several Asian countries, as well as Australia and New Zealand. Data from APCSC have demonstrated that the nature and magnitude of the associations between cholesterol [75] and blood pressure [76] are broadly sim-

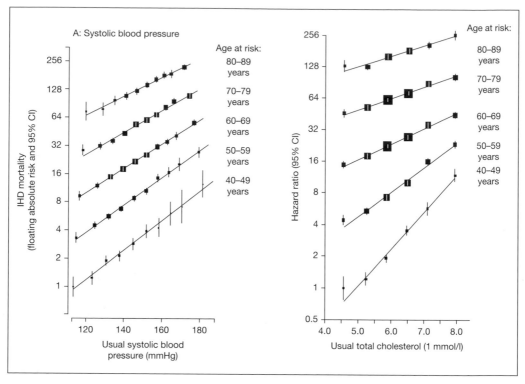

Figure 1.2 Associations between (A) usual systolic blood pressure and (B) usual total cholesterol, and ischaemic heart disease in the Prospective Studies Collaboration (with permission from [70, 71]).

ilar in East Asian countries (including China, Japan, Korea, Singapore, Thailand and Taiwan) compared with populations in Australia and New Zealand (Figure 1.3). Absence of regional heterogeneity in the associations with cardiovascular diseases was also demonstrated for other risk factors including HDL-C [77], triglycerides [78], tobacco use [79], blood glucose levels [80] and measures of adiposity [81].

As might be anticipated, a relatively high proportion of cardiovascular events among the Asian cohorts included in APCSC were haemorrhagic strokes. Analysis of APCSC data demonstrated a significant positive log-linear association between total cholesterol levels and ischaemic stroke (25% higher risk of ischaemic stroke for each 1 mmol/l higher level of usual total cholesterol), but also a significant inverse log-linear association between total cholesterol and haemorrhagic stroke (20% higher risk of haemorrhagic stroke death for each 1 mmol/l lower level of usual total cholesterol) [75]. While these findings are important, the implications of differences in the associations between cholesterol and stroke subtypes results should be interpreted in the light of a rapid transition in most developing regions of the world towards a strong preponderance of atherothrombotic vascular diseases.

GLOBAL PERSPECTIVES ON ATTRIBUTABLE RISKS

A frequent claim in the literature is that established cardiovascular risk factors explain only about one-half or less of cardiovascular diseases [82]. Such claims suggest that important discoveries could be made if priority were given to research identifying new determinants of cardiovascular diseases. To what extent can these claims be justified?

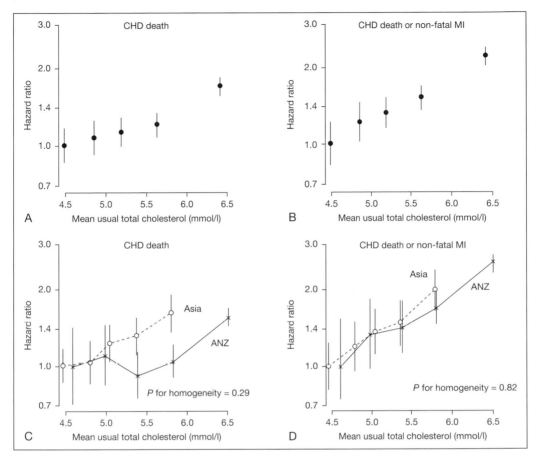

Figure 1.3 Association between usual cholesterol level and coronary heart disease in APCSC. (A) Death due to coronary heart disease (CHD) in the entire study population. (B) Death due to fatal or non-fatal CHD in the entire study population. (C) Death due to CHD stratified by region. (D) Death due to fatal or non-fatal CHD stratified by region. In parts (C) and (D), the hazard ratio for the lowest fifth of cholesterol is fixed at 1.0 separately for Asia and ANZ. *P* values for test of homogeneity are shown (with permission from [75]).

In fact, data that strongly contradict this view have been available for at least two decades. Using data from the Multiple Risk Factor Intervention Trial (MRFIT) cohort, Stamler and colleagues [82, 83] illustrated that individuals with the most favourable levels of cholesterol and blood pressure, who did not smoke and did not have diabetes or previous coronary disease, had approximately 75% fewer coronary heart disease events and a lower rate of long-term mortality compared to the rest of the population. These findings suggest that the majority of coronary events can be attributed to a short list of established major risk factors. Fewer than 10% of the MRFIT cohort contributed to this 'lowest' risk category, indicating large potential for achieving substantial reductions in cardiovascular events if a greater proportion of the population were exposed to a lifetime of lower levels of 'traditional' risk factors.

More recently, similar conclusions have been drawn from the results of the INTERHEART study. This study examined the contribution of nine risk factors to acute myocardial infarction (MI) in a large global case-control study involving about 28 000 individuals (14 000

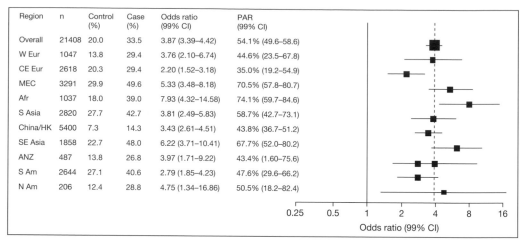

Region	n	Control (%)	Case (%)	Odds ratio (99% CI)	PAR (99% CI)
Overall	21408	20.0	33.5	3.87 (3.39–4.42)	54.1% (49.6–58.6)
W Eur	1047	13.8	29.4	3.76 (2.10–6.74)	44.6% (23.5–67.8)
CE Eur	2618	20.3	29.4	2.20 (1.52–3.18)	35.0% (19.2–54.9)
MEC	3291	29.9	49.6	5.33 (3.48–8.18)	70.5% (57.8–80.7)
Afr	1037	18.0	39.0	7.93 (4.32–14.58)	74.1% (59.7–84.6)
S Asia	2820	27.7	42.7	3.81 (2.49–5.83)	58.7% (42.7–73.1)
China/HK	5400	7.3	14.3	3.43 (2.61–4.51)	43.8% (36.7–51.2)
SE Asia	1858	22.7	48.0	6.22 (3.71–10.41)	67.7% (52.0–80.2)
ANZ	487	13.8	26.8	3.97 (1.71–9.22)	43.4% (1.60–75.6)
S Am	2644	27.1	40.6	2.79 (1.85–4.23)	47.6% (29.6–66.2)
N Am	206	12.4	28.8	4.75 (1.34–16.86)	50.5% (18.2–82.4)

Figure 1.4 Risk of acute myocardial infarction associated with apo(a)/apoAI ratio (top vs. lowest quintile), overall and by region after adjustment for age, sex and smoking. PAR is for the top four quintiles vs. the lowest quintile (with permission from [84]). PAR = population attributable risk.

cases of first MI and 14 000 matched controls) from 52 countries [84]. The principal findings of this study were that nine risk factors (abnormal lipids, smoking, hypertension, diabetes, abdominal obesity, psychosocial factors, consumption of fruits, vegetables and alcohol, and regular physical activity) account for over 90% of cases of acute MI. The combination of smoking and abnormal lipids accounted for approximately 70% of MIs, and the combination of five risk factors (smoking, lipids, hypertension, diabetes and obesity) accounts for approximately 85% of MIs. However, for a number of reasons, it is likely that these risk factors account for substantially more, if not nearly all, of the risk of developing acute MI. First, hypertension and diabetes were self-reported in this study. This was likely to have resulted in an underestimate of the prevalence of these risks. Second, the consideration of major risk factors as categorical predictors, despite known continuous relationships between levels of blood pressure, blood lipids, blood glucose and adiposity with the risk of MI, would underestimate their contribution to the disease burden. Finally, the inability to correct for regression dilution biases is likely to have resulted in underestimation of the strength of each of the associations with MI.

The apparent contribution of abnormal lipid levels (apoB/apoAI ratio) in INTERHEART was large, with this risk factor accounting for about half of the risk of MI globally. The apoB/apoAI ratio showed a graded relation with MI risk, with no evidence of a threshold, and an odds ratio of 4.73 (99% confidence interval [CI] 3.93–5.69) for the highest vs. the lowest decile of apoB/apoAI ratio. The findings in relation to abnormal lipids were broadly similar across all major (developed and developing) regions of the world, both in terms of the magnitude of the associations and population attributable risks (Figure 1.4). The findings were also generalisable among men and women, and in younger and older individuals.

Analyses that contributed to the 2002 World Health Report [85] also attempted to quantify selected major risks to vascular health from a global perspective. Globally, 62% of cerebrovascular disease and 49% of ischaemic heart disease were estimated to be attributable to non-optimal blood pressure (systolic >115 mmHg). The corresponding estimates for non-optimal cholesterol levels (total cholesterol >3.8 mmol/l) were 18% and 56%, respectively. The attributable fraction for vascular disease associated with tobacco use was estimated to be 12%, while approximately 21% of ischaemic heart disease was attributed to overweight

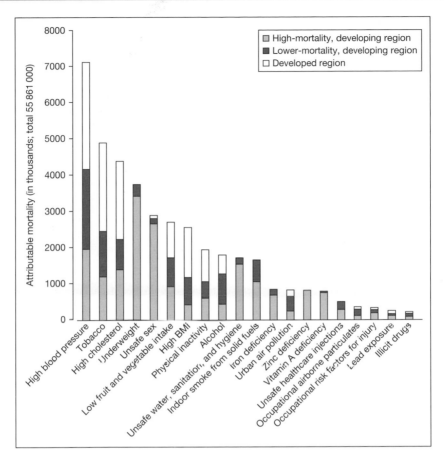

Figure 1.5 Mortality due to leading global risk factors (modified with permission from [43]).

and obesity. Physical inactivity was estimated to cause, globally, about 22% of ischaemic heart disease. Importantly, the effects of the 'epidemiological transition' were clearly apparent in these analyses, with overall mortality substantially attributable to the major risk factors of non-optimal blood pressure, non-optimal cholesterol levels and tobacco use not only in highly developed economies, but also in low-mortality and high-mortality developing regions of the world (Figure 1.5).

CONCLUSIONS

Cardiovascular diseases represent a major and increasing global health challenge. While a number of modifiable risk factors for cardiovascular diseases have been discovered over the past several decades, only a few have consistently been found to be of major importance across multiple populations defined by geographic, ethnic and socioeconomic criteria. These are non-optimal blood cholesterol, non-optimal blood pressure (and their proximal determinants) and tobacco use. For each of these, there are extensive data from long-term observational studies that have established their role as major risk factors for the development of cardiovascular diseases. Furthermore, there is increasing evidence to indicate that the associations between these risk factors and cardiovascular diseases are broadly similar in diverse populations across more and less developed regions of the world. In light of these findings, the large unfavourable shifts occurring in the population distribution of risk factors within middle- and low-income countries, as well as a possible levelling-off in the positive trends that have been observed in higher-income countries, herald a future burden of cardiovascular diseases even greater than current projections that are primarily based on sociodemographic changes alone. A global perspective dictates preventative and therapeutic approaches that recognise this rapidly evolving epidemiology of cardiovascular diseases and their risk factors.

REFERENCES

1. Murray CJ, Lopez AD. Alternative projections of mortality and disability by cause 1990–2020: Global Burden of Disease Study. *Lancet* 1997; 349:1498–1504.
2. Yusuf S, Reddy KS, Ounpuu S, Anand S. Global burden of cardiovascular diseases: Part II: variations in cardiovascular disease by specific ethnic groups and geographic regions and prevention strategies. *Circulation* 2001; 104:2855–2864.
3. Reddy KS, Yusuf S. Emerging epidemic of cardiovascular disease in developing countries. *Circulation* 1998; 97:596–604.
4. Benfante R. Studies of cardiovascular disease and cause-specific mortality trends in Japanese-American men living in Hawaii and risk factor comparisons with other Japanese populations in the Pacific region: a review. *Hum Biol* 1992; 64:791–805.
5. Bhatnagar D, Anand IS, Durrington PN *et al.* Coronary risk factors in people from the Indian subcontinent living in west London and their siblings in India. *Lancet* 1995; 345:405–409.
6. Harding S. Mortality of migrants from the Indian subcontinent to England and Wales: effect of duration of residence. *Epidemiology* 2003; 14:287–292.
7. World Health Organization. The World Health Report 2000. Health systems: improving performance. WHO, Geneva, 2000.
8. Chen D, Roman GC, Wu GX *et al.* Stroke in China (Sino-MONICA-Beijing study) 1984–1986. *Neuroepidemiology* 1992; 11:15–23.
9. Kimura Y, Takishita S, Muratani H *et al.* Demographic study of first-ever stroke and acute myocardial infarction in Okinawa, Japan. *Intern Med* 1998; 37:736–745.
10. Hong Y, Bots ML, Pan X, Hofman A, Grobbee DE, Chen H. Stroke incidence and mortality in rural and urban Shanghai from 1984 through 1991. Findings from a community-based registry. *Stroke* 1994; 25:1165–1169.
11. Shi FL, Hart RG, Sherman DG, Tegeler CH. Stroke in the People's Republic of China. *Stroke* 1989; 20:1581–1585.
12. Sudlow CL, Warlow CP. Comparable studies of the incidence of stroke and its pathological types: results from an international collaboration. International Stroke Incidence Collaboration. *Stroke* 1997; 28:491–499.
13. Thrift AG, Dewey HM, Macdonell RA, McNeil JJ, Donnan GA. Incidence of the major stroke subtypes: initial findings from the North East Melbourne stroke incidence study (NEMESIS). *Stroke* 2001; 32:1732–1738.
14. Critchley J, Liu J, Zhao D, Wei W, Capewell S. Explaining the increase in coronary heart disease mortality in Beijing between 1984 and 1999. *Circulation* 2004; 110:1236–1244.
15. Zhang LF, Yang J, Hong Z *et al.* Proportion of different subtypes of stroke in China. *Stroke* 2003; 34:2091–2096.
16. Suh I. Cardiovascular mortality in Korea: a country experiencing epidemiologic transition. *Acta Cardiol* 2001; 56:75–81.
17. Kitamura A, Iso H, Iida M *et al.* Trends in the incidence of coronary heart disease and stroke and the prevalence of cardiovascular risk factors among Japanese men from 1963 to 1994. *Am J Med* 2002; 112:104–109.
18. Gupta R, Gupta VP. Meta-analysis of coronary heart disease prevalence in India. *Indian Heart J* 1996; 48:241–245.
19. Terris M. The development and prevention of cardiovascular disease risk factors: socioenvironmental influences. *Prev Med* 1999; 29:S11–S17.

20. Winkleby M, Sundquist K, Cubbin C. Inequities in CHD incidence and case fatality by neighbourhood deprivation. *Am J Prev Med* 2007; 32:97–106.

21. Pell JP, Pell AC, Norrie J, Ford I, Cobbe SM. Effect of socioeconomic deprivation on waiting time for cardiac surgery: retrospective cohort study. *Br Med J* 2000; 320:15–18.

22. Ward PR, Noyce PR, St Leger AS. How equitable are GP practice prescribing rates for statins?: an ecological study in four primary care trusts in North West England. *Int J Equity Health* 2007; 6:2.

23. Winkler E, Turrell G, Patterson C. Does living in a disadvantaged area mean fewer opportunities to purchase fresh fruit and vegetables in the area? Findings from the Brisbane food study. *Health Place* 2006; 12:306–319.

24. Macdonald L, Cummins S, Macintyre S. Neighbourhood fast food environment and area deprivation-substitution or concentration? *Appetite* 2007; 49:251–254.

25. Frank LD, Schmid TL, Sallis JF, Chapman J, Saelens BE. Linking objectively measured physical activity with objectively measured urban form: findings from SMARTRAQ. *Am J Prev Med* 2005; 28(2 suppl 2):117–125.

26. Laurent O, Bard D, Filleul L, Segala C. Effect of socioeconomic status on the relationship between atmospheric pollution and mortality. *J Epidemiol Community Health* 2007; 61:665–675.

27. Chaix B, Rosvall M, Merlo J. Neighborhood socioeconomic deprivation and residential instability: effects on incidence of ischemic heart disease and survival after myocardial infarction. *Epidemiology* 2007; 18:104–111.

28. Greenberg H, Raymond SU, Leeder SR. Cardiovascular disease and global health: threat and opportunity. *Health Aff (Millwood)* 2005; (suppl Web Exclusives):W-5-31–W-5-41.

29. Janus ED, Postiglione A, Singh RB, Lewis B. The modernization of Asia. Implications for coronary heart disease. Council on Arteriosclerosis of the International Society and Federation of Cardiology. *Circulation* 1996; 94:2671–2673.

30. Murray C, Lopez A. The Global Burden of Disease: A Comprehensive Assessment of Mortality and Disability from Disease, Injuries and Risk Factors in 1990 and Projected to 2020. Harvard School of Public Health, Boston, Mass, 1996.

31. Yusuf S, Reddy S, Ounpuu S, Anand S. Global burden of cardiovascular diseases: Part I: general considerations, the epidemiologic transition, risk factors, and impact of urbanization. *Circulation* 2001; 104:2746–2753.

32. Rodriguez T, Malvezzi M, Chatenoud L et al. Trends in mortality from coronary heart and cerebrovascular diseases in the Americas: 1970–2000. *Heart* 2006; 92:453–460.

33. Singh RB, Sharma JP, Rastogi V et al. Prevalence of coronary artery disease and coronary risk factors in rural and urban populations of north India. *Eur Heart J* 1997; 18:1728–1735.

34. India at a glance: rural urban distribution. Census of India, 1991.

35. Hunink MG, Goldman L, Tosteson AN et al. The recent decline in mortality from coronary heart disease, 1980–1990. The effect of secular trends in risk factors and treatment. *JAMA* 1997; 277:535–542.

36. Critchley JA, Capewell S, Unal B. Life-years gained from coronary heart disease mortality reduction in Scotland: prevention or treatment? *J Clin Epidemiol* 2003; 56:583–590.

37. Kuulasmaa K, Tunstall-Pedoe H, Dobson A et al. Estimation of contribution of changes in classic risk factors to trends in coronary-event rates across the WHO MONICA Project populations. *Lancet* 2000; 355:675–687.

38. Unal B, Critchley JA, Fidan D, Capewell S. Life-years gained from modern cardiological treatments and population risk factor changes in England and Wales, 1981–2000. *Am J Public Health* 2005; 95:103–108.

39. Ford ES, Ajani UA, Croft JB et al. Explaining the decrease in U.S. deaths from coronary disease, 1980–2000. *N Engl J Med* 2007; 356:2388–2398.

40. Ford ES, Capewell S. Coronary heart disease mortality among young adults in the U.S. from 1980 through 2002: concealed leveling of mortality rates. *J Am Coll Cardiol* 2007; 50:2128–2132.

41. Wu X, Duan X, Gu D, Hao J, Tao S, Fan D. Prevalence of hypertension and its trends in Chinese populations. *Int J Cardiol* 1995; 52:39–44.

42. Gupta R. Trends in hypertension epidemiology in India. *J Hum Hypertens* 2004; 18:73–78.

43. Ezzati M, Lopez AD. Estimates of global mortality attributable to smoking in 2000. *Lancet* 2003; 362:847–852.

44. Perlman F, Bobak M, Gilmore A, McKee M. Trends in the prevalence of smoking in Russia during the transition to a market economy. *Tob Control* 2007; 16:299–305.

45. Guindon GE, Tobin S, Yach D. Trends and affordability of cigarette prices: ample room for tax increases and related health gains. *Tob Control* 2002; 11:35–43.
46. Popkin BM, Gordon-Larsen P. The nutrition transition: worldwide obesity dynamics and their determinants. *Int J Obes Relat Metab Disord* 2004; 28(suppl 3):S2–S9.
47. Lipoeto NI, Wattanapenpaiboon N, Malik A, Wahlqvist ML. Nutrition transition in west Sumatra, Indonesia. *Asia Pac J Clin Nutr* 2004; 13:312–316.
48. Batista Filho M, Rissin A. Nutritional transition in Brazil: geographic and temporal trends. *Cad Saude Publica* 2003; 19(suppl 1):S181–S191.
49. Popkin BM. Global nutrition dynamics: the world is shifting rapidly toward a diet linked with noncommunicable diseases. *Am J Clin Nutr* 2006; 84:289–298.
50. Bell AC, Ge K, Popkin BM. The road to obesity or the path to prevention: motorized transportation and obesity in China. *Obes Res* 2002; 10:277–283.
51. Wild S, Roglic G, Green A, Sicree R, King H. Global prevalence of diabetes: estimates for the year 2000 and projections for 2030. *Diabetes Care* 2004; 27:1047–1053.
52. Ramachandran A, Snehalatha C, Latha E, Vijay V, Viswanathan M. Rising prevalence of NIDDM in an urban population in India. *Diabetologia* 1997; 40:232–237.
53. Ramachandran A, Snehalatha C, Kapur A *et al.* High prevalence of diabetes and impaired glucose tolerance in India: National Urban Diabetes Survey. *Diabetologia* 2001; 44:1094–1101.
54. Ramachandran A, Snehalatha C, Baskar AD *et al.* Temporal changes in prevalence of diabetes and impaired glucose tolerance associated with lifestyle transition occurring in the rural population in India. *Diabetologia* 2004; 47:860–865.
55. Barnes R. Comparisons of Blood Pressures and Blood Cholesterol Levels of New Guineans and Australians. *Med J Aust* 1965; 1:611–617.
56. Page LB, Damon A, Moellering RC Jr. Antecedents of cardiovascular disease in six Solomon Islands societies. *Circulation* 1974; 49:1132–1146.
57. Hodge AM, Dowse GK, Erasmus RT *et al.* Serum lipids and modernization in coastal and highland Papua New Guinea. *Am J Epidemiol* 1996; 144:1129–1142.
58. Fan WX, Parker R, Parpia B *et al.* Erythrocyte fatty acids, plasma lipids, and cardiovascular disease in rural China. *Am J Clin Nutr* 1990; 52:1027–1036.
59. Xie J, Liu L, Huang J, Hu H, Kesteloot H. Nutritional habits and serum lipid levels in a low-fat intake Chinese population sample. *Acta Cardiol* 1998; 53:359–364.
60. Lubree HG, Rege SS, Bhat DS *et al.* Body fat and cardiovascular risk factors in Indian men in three geographical locations. *Food Nutr Bull* 2002; 23(4 suppl):146–149.
61. Li YH, Li Y, Davis CE *et al.* Serum cholesterol changes from 1983–1984 to 1993–1994 in the People's Republic of China. *Nutr Metab Cardiovasc Dis* 2002; 12:118–126.
62. He J, Gu D, Reynolds K *et al.* Serum total and lipoprotein cholesterol levels and awareness, treatment, and control of hypercholesterolemia in China. *Circulation* 2004; 110:405–411.
63. Watkins LO. Coronary heart disease and coronary disease risk factors in black populations in underdeveloped countries: the case for primordial prevention. *Am Heart J* 1984; 108:850–862.
64. Singh RB, Sharma JP, Rastogi V *et al.* Social class and coronary disease in rural population of north India. The Indian Social Class and Heart Survey. *Eur Heart J* 1997; 18:588–595.
65. Gupta R, Gupta VP, Sarna M, Prakash H, Rastogi S, Gupta KD. Serial epidemiological surveys in an urban Indian population demonstrate increasing coronary risk factors among the lower socioeconomic strata. *J Assoc Physicians India* 2003; 51:470–477.
66. Chow CK, Naidu S, Raju K *et al.* Significant lipid, adiposity and metabolic abnormalities amongst 4535 Indians from a developing region of rural Andhra Pradesh. *Atherosclerosis* 2008; 196:943–952.
67. Pajak A, Williams OD, Broda G *et al.* Changes over time in blood lipids and their correlates in Polish rural and urban populations: the Poland-United States Collaborative Study in cardiopulmonary disease epidemiology. *Ann Epidemiol* 1997; 7:115–124.
68. WHO Global Infobase Surf 2 Country Profiles. In: World Health Organization. *WHO Global InfoBase*, 2005.
69. Azizi F, Rahmani M, Emami H *et al.* Cardiovascular risk factors in an Iranian urban population: Tehran lipid and glucose study (phase 1). *Soz Praventivmed* 2002; 47:408–426.
70. Lewington S, Clarke R, Qizilbash N, Peto R, Collins R. Age-specific relevance of usual blood pressure to vascular mortality: a meta-analysis of individual data for one million adults in 61 prospective studies. *Lancet* 2002; 360:1903–1913.

71. Lewington S, Whitlock G, Clarke R *et al*. Blood cholesterol and vascular mortality by age, sex, and blood pressure: a meta-analysis of individual data from 61 prospective studies with 55 000 vascular deaths. *Lancet* 2007; 370:1829–1839.

72. Hokanson JE, Austin MA. Plasma triglyceride level is a risk factor for cardiovascular disease independent of high-density lipoprotein cholesterol level: a meta-analysis of population-based prospective studies. *J Cardiovasc Risk* 1996; 3:213–219.

73. Sarwar N, Danesh J, Eiriksdottir G *et al*. Triglycerides and the risk of coronary heart disease: 10 158 incident cases among 262 525 participants in 29 Western prospective studies. *Circulation* 2007; 115:450–458.

74. Bansal S, Buring JE, Rifai N, Mora S, Sacks FM, Ridker PM. Fasting compared with nonfasting triglycerides and risk of cardiovascular events in women. *JAMA* 2007; 298:309–316.

75. Zhang X, Patel A, Horibe H *et al*. Cholesterol, coronary heart disease, and stroke in the Asia Pacific region. *Int J Epidemiol* 2003; 32:563–572.

76. Lawes CM, Rodgers A, Bennett DA *et al*. Blood pressure and cardiovascular disease in the Asia Pacific region. *J Hypertens* 2003; 21:707–716.

77. Woodward M, Barzi F, Feigin V *et al*. Associations between high density lipoprotein cholesterol and both stroke and coronary heart disease in the Asia Pacific region. *Eur Heart J* 2007; 28:2653–2660.

78. Patel A, Barzi F, Jamrozik K *et al*. Asia Pacific Cohort Studies Collaboration. Serum triglycerides as a risk factor for cardiovascular diseases in the Asia-Pacific region. *Circulation* 2004; 110:2678–2686.

79. Woodward M, Lam TH, Barzi F *et al*. Smoking, quitting, and the risk of cardiovascular disease among women and men in the Asia-Pacific region. *Int J Epidemiol* 2005; 34:1036–1045.

80. Lawes CM, Parag V, Bennett DA *et al*. Blood glucose and risk of cardiovascular disease in the Asia Pacific region. *Diabetes Care* 2004; 27:2836–2842.

81. Ni Mhurchu C, Rodgers A, Pan WH, Gu DF, Woodward M. Body mass index and cardiovascular disease in the Asia-Pacific Region: an overview of 33 cohorts involving 310 000 participants. *Int J Epidemiol* 2004; 33:751–758.

82. Magnus P, Beaglehole R. The real contribution of the major risk factors to the coronary epidemics: time to end the "only-50%" myth. *Arch Intern Med* 2001; 161:2657–2660.

83. Stamler J, Stamler R, Neaton JD *et al*. Low risk-factor profile and long-term cardiovascular and noncardiovascular mortality and life expectancy: findings for 5 large cohorts of young adult and middle-aged men and women. *JAMA* 1999; 282:2012–2018.

84. Yusuf S, Hawken S, Ounpuu S *et al*. Effect of potentially modifiable risk factors associated with myocardial infarction in 52 countries (the INTERHEART study): case-control study. *Lancet* 2004; 364:937–952.

85. World Health Organization. The World Health Report 2002. Reducing risks, promoting healthy life. WHO, Geneva, 2002.

2

Low-density lipoprotein cholesterol as a therapeutic target

J. Armitage, L. Bowman

WHAT IS LOW-DENSITY LIPOPROTEIN?

Lipoprotein particles are macromolecular complexes consisting of cholesterol, cholesteryl esters, triglycerides, phospholipids and proteins. The relative proportions of these constituents vary considerably between types of lipoprotein: chylomicrons and very low-density lipoprotein (VLDL) are triglyceride-rich, whereas the smaller low-density lipoprotein (LDL) and high-density lipoprotein (HDL) particles are cholesterol-rich (Figure 2.1).

Most of the cholesterol present in plasma is found in LDL particles which vary in size according to the amount of cholesterol they contain. The smaller particles contain less cholesterol and, since lipids are less dense than proteins, are denser than larger ones. As a result, measurement of the LDL cholesterol level does not provide an accurate assessment of the number of LDL particles. Moreover, small dense LDLs appear to be particularly atherogenic [1]. Therefore, in order to accurately evaluate the role of LDL in atherosclerosis, it is necessary to measure not only the amount of LDL cholesterol, but also the number of particles and their size. Unfortunately, however, laboratory techniques for the assessment of particle size and number are not readily available in current clinical practice (although measurement of apolipoproteins is an important step towards this) and treatment decisions at present are based largely on LDL cholesterol levels.

In most laboratories LDL cholesterol is a calculated value rather than a direct measurement. The Friedewald equation [2] uses measures of total cholesterol, HDL cholesterol and fasting triglycerides. Inaccuracies in the measurement of any of these (or the use of non-fasting samples) will therefore affect the calculation of LDL cholesterol.

For concentrations in mmol/l:

[LDL cholesterol] = [total cholesterol] − [HDL cholesterol] − [triglycerides]/2.2

For concentrations in mg/dl:

[LDL cholesterol] = [total cholesterol] − [HDL cholesterol] − [triglycerides]/5

Jane Armitage, FRCP, FFPH, Professor of Clinical Trials and Epidemiology, University of Oxford; Honorary Consultant in Public Health Medicine, Oxford Radcliffe Trust, Oxford, UK

Louise Bowman, MBBS, MRCP, Clinical Research Fellow, University of Oxford, Oxford, UK

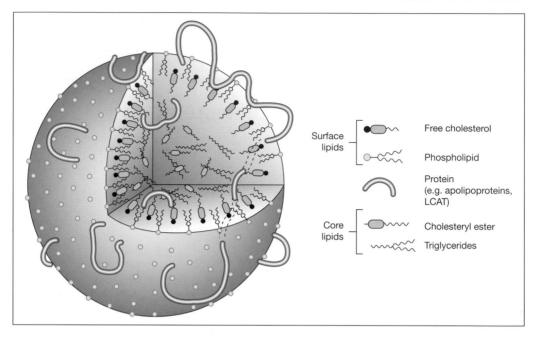

Figure 2.1 The structure of a typical lipoprotein consisting of a droplet core of triglycerides and/or cholesteryl esters and a surface monolayer of phospholipid, unesterified cholesterol and specific proteins (apolipoproteins; e.g. apoB in low-density lipoprotein).

This formula is invalid if triglyceride concentrations are >4.5 mmol/l (445 mg/dl) and becomes less reliable as levels of fasting triglycerides increase above the normal range. Thus the 'measurement' of LDL cholesterol is imprecise. Furthermore, there is considerable overlap in the values of LDL cholesterol between those with cardiovascular disease and those without and as a risk factor in isolation: LDL cholesterol is of limited value in determining risk.

Nevertheless, LDL cholesterol is clearly important in the development of atherosclerosis and remains the primary target of therapy for disease prevention. It may be, however, that future improvements in assays to characterise subfractions of LDL may enable treatment decisions to be refined.

THE ROLE OF LDL IN ATHEROGENESIS

PATHOPHYSIOLOGY

A causal role for cholesterol in atherosclerosis was suggested by Anitschkow in 1913 [3]. The observation that plaques developed in the arteries of cholesterol-fed rabbits led to the conclusion that *'there can be no atheroma without cholesterol'*. In the subsequent 100 years, the pathophysiological mechanisms behind this observation have been explored in great detail and this early description still appears to hold true.

Early lesions, known as fatty streaks, that later give rise to atheroma have been observed in children in populations with high rates of coronary heart disease (CHD). The fatty streak is characterised by lipid-laden macrophages, known as foam cells. These are derived from monocytes which migrate from the blood into the vessel wall where

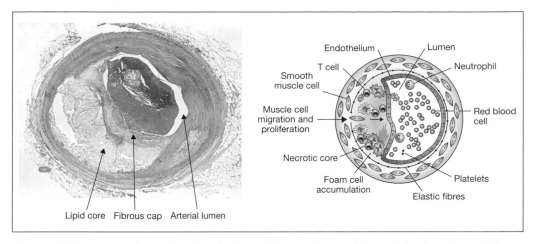

Figure 2.2 The structure of an atherosclerotic plaque (diagram redrawn with permission from *Expert Reviews in Molecular Medicine* ©2005, Cambridge University Press).

they accumulate cholesterol (in particular derived from oxidatively modified LDL) and transform into macrophages. Foam cells produce growth factors that recruit smooth muscle cells which subsequently differentiate into fibroblasts and lay down collagen. The process repeats and, as the lesion progresses, necrosis of the foam cells leaves behind a pool of extracellular cholesterol trapped beneath a fibrous cap. Certain conditions predispose to accelerated accumulation of LDL cholesterol and the formation of such 'plaques'. These include sites of turbulent blood flow, high circulating levels of LDL cholesterol and damage to the endothelium, for example, by hypertension, oxidation or glycation.

Cholesterol-rich plaques are particularly liable to rupture of their overlying fibrous cap, leading to discharge of the cholesterol pool from beneath it. Thrombosis occurs at the raw endothelial surface of such sites of rupture and may cause acute occlusion of the arterial lumen (leading to unstable angina or myocardial infarction, or cerebral infarction if in the brain) (Figure 2.2).

EPIDEMIOLOGY

The pathophysiological role of cholesterol in the development of atherosclerosis is supported by consistent evidence from prospective observational studies. A continuous positive relationship is seen between blood cholesterol levels and CHD risk, extending well below the range commonly seen in western populations [4, 5]. There appears to be no threshold below which a lower level is not associated with a lower risk.

When considered in relation to other risk factors for CHD, the association between cholesterol and CHD risk is somewhat attenuated in older age and at higher systolic blood pressure (SBP) levels [6]. For example, 1 mmol/l (39 mg/dl) higher usual total cholesterol is associated with a doubling in CHD mortality at ages 40–49 years but with just one-sixth higher mortality at ages 80–89 years. Nonetheless, the positive associations in old age (and, similarly, with increasing SBP) are definite and, because of the higher CHD mortality rates in older individuals, the absolute increase in CHD mortality for a given absolute higher level of usual total cholesterol is greater in old than middle age (Figure 2.3).

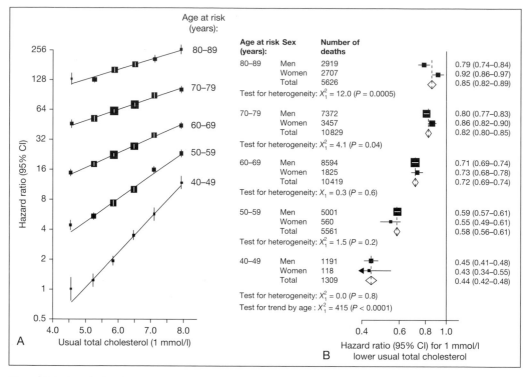

Figure 2.3 Association between CHD mortality and baseline usual total cholesterol (based on 900 000 adults in 61 prospective studies) [6]. (A) Age-specific associations between usual total cholesterol and death from CHD. (B) Age-specific and sex-specific hazard ratios for death from CHD for 1 mmol/l lower usual total cholesterol. Hazard ratios are plotted on a floating absolute scale of risk. The area of each square (A or B) is proportional to the amount of statistical information in that category. Mean time to any death is 12 years.

By contrast, prospective observational studies have generally found no evidence of an association between total cholesterol and risk of death from stroke, despite such studies having consistently reported strong positive associations for CHD risk, and despite large randomised trials clearly showing that cholesterol-lowering statin therapy prevents ischaemic stroke [6]. Reasons for this lack of association may include the heterogeneous nature of stroke and the use of total cholesterol rather than subfractions in most observational studies. However, studies including data on non-fatal strokes (which are more likely to be ischaemic) as well as death from cerebrovascular disease have tended to show a somewhat clearer association between cholesterol levels and stroke risk, particularly when imaging data is available to reliably differentiate ischaemic from haemorrhagic strokes [7, 8].

LDL-LOWERING TREATMENTS

There are currently several treatments available, including dietary intervention, which will lower blood LDL cholesterol. In the last 25 years the clinical effectiveness of these treatments has been subject to careful examination and it is now clear that, irrespective of the therapy used, lowering LDL cholesterol reduces cardiovascular risk. The relative reduction in risk depends on the magnitude of the LDL reduction achieved and is remarkably constant irrespective of other patient characteristics (e.g. age, gender, other treatments) [9, 10]. The absolute risk reduction for an individual patient will therefore depend on their overall cardiovascular risk before treatment, and the LDL reduction achieved (and maintained) as a result of cholesterol-lowering therapy. As will be discussed in other chapters on management, current guidelines now highlight LDL lowering as a top priority in the prevention of cardiovascular disease [11, 12]. A variety of strategies are available and it is often appropriate to use combinations of treatments to achieve the maximum safe benefits.

DIETARY INTERVENTION

The chief dietary determinants of blood cholesterol are intake of saturated fat, polyunsaturated fat and dietary cholesterol [13–15]. Blood cholesterol concentrations are also affected by reduced energy intakes resulting in weight loss [16] and possibly by specific dietary constituents such as fibre and soya. In addition, certain dietary supplements, including fish oils and plant stanols and sterols (phytosterols), have become popular in recent years, although the doses routinely used are probably too small to have significant effects on lipids.

Metabolic ward studies have suggested that, in a typical western diet, replacing 60% of saturated fats by mono- or polyunsaturates and avoiding 60% of dietary cholesterol would reduce blood total cholesterol by about 10–15% (typically about 0.5 mmol/l) [15]. Individualised intensive dietary advice has a more modest effect in free-living subjects with typical reductions of only about 4–6% which tend to decrease over time [17]. Failure to comply fully with dietary recommendations is the likely explanation for the limited efficacy seen. However, if such improvements can be sustained, then the cardiovascular benefits are, as with other treatment strategies, dependent on the degree of LDL lowering achieved [18].

Dietary intervention is a widely applicable strategy and should be considered for all patients for the prevention of cardiovascular disease. Indeed, with the alarming increase in obesity worldwide in the last few decades, this strategy should be applied at a population, rather than only at an individual, level. However, without intensive (and hence costly) professional support, cholesterol reductions as a result of dietary changes are, at best, modest. For patients with established cardiovascular disease, or at high risk due to other factors, dietary measures alone are usually insufficient and additional drug treatments are generally recommended to achieve greater reductions in LDL cholesterol.

STATINS

Mode of action
The 'statins' represent the most important and best-studied class of LDL-lowering drug. They competitively inhibit the rate-limiting enzyme, 3-hydroxy 3-methylglutaryl coenzymeA (HMG CoA) reductase in the metabolic pathway of cholesterol synthesis in the liver [19]. Their principal effect is to reduce total and LDL cholesterol (and, importantly, LDL particle number) with a constant proportional effect across the dose range. Typically doubling the dose of an individual statin is associated with a 6% greater reduction in LDL cholesterol. The statins also vary in their potency in lowering LDL cholesterol across their usual dose range. In addition, statins produce modest increases in HDL cholesterol and variable decreases in plasma triglycerides. By altering the balance of cholesterol and cholesteryl ester within the hepatocyte, statins promote the removal of intermediate-density lipoprotein (IDL) and LDL, and reduce the production of VLDL and LDL.

Efficacy
Six statins are available in most parts of the world: lovastatin (first licensed in 1987 but not available in the UK), simvastatin (1988), pravastatin (1991), fluvastatin (1994), atorvastatin

Table 2.1 Efficacy and safety characteristics of statins [20]

	Licensed dose range (% LDL cholesterol reduction)*	Metabolism	Most important drug interactions increasing myopathy risk[†]
Lovastatin	20–80 mg daily (30% with 40 mg)	Mainly CYP3A4	Potent inhibitors of CYP3A4[‡]
Simvastatin	10–80 mg (41% with 40 mg)	Mainly CYP3A4	Potent inhibitors of CYP3A4
Pravastatin	20–80 mg daily (34% with 40 mg)	Sulphation, biliary, and urinary excretion	
Fluvastatin	40–80 mg daily (23% with 40 mg)	CYP2C9 (some CYP2C8 and CYP3A4)	Inhibitors of CYP2C9
Atorvastatin	10–80 mg daily (38% with 10 mg)	CYP3A4	Potent inhibitors of CYP3A4
Rosuvastatin	5–40 mg daily (45% with 10 mg)	Minimal metabolism (via CYP2CP and some CYP2C19) and biliary excretion	
Pitavastatin	2–4 mg daily (42% with 2 mg)	Minimal metabolism (via CYP2C8 and CYP2C9), lactonisation, and bilary excretion	Unclear

*Typically, doubling of a statin dose produces an additional 6% absolute decrease in LDL cholesterol – e.g., simvastatin 20 mg daily reduces LDL by 35% and 40 mg daily by 41%.
[†]With all statins, the risk of myopathy is also increased by ciclosporin and gemfibrozil, and possibly other fibrates; prescribing information will provide further details and other interactions.
[‡]Including itraconazole, ketoconazole, erythromycin, clarithromycin, telithromycin, nefazodone, HIV protease inhibitors, and regular ingestion of grapefruit juice.

(1997), and rosuvastatin (2003). Pitavastatin (2003) is available in Japan and India only. Cerivastatin was approved in 1998 but then withdrawn in 2001 because of an unacceptably high risk of rhabdomyolysis. Statins are very effective LDL-lowering agents with excellent clinical trial evidence to support their use (see below). The vast majority of patients requiring lipid-lowering treatment will be adequately managed using statins alone. The relative potency of the statins is shown in Table 2.1.

Safety

Statins appear safe and well tolerated at the standard doses tested in the large randomised trials (atorvastatin 10 mg, fluvastatin 40–80 mg, pravastatin 40 mg and simvastatin 20–40 mg) and are safe in the elderly with no need for dose adjustment or any special consideration [20]. The only important side-effect of statins is myopathy [21], but this is rare and, currently, largely unpredictable. In the randomised trials no other side-effects were found to be more common in those allocated statin compared with placebo. Importantly, there is no convincing evidence that statins cause muscle pain – if creatine kinase (CK) is normal – and given that muscle pain is common, it is extremely important that muscle symptoms in the absence of myopathy do not lead to people having their statin inappropriately stopped. Myopathy or myositis is defined as muscle pain or weakness with a raised CK more than 10 times upper limit of normal (ULN). If unrecognised, this can lead to rhabdomyolysis (arbitrarily defined as a CK greater than 10 000 IU/l) with myoglobinuria and risk of acute renal failure. With simvastatin 40 mg daily in the Heart Protection Study the excess myopathy risk was about 1 in 10 000 per annum and the risk is probably similar or somewhat lower with other statins [22]. Myopathy risk with statins is dose-related, and seems to be more likely to occur in the elderly and those with other diseases. Certain other concomitant medications are also recognised to increase the risk of myopathy when given with statins, the most important of these being ciclosporin, systemic azole antifungals such as ketoconazole and itraconazole, macrolide antibiotics (erythromycin and clarithromycin), the calcium-channel blocker verapamil and certain other lipid-lowering agents (in particular fibrates). Amiodarone in combination with 80 mg simvastatin also increases the risk of myopathy but this interaction has not been documented with other statins.

Statins are contraindicated in the presence of active hepatic disease. Reversible increases in liver transaminases – aspartate transaminase (AST) and alanine transaminase (ALT) – are seen in 1–2% of patients after starting statins [23] and a similar effect is seen with other classes of cholesterol-lowering drugs. However, there is no clear evidence from the large randomised trials that statins are hepatotoxic, suggesting that the observed liver enzyme effects may reflect some reaction by the liver to cholesterol lowering.

Some statins (simvastatin and atorvastatin) have a small effect on anticoagulant control in patients taking warfarin and additional testing of International Normalized Ratio (INR) is recommended when statin treatment is started or stopped or the dose altered. Statins are generally considered safe in patients with impaired renal function and may even limit deterioration in renal function over time [24]. Rosuvastatin has been associated with proteinuria at high doses, an effect not seen with any other statin. However this effect most likely reflects a tubular effect rather than glomerular damage [25].

Clinical trials

Since their introduction about 20 years ago, statins have been extensively studied in a number of well-designed large-scale randomised trials [10]. These have reliably shown that the use of statins produces clear reductions in coronary and cardiovascular events that are roughly proportional to the average cholesterol difference achieved during the trial, consistent with a log-linear relationship between cholesterol level and risk. Indirectly, this supports the idea that more intensive cholesterol lowering will produce greater benefits. Four studies that compared the effects on clinical endpoints of intensive versus standard statin regimens have more recently reported their results [26–29]. When considered together, these studies suggest that more intensive cholesterol lowering may well reduce the risk of further cardiovascular disease in high-risk groups [30]. However, concerns remain about the balance of benefits versus risks of this approach. The SEARCH trial (Study of the Effectiveness of Additional Reductions in Cholesterol and Homocysteine) reported preliminary results in 2008, and these support the use of more intensive LDL lowering (although simvastatin 80 mg daily was associated with a significant excess risk of myopathy [31–33]). With the large amount of trial data to support their use, statins are the drug of choice for patients requiring LDL cholesterol-lowering treatment, either because of their increased cardiovascular risk or because of high cholesterol levels. A 1 mmol/l (39 mg/dl) reduction in total or LDL cholesterol reduces the risk of coronary and cardiovascular events by about one-fifth, and similar proportional benefits are seen regardless of starting total cholesterol, LDL cholesterol or HDL level and regardless of age, gender, other treatment or any other characteristic of the patient [10] (Figure 2.4).

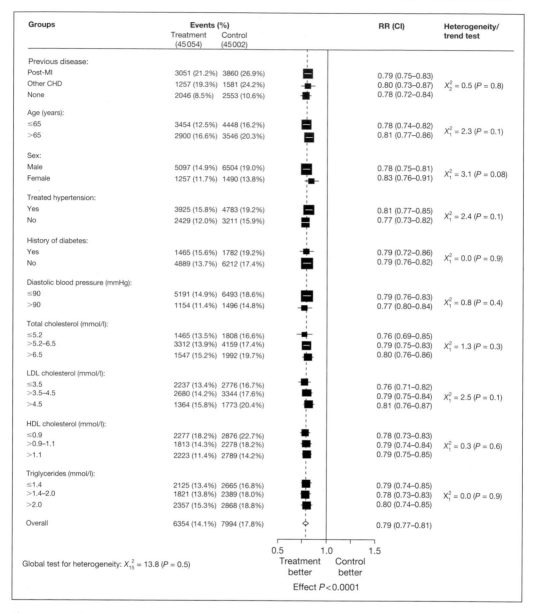

Figure 2.4 Reduction in major vascular events per 1 mmol/l reduction in LDL cholesterol achieved with standard statin doses (meta-analysis of 14 randomised trials of statins) [10].

OTHER LDL-LOWERING THERAPIES

EZETIMIBE

Mode of action

Ezetimibe is the only currently available drug which inhibits the absorption of cholesterol from the intestine. It selectively blocks the Niemann–Pick C1-like 1 (NPC1L1) intestinal transporter, which is responsible for the uptake of cholesterol and phytosterols from the intestinal lumen. Only about one-third of the cholesterol delivered to the gut is dietary in origin, with the remainder from bile and/or released from cell destruction [34]. Ezetimibe reduces both dietary and biliary cholesterol absorption by about one-half, resulting in reduced cholesterol delivery to the liver, upregulation of LDL receptors and, as a consequence, a reduction in circulating LDL cholesterol levels. It has no effect on the absorption of triglycerides, fatty acids, bile acids, steroid hormones or fat-soluble vitamins.

Efficacy

Used alone, in comparison with placebo, ezetimibe reduces total and LDL cholesterol by an average of about 12% and 18% respectively, with a very small (~3%) increase in HDL cholesterol and a moderate decrease (~8%) in triglycerides [35–37]. When given alone, the LDL lowering effect may seem modest and is comparable to very low-dose statin (e.g. ~2.5 mg simvastatin or 5 mg pravastatin) or to that achieved with a bile acid sequestrant such as cholestyramine, but such an effect may nevertheless be clinically valuable. When ezetimibe is added to a statin, a similar additional 15–18% reduction is seen in LDL cholesterol over and above the effect of statin. Adding ezetimibe to a particular statin dose is therefore comparable to about three doublings of that dose of statin (since typically each doubling of statin dose produces about 6% absolute additional LDL lowering [38]). Its effect is similar irrespective of the amount of cholesterol in the diet but polymorphisms in the NPC1L1 gene may account for variability in the response to ezetimibe [39]. Ezetimibe has been studied in combination with fibrates, niacin and bile acid sequestrants and, in all cases, similar additional reductions in LDL cholesterol are seen [36]. Ezetimibe is neither an inhibitor nor inducer of cytochrome P450 enzymes implying that drug/drug interactions through this mechanism are unlikely. Neither does ezetimibe appear to alter the pharmacokinetics of other drugs.

Safety

Ezetimibe is well tolerated. Rates of adverse events on ezetimibe reported in short-term and small clinical studies generally show no difference compared with rates on placebo or statin alone [36, 39]. Large-scale randomised comparisons are ongoing, and one year safety data from the Study of Heart and Renal Protection (SHARP) comparing ezetimibe 10 mg plus simvastatin 20 mg versus placebo in over 9000 patients with chronic kidney disease, provides substantial reassurance about safety, with no excess of myopathy or in elevations of muscle or liver enzymes [40]. No dose adjustment is required either for the elderly or in renal disease although caution is required with concomitant ciclosporin because of significant increases in ciclosporin blood levels [36]. As ezetimibe is usually given with statins, disentangling the effects on skeletal muscle has been difficult. Although there are rare reports of rhabdomyolysis with ezetimibe alone (there is also a background rate), the body of evidence does not support ezetimibe causing muscle toxicity [41].

Like other lipid-lowering agents, ezetimibe increases liver transaminases in a small proportion of people, although as with the statins these changes have not been implicated in more serious liver damage. It can very rarely cause allergic reactions such as angio-oedema and rashes, but the more commonly reported side-effects are headaches and gastrointestinal symptoms. Ezetimibe is contraindicated in active liver disease and, like statins, in pregnancy and during breast-feeding.

Clinical trials

No trials have yet been completed in which cholesterol lowering with ezetimibe has been shown to prevent cardiovascular events. One large trial is ongoing in which ezetimibe or placebo is being used with statins in high-risk patients (for whom statins are already clearly indicated) [42]. Another trial of several hundred patients with familial hypercholesterolaemia (FH) recently failed to demonstrate any effect of the addition of ezetimibe to simvastatin

80 mg daily on carotid intima-media thickness (IMT) [43], but it seems this group of FH patients were already well treated with almost normal IMT and this may account for the lack of demonstrable effect [44]. In another small study of simvastatin plus ezetimibe in 1900 patients with aortic stenosis, a secondary endpoint of ischaemic events was reduced with this lipid lowering combination, although no effect was seen on aortic valve replacement [45]. The largest ongoing study, SHARP [40] should provide valuable efficacy and safety information about regimens containing ezetimibe.

Resins

The bile acid sequestrants colestyramine, colestipol and colesevalam – also known as resins – bind bile acids in the small intestine and interrupt the enterohepatic circulation of cholesterol. This leads to upregulation of LDL receptors to maintain the cholesterol pool within the liver and produces dose-dependent reductions in LDL cholesterol of 15–20%, but with a tendency to increase triglyceride levels. They are not significantly absorbed but can interfere with the absorption of fat-soluble vitamins (especially vitamin K). Bile acid sequestrants can decrease serum folate levels and may decrease absorption of other drugs such as digoxin. Gastrointestinal side-effects are common (particularly constipation) and compliance may therefore be poor. Furthermore the older agents, cholestyramine and colestipol, are unpalatable and must be given in large doses (typically 20–30 g daily) to have a worthwhile lipid-lowering effect. The newer bile acid sequestrant, colesevalam, was designed to combat the limitations of the traditional resins. It is available in tablet form and appears to be better tolerated, while still lowering LDL cholesterol to the same degree as its predecessors. These agents have some role in the management of children with familial hypercholesterolaemia (see chapter 9), but their use has largely been superseded by statins (and ezetimibe) which lower LDL cholesterol to a greater extent and are more palatable.

Niacin (formerly called nicotinic acid)

Since the 1950s, niacin has been known to be an effective cholesterol-lowering drug with a reduction in coronary events seen with 3 g daily in the Coronary Drug Project [48]. However, its use has been limited because side-effects (especially flushing and itching) are frequent and unpleasant. Internationally, use varies widely with very little use in Europe but much more in the USA. The derivative acipimox is probably better tolerated but still not widely prescribed. Niacin is thought to act by reducing the release of non-esterified fatty acids from adipose tissue, which diminishes hepatic triglyceride synthesis and VLDL secretion from the liver. This may in turn decrease triglyceride/cholesterol exchange via cholesteryl ester transfer protein (CETP), resulting in increased HDL cholesterol [49]. It may also upregulate the ABCA1 transporter. Although the exact mechanism remains unclear, the effect is to lower LDL cholesterol and triglycerides, and increase HDL cholesterol. Doses of 2 g daily (of extended release preparation) result in a reduction of about 15% in LDL cholesterol and an increase in HDL cholesterol of about 20%. These reductions are similar in the presence and absence of statins.

Various sustained-release preparations of niacin have been developed but the side-effects have not been eliminated and some of these products were found to be hepatotoxic. The modified-release preparation marketed as Niaspan appears to be better tolerated than either the crystalline, immediate-release formulation or the sustained-release preparations, with tolerance to the flushing said to develop over time [50]. A careful upward dose titration is recommended to minimise the side-effect profile, starting at 375 mg once daily at night, increasing to a maximum of 2000 mg taken as a single dose at night. Monitoring of liver function is recommended during treatment.

Niaspan has been extensively used in the USA and produces additive effects on the lipid profile when combined with a statin. A large-scale trial of this combination (AIM-HIGH) is ongoing and will assess the comparative efficacy, safety and tolerability of this combination [51]. One concern has been the increased risk of myopathy with the combination of statins and high-dose niacin (>1 g per day), but the magnitude of this risk is at present unclear and this combination is widely used in the USA.

A new product, laropiprant, is a selective prostaglandin D receptor antagonist that substantially reduces the frequency and intensity of niacin-induced flushing [52]. Daily oral doses of the combined extended-release niacin/laropiprant 2 g have been well tolerated in early studies and a further large-scale randomised trial (HPS2-THRIVE) is ongoing to assess the benefits and safety of this combined preparation in addition to routine statin therapy in high-risk patients [53].

CONCLUSIONS

There is now overwhelming evidence that LDL cholesterol is one of the most important causes of atherosclerosis and that lowering it produces clinical benefit. LDL-lowering treatment is one of the cornerstones of prevention of cardiovascular disease. For most patients a statin will be the drug of first choice but, for some people at high risk, standard statin doses may not be sufficient to produce an appropriately large reduction in LDL cholesterol. Ezetimibe offers the opportunity to safely lower LDL cholesterol further and to minimise the need for the use of higher, perhaps less well-tolerated, statin doses as well as providing a valuable moderately effective but well-tolerated LDL-lowering therapy for those unable to take a statin. Niacin may have an additional role in those patients for whom both LDL lowering and HDL raising are required, and trials are ongoing to assess its use in combination with a statin. The efficacy of statins has been clearly demonstrated in a wide range of people at risk of cardiovascular disease and, within a few years, such trial evidence may be available to support the additional use of ezetimibe and niacin. The introduction and widespread use of these LDL-lowering treatments is likely to have a huge impact on the worldwide epidemic of cardiovascular disease.

REFERENCES

1. Lamarche B, St-Pierre AC, Ruel IL, Cantin B, Dagenais GR, Després JP. A prospective, population-based study of low density lipoprotein particle size as a risk factor for ischemic heart disease in men. *Can J Cardiol* 2001; 17:859–865.
2. Friedewald WT, Levy RI, Fredrickson DS. Estimation of the concentration of low-density lipoprotein cholesterol in plasma, without use of the preparative ultracentrifuge. *Clin Chem* 1972; 18:499–502.
3. Anitschow N, Chatalow S. *Centralblatt Für Allgemeine Pathologie Und Pathologische Anatomie* 1913; 1–9.
4. Stamler J, Vaccaro O, Neaton JD, Wentworth D. Diabetes, other risk factors, and 12-yr cardiovascular mortality for men screened in the Multiple Risk Factor Intervention Trial. *Diabetes Care* 1993; 16:434–444.
5. Chen J, Campbell TC, Li J, Peto R. *Diet, lifestyle and mortality in China.* Oxford University Press, Oxford, 1990.
6. Lewington S, Whitlock G, Clarke R *et al.* Blood cholesterol and vascular mortality by age, sex, and blood pressure: a meta-analysis of individual data from 61 prospective studies with 55 000 vascular deaths. *Lancet* 2007; 370:1829–1839.
7. Iso H, Jacobs DR Jr, Wentworth D, Neaton JD, Cohen JD. Serum cholesterol levels and six-year mortality from stroke in 350 977 men screened for the multiple risk factor intervention trial. *N Engl J Med* 1989; 320:904–910.
8. Zhang X, Patel A, Horibe H *et al.* Cholesterol, coronary heart disease, and stroke in the Asia Pacific region. *Int J Epidemiol* 2003; 32:563–572.
9. Law MR, Wald NJ, Thompson SG. By how much and how quickly does reduction in serum cholesterol concentration lower risk of ischaemic heart disease? *Br Med J* 1994; 308:367–372.

10. Cholesterol Treatment Trialists' (CTT) Collaborators. Efficacy and safety of cholesterol-lowering treatment: prospective meta-analysis of data from 90 056 participants in 14 randomised trials of statins. *Lancet* 2005; 366:1267–1278.

11. JBS 2: Joint British Societies' guidelines on prevention of cardiovascular disease in clinical practice. *Heart* 2005; 91(suppl 5):v1–v52.

12. Executive Summary of The Third Report of The National Cholesterol Education Program (NCEP) Expert Panel on Detection, Evaluation, And Treatment of High Blood Cholesterol In Adults (Adult Treatment Panel III). *JAMA* 2001; 285(19):2486–2497.

13. Hegsted DM, Ausman LM, Johnson JA, Dallal GE. Dietary fat and serum lipids: an evaluation of the experimental data. *Am J Clin Nutr* 1993; 57:875–883.

14. Keys A, Anderson JT, Grande F. Prediction of serum-cholesterol responses of man to changes in fats in the diet. *Lancet* 1957; 273:959–966.

15. Clarke R, Frost C, Collins R, Appleby P, Peto R. Dietary lipids and blood cholesterol: quantitative meta-analysis of metabolic ward studies. *Br Med J* 1997; 314:112–117.

16. Dattilo AM, Kris-Etherton PM. Effects of weight reduction on blood lipids and lipoproteins: a meta-analysis. *Am J Clin Nutr* 1992; 56:320–328.

17. Tang JL, Armitage JM, Lancaster T, Silagy CA, Fowler GH, Neil HA. Systematic review of dietary intervention trials to lower blood total cholesterol in free-living subjects. *Br Med J* 1998; 316:1213–1220.

18. Hooper L, Summerbell CD, Higgins JP *et al*. Dietary fat intake and prevention of cardiovascular disease: systematic review. *Br Med J* 2001; 322:757–763.

19. Brown MS, Goldstein JL. Multivalent feedback regulation of HMG CoA reductase, a control mechanism coordinating isoprenoid synthesis and cell growth. *J Lipid Res* 1980; 21:505–517.

20. Armitage J. The safety of statins in clinical practice. *Lancet* 2007; 370:1781–1790.

21. Thompson PD, Clarkson P, Karas RH. Statin-associated myopathy. *JAMA* 2003; 289:1681–1690.

22. Law M, Rudnicka AR. Statin safety: a systematic review. *Am J Cardiol* 2006; 97:52C–60C.

23. Grundy SM. HMG-CoA reductase inhibitors for treatment of hypercholesterolemia. *N Engl J Med* 1988; 319:24–33.

24. Fried LF, Orchard TJ, Kasiske BL. Effect of lipid reduction on the progression of renal disease: a meta-analysis. *Kidney Int* 2001; 59:260–269.

25. Brewer HB Jr. Benefit-risk assessment of rosuvastatin 10 to 40 milligrams. *Am J Cardiol* 2003; 92:23K–29K.

26. de Lemos JA, Blazing MA, Wiviott SD *et al*. Early intensive vs a delayed conservative simvastatin strategy in patients with acute coronary syndromes: phase Z of the A to Z trial. *JAMA* 2004; 292:1307–1316.

27. LaRosa JC, Grundy SM, Waters DD *et al*. Intensive Lipid Lowering with Atorvastatin in Patients with Stable Coronary Disease. *N Engl J Med* 2005; 352:1425–1435.

28. Pedersen TR, Faergeman O, Kastelein JJP *et al*. High-dose atorvastatin vs usual-dose simvastatin for secondary prevention after myocardial infarction: the IDEAL study: a randomized controlled trial. *JAMA* 2005; 294:2437–2445.

29. Cannon CP, Braunwald E, McCabe CH *et al*. Intensive versus moderate lipid lowering with statins after acute coronary syndromes. *N Engl J Med* 2004; 350:1495–1504.

30. Cannon CP, Steinberg BA, Murphy SA, Mega JL, Braunwald E. Meta-analysis of cardiovascular outcomes trials comparing intensive versus moderate statin therapy. *J Am Coll Cardiol* 2006; 48:438–445.

31. Bowman L, Armitage J, Bulbulia R, Parish S, Collins R. Study of the Effectiveness of Additional Reductions in Cholesterol and Homocysteine (SEARCH): characteristics of a randomized trial among 12064 myocardial infarction survivors. *Am Heart J* 2007; 154:815–823.

32. Collins RE on behalf of the SEARCH Study Collaborative Group. SEARCH (Study of the Effectiveness of Additional Reduction in Cholesterol and Homocysteine): randomized comparison of simvastatin 80 mg versus 20 mg daily for 7 years in 12 064 myocardial infarction survivors. *Circulation* 2008; 118:No. 22 168.

33. Link E, Parish S, Armitage J *et al*. SLCO1B1 variants and statin-induced myopathy – a genome wide study. *N Engl J Med* 2008; 359:789–799.

34. Bays H. Ezetimibe. *Expert Opin Investig Drugs* 2002; 11:1587–1604.

35. Knopp RH, Gitter H, Truitt T *et al*. Effects of ezetimibe, a new cholesterol absorption inhibitor, on plasma lipids in patients with primary hypercholesterolemia. *Eur Heart J* 2003; 24:729–741.

36. Sweeney ME, Johnson RR. Ezetimibe: an update on the mechanism of action, pharmacokinetics and recent clinical trials. *Expert Opin Drug Metab Toxicol* 2007; 3:441–450.
37. Bays HE, Moore PB, Drehobl MA *et al*. Effectiveness and tolerability of ezetimibe in patients with primary hypercholesterolemia: pooled analysis of two phase II studies. *Clin Ther* 2001; 23:1209–1230.
38. Roberts WC. The rule of 5 and the rule of 7 in lipid-lowering by statin drugs. *Am J Cardiol* 1997; 80:106–107.
39. Huff MW, Pollex RL, Hegele RA. NPC1L1: evolution from pharmacological target to physiological sterol transporter. *Arterioscler Thromb Vasc Biol* 2006; 26:2433–2438.
40. SHARP collaborative group. SHARP: An international randomized placebo-controlled trial of lipid-lowering in chronic kidney disease – 1 year safety and biochemical efficacy. *J Am Soc Nephrol* 2007; 18:P817A.
41. Davidson MH, Robinson JG. Safety of aggressive lipid management. *J Am Coll Cardiol* 2007; 49:1753–1762.
42. IMPROVE-IT: examining outcomes in subjects with acute coronary syndrome:vytorin (ezetimibe/simvastatin) vs simvastatin [web page]. Available at http://www.controlled-trials.com/mrct/trial/120167/IMPROVE-IT (accessed 16 January 2007).
43. Kastelein JJ, Sager PT, de Groot E, Veltri E. Comparison of ezetimibe plus simvastatin versus simvastatin monotherapy on atherosclerosis progression in familial hypercholesterolemia. Design and rationale of the Ezetimibe and Simvastatin in Hypercholesterolemia Enhances Atherosclerosis Regression (ENHANCE) trial. *Am Heart J* 2005; 149:234–239.
44. Kastelein JJ, Akdim F, Stroes ES *et al*. Simvastatin with or without ezetimibe in familial hypercholesterolemia. *N Engl J Med* 2008; 358:1431–1433. Erratum in *N Engl J Med* 2008; 358:1977.
45. Rossebø AB, Pedersen TR, Borman K *et al*. Intensive lipid lowering with simvastatin and ezetimibe in aortic stenosis. *N Engl J Med* 2008; 359:1343–1356.
46. Rossebø AB, Pedersen TR, Allen C *et al*. Design and baseline characteristics of the Simvastatin and Ezetimibe in Aortic Stenosis (SEAS) Study. *Am J Cardiol* 2007; 99:970–973.
47. Baigent C, Landray M. Study of Heart and Renal Protection (SHARP). *Kidney Int Suppl* 2003; 84:S207–S210.
48. Clofibrate and niacin in coronary heart disease. *JAMA* 1975; 231:360–381.
49. Hernandez M, Wright SD, Cai TQ. Critical role of cholesterol ester transfer protein in nicotinic acid-mediated HDL elevation in mice. *Biochem Biophys Res Commun* 2007; 355:1075–1080.
50. Capuzzi DM, Guyton JR, Morgan JM *et al*. Efficacy and safety of an extended-release niacin (Niaspan): a long-term study. *Am J Cardiol* 1998; 82(12A):74U–81U; discussion 85U–86U.
51. AIM-HIGH: Niacin plus statin to prevent vascular events [web page]. Available at http://www.controlled-trials.com/mrct/trial/100817/aim-high (accessed 16 January 2007).
52. Cheng K, Wu TJ, Wu KK *et al*. Antagonism of the prostaglandin D2 receptor 1 suppresses nicotinic acid-induced vasodilation in mice and humans. *Proc Natl Acad Sci USA* 2006; 103:6682–6687.
53. HPS2-THRIVE: Treatment of High density lipoprotein to Reduce the Incidence of Vascular Events [web page]. Available at http://www.controlled-trials.com/mrct/trial/258393/HPS2-THRIVE. (Accessed 16 January 2007).

3

High-density lipoprotein as a therapeutic target

P. Barter, K.-A. Rye

INTRODUCTION

The concentration of high-density lipoprotein cholesterol (HDL-C) is a strong, independent, inverse predictor of atherosclerotic coronary heart disease (CHD) [1–5]. The relationship between HDL-C level and CHD risk has been assessed in several population studies where it has been found that for every 0.026 mmol/l (1 mg/dl) increase in HDL-C there is a 2–3% decrease in the risk of future CHD [6]. To date, however, there is no conclusive evidence from clinical trials that interventions which raise HDL-C translate into a reduced CHD risk. This contrasts with the massive evidence base showing the cardioprotective effects of reducing low-density lipoprotein cholesterol (LDL-C) with statins.

Human trials using statins to lower LDL-C have shown consistent and substantial reductions in major cardiovascular events (MCVEs) in the treated group. Furthermore, the magnitude of the event reduction is a function of how much the level of LDL-C is lowered. Each 1 mmol/l (39 mg/dl) decrease in LDL-C equates with a 24% reduction in MCVEs [7]. However, in all of the statin trials reported to date there remains a substantial residual risk in the treated groups. One predictor of this residual risk in people treated with statins is the presence of a low baseline level of HDL-C [8–10]. This is apparent even when the level of LDL-C is reduced by aggressive statin treatment to levels below 1.7 mmol/l (70 mg/dl) [11] (Figure 3.1). This supports the proposition that raising the level of HDL-C should be considered as a therapeutic strategy independent of LDL-C lowering.

In support of the human epidemiological observations suggesting a protective role of HDLs, there are numerous studies in animal models showing that HDL-raising interventions inhibit the development of atherosclerosis. In humans, however, the evidence of a protective effect of HDL is still circumstantial and, although strengthening, awaits direct confirmation. This chapter addresses potential mechanisms by which HDLs protect against cardiovascular disease. The as yet incomplete evidence base that HDLs protect against cardiovascular disease is also summarised.

PROTECTIVE FUNCTIONS OF HDLs

HDLs have several functions which have the potential to protect against the development of atherosclerosis and its sequelae (Table 3.1). These include promoting the efflux of choles-

Philip Barter, MBBS, PhD, FRACP, Director and Chief Executive Officer, The Heart Research Institute, Camperdown, New South Wales, Australia

Kerry-Anne Rye, BSc(Hons), PhD, Head, Lipid Research Group, The Heart Research Institute, Camperdown, New South Wales, Australia

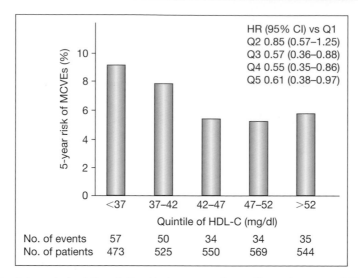

Figure 3.1 Multivariate analysis of the relationship between major cardiovascular events (MCVEs) and HDL-C concentration in 2571 people in the Treatment to New Targets (TNT) trial whose LDL-C had been reduced to <70 mg/dl by treatment with atorvastatin [11]. Results were analysed according to quintile of HDL-C level during treatment and included the following covariates: baseline LDL-C level, treatment, gender, age as a continuous variable, smoking status, body mass index, systolic blood pressure, fasting glucose level, triglyceride level at month 3, and the presence or absence of diabetes, myocardial infarction, cardiovascular disease, and hypertension (adapted with permission from [11]).

terol from cells in the artery wall [12]. HDLs also have potentially protective properties that may be unrelated to their role in cholesterol metabolism (Table 3.1). For example, HDLs bind lipopolysaccharide [13], promote endothelial repair [14, 15] and inhibit the synthesis of platelet-activating factor by endothelial cells [16]. HDLs are also antithrombotic [17] and modulate endothelial function by stimulating endothelial nitric oxide (NO) production [18]. In addition, they show antioxidant and anti-inflammatory activities [19].

ROLE OF HDLs IN PROMOTING CHOLESTEROL EFFLUX

There are at least four documented processes that promote the efflux of cholesterol from cell membranes to HDL acceptors in the extracellular space [20] (Figure 3.2). These include:

1. An interaction of HDL apolipoproteins with the adenosine triphosphate (ATP) binding cassette transporter A1 (ABCA1).
2. An interaction of HDLs with the ATP binding cassette transporter G1 (ABCG1).
3. An interaction of HDLs with the scavenger receptor-B1 (SR-B1).
4. A process of passive diffusion of cholesterol from cell membranes to HDLs in the extra-cellular space.

ABCA1 translocates phospholipids and cholesterol from the inner to the outer leaflets of cell membranes where they associate with apolipoprotein AI (apoAI) or other HDL apolipo-proteins [21]. This interaction is largely confined to apolipoproteins that contain no or very little lipid and mediates apolipoprotein lipidation in a process that results in the formation of discoidal HDL particles. Discoidal HDL particles are excellent substrates for the plasma

Table 3.1 HDL functions with the potential to protect against vascular disease

- Promotion of cholesterol efflux from macrophages in artery wall
- Inhibition of oxidation
- Inhibition of vascular inflammation
- Binding of lipopolysaccharide
- Promotion of endothelial repair
- Stimulation of NO production by endothelium
- Inhibition of synthesis of platelet-activating factor by endothelial cells
- Promotion of angiogenesis

enzyme lecithin:cholesterol acyltransferase (LCAT) which esterifies their cholesterol in a process that converts the discs into spherical HDL particles that are typical of those found in plasma. Both discoidal and spherical HDLs function as acceptors of the cholesterol that is released from cells by ABCG1. ABCG1 promotes a unidirectional transfer of cholesterol from cells, including macrophages, to HDL particles outside the cell [22, 23]. A third efflux mechanism involves binding of discoidal and spherical HDLs to SR-B1 on the surface of cells [20] in a process that facilitates bidirectional transfers of unesterified cholesterol between cells and HDLs. This results in a net efflux of cholesterol from the cell so long as there is a concentration gradient of unesterified cholesterol from the donor cell to the acceptor HDL particle. Both discoidal and spherical HDLs in the extracellular space are also capable of accepting unesterified cholesterol from cell membranes in a process of passive aqueous diffusion that is independent of ABCA1, ABCG1 or SR-B1 [20]. In this diffusion process, unesterified cholesterol in cell membranes is spontaneously released into the extracellular fluid, where it collides with and is incorporated into any pre-existing HDL particles that are present. As is the case for SR-B1-mediated cholesterol efflux, this is a bi-directional process in which unesterified cholesterol exchanges between HDLs and cell membranes. However, a net transfer of cholesterol into HDLs may result when LCAT-mediated esterification of cholesterol on the HDL surface generates a concentration gradient between the cell surface and the HDL particle down which cholesterol flows into HDLs. The relative contributions of these different processes to the net efflux of cholesterol from macrophages in the artery wall are not known.

Once cholesterol has been transferred from cells to HDLs in the extracellular space, it is transported to the liver for recycling or for elimination from the body. Delivery of HDL cholesterol to the liver may be achieved either via a direct pathway in a process involving binding of HDLs to hepatic SR-B1, or via an indirect pathway after being transferred to very low-density lipoproteins (VLDLs) and LDLs by the cholesteryl ester transfer protein (CETP).

ANTI-OXIDANT ACTIVITY OF HDLs

HDLs possess anti-oxidant properties [24] and inhibit the pro-atherogenic oxidative modification of LDLs. The mechanism by which HDLs inhibit oxidation is uncertain, although it may involve paraoxonase that is known to be transported by HDLs in plasma [25]. However, several of the major HDL apolipoproteins have been shown to have anti-oxidant properties that are independent of paraoxonase [26]. The clinical relevance of the anti-oxidant properties of HDLs is not known.

ANTI-INFLAMMATORY ACTIVITY OF HDLs

Inflammation plays a role in the genesis and instability of atherosclerotic plaques. HDLs have the capacity to inhibit this inflammation. They inhibit binding of monocytes to endothelial

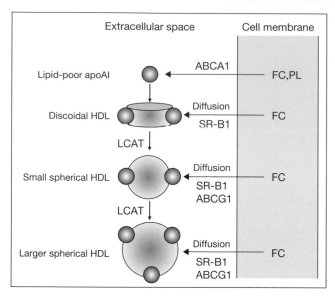

Figure 3.2 Efflux of free cholesterol (FC) from macrophages. FC in macrophage cell membranes is transferred (with phospholipids) to lipid-free apolipoprotein AI (apoAI) or other HDL apolipoproteins in the extracellular space to form discoidal high-density lipoproteins (HDLs). Discoidal HDLs are sequentially converted into small and then larger spherical HDLs by lecithin:cholesterol acyltransferase (LCAT) that esterifies FC on the particle surface to form cholesteryl esters that move into the hydrophobic core of the expanding HDL particle. Discoidal and the spherical HDLs may acquire additional FC from cells by either passive diffusion or by diffusion facilitated by the scavenger receptor type B1 (SR-B1) (reproduced with permission from: Barter PJ. Overview of HDL and reverse cholesterol transport. In: Packard CJ, Rader RJ (eds). *Lipids and Atherosclerosis.* Taylor & Francis, London, 2006, pp 81–92).

cells growing in culture [27]. They also inhibit the cytokine-induced expression of vascular cell adhesion molecule-1 (VCAM-1) (Figure 3.3), intercellular adhesion molecule-1 (ICAM-1) and E-selectin in cultured endothelial cells in a concentration-dependent manner [28], possibly by inhibiting endothelial cell sphingosine kinase [29]. The anti-inflammatory properties of HDLs are dependent on the presence and type of phospholipids in the particles [30, 31].

The anti-inflammatory properties of HDLs are also apparent *in vivo*. For example, intravenous infusions of reconstituted HDLs (rHDLs) consisting of apoAI complexed with phospholipid, reduce the expression of endothelial adhesion molecules that are induced by insertion of carotid periarterial cuffs in cholesterol-fed, apoE-knockout mice [32]. In another study of apoE-knockout mice, expression of the human apoAI gene increased the concentration of HDL and reduced macrophage accumulation in the aortic root by more than 3-fold [32]. This was associated with lower ICAM-1 and VCAM-1 expression and diminished *ex vivo* leukocyte adhesion. In a study conducted in rabbits in which aortic atherosclerosis was induced by a balloon injury followed by 17 weeks of a high cholesterol diet, injections of relatively small amounts of HDLs given during the last week of the study significantly reduced inflammation in the aortic wall [33].

HDLs also have anti-inflammatory properties *in vivo* in the absence of atherosclerosis. For example, injection of rHDLs inhibits the development of a local inflammatory infiltrate following the subcutaneous administration of interleukin-1 in a porcine model [34]. In studies of experimental stroke in rats, pre-treatment with rHDLs substantially reduces the brain necrotic area [34]. In a study of haemorrhagic shock in rats, the resulting multiple organ dysfunction syndrome was largely abolished by an injection of human HDLs given 90 min-

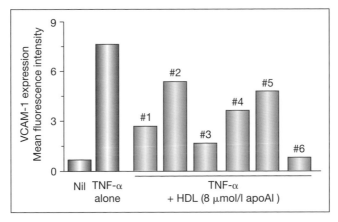

Figure 3.3 Inhibition of cytokine-induced endothelial cell vascular cell adhesion molecule-1 (VCAM-1) expression by HDL isolated from six different human subjects. Human umbilical vein endothelial cells were pre-incubated for 1 hour with HDLs isolated from each of six subjects before being activated with tumour necrosis factor-alpha (TNF-α) and incubated for a further 4.5 hours. 'Nil' depicts a control incubation in which TNF-α was not added. Expression of VCAM-1 was quantified by flow cytometry. Values are expressed relative to the samples that were pre-incubated in the absence of HDL before being activated with TNF-α (with permission from [19, 71]).

utes after the haemorrhage and 1 minute before resuscitation [34]. In other *in vivo* studies conducted in normocholesterolaemic rabbits in which arterial inflammation was induced by application of a non-occlusive silastic collar around a carotid artery, it was found that infusions of rHDLs containing apoAI complexed with phosphatidylcholine markedly inhibited the infiltration of neutrophils into the carotid arterial wall [35]. There was also an inhibition of collar-induced reactive oxygen species formation by the vascular wall, as well as an inhibition of the expression of adhesion molecules and chemokines on the endothelial surface. This inhibition of acute vascular inflammation in rabbits fitted with periarterial collars was achieved with a single injection of remarkably small amounts (2 mg/kg) of apoAI [36].

HDLs appear also to have acute anti-inflammatory effects when infused intravenously into humans. A single infusion of apoAI rHDLs into human subjects with hypercholesterolaemia [37] or with low levels of HDLs secondary to partial deficiency of ABCA1 [18] resulted in normalisation of endothelial function.

INHIBITION OF THROMBOSIS BY HDLs

HDLs inhibit thrombosis by attenuating the expression of tissue factor and selectins, by downregulating thrombin generation via the protein C pathway and by directly and indirectly blunting platelet activation [17]. HDLs also have the potential to protect against arterial and venous thrombosis by activating prostacyclin synthesis [17].

HDLs AND ENDOTHELIAL REPAIR

HDLs enhance endothelial repair by at least two distinct mechanisms. They stimulate endothelial cell migration in a nitric oxide-independent manner via SR-B1-mediated activation of Rac GTPase in a process that depends on the activation of Src kinases, phosphatidylinositol 3-kinase, and p44/42 mitogen-activated protein kinases [14]. In addition, HDLs have the capacity to promote endothelial repair by enhancing the engraftment of endothelial progenitor cells into the endothelium [15, 38]. HDLs also promote angiogenesis [38].

HDL SUBPOPULATIONS

Human plasma HDLs are heterogeneous in terms of their shape, size, density, composition and surface charge [39]. When isolated on the basis of density by ultracentrifugation human HDLs are separated into two major subfractions, HDL_2 and HDL_3. Non-denaturing polyacrylamide gradient gel electrophoresis separates human HDLs on the basis of particle size into at least five distinct subpopulations. HDLs can also be divided into two main subpopulations on the basis of their apolipoprotein composition: HDLs that contain apoAI but no apoAII (AI HDLs) and HDLs that contain both apoAI and apoAII (AI/AII HDLs). apoAI is divided approximately equally between AI HDL and AI/AII HDLs in most subjects, while almost all of the apoAII is in AI/AII HDLs. When subjected to agarose gel electrophoresis, HDLs have either alpha, pre-alpha, pre-beta or gamma migration [39]. The alpha-migrating particles are spherical lipoproteins and predominate in plasma. They include the HDL_2 and HDL_3 subfractions as well as the AI HDL and AI/AII HDL subpopulations. Pre-beta HDLs consist of either a single molecule of lipid-poor apoAI or discoidal particles that contain two or three molecules of apoAI complexed with phospholipids and a small amount of unesterified cholesterol. Gamma-HDLs are spherical particles that contain apoE without apoAI.

Some human population and transgenic animal studies have suggested that AI HDLs may be superior to AI/AII HDLs in their ability to protect against atherosclerosis [40, 41]. Other studies, however, have suggested that the protection conferred by AI HDLs and AI/AII HDLs is similar [42]. Some reports have suggested that populations of larger HDLs are more protective than smaller HDLs [43]. On the other hand, it has been reported that an increase in the concentration of large, cholesterol-rich HDLs is associated with increased rather than decreased cardiovascular risk unless it is accompanied by a high level of apoAI [44]. Overall, therefore, at this time it must be concluded that the evidence linking protection against CHD in humans to specific HDL subpopulations in humans is conflicting and confusing.

EVIDENCE THAT HDLs PROTECT AGAINST ATHEROSCLEROSIS

HDL-RAISING INTERVENTIONS AND ATHEROSCLEROSIS IN ANIMALS

Animal studies have provided powerful evidence that interventions which raise HDL-C protect against atherosclerosis. Badimon and colleagues [45] found in a rabbit model of experimental atherosclerosis that weekly infusions of HDLs significantly reduced the development of aortic fatty streaks. A similar beneficial effect has since been observed in rabbits infused with rHDLs containing either apoAI$_{Milano}$ [46] or native apoAI [33]. However, the most compelling evidence has come from studies in a range of genetically modified animals.

Expression of the human apoAI gene in transgenic rabbits [47] and mice [48, 49] increases the concentration of HDL-C and inhibits the development of atherosclerosis. Increasing the concentration of HDLs in rabbits by inhibiting CETP is also anti-atherogenic [50, 51].

Inhibition of CETP increases the concentration of HDL-C by preventing the transfer of cholesteryl esters from HDLs to VLDLs and LDLs. Such inhibition protects against the development of atherosclerosis in rabbits, regardless of whether the CETP is inhibited by injection of antisense oligodeoxynucleotides against CETP [52], by an anti-CETP vaccine [53] or by the use of small molecule chemical inhibitors of CETP [50, 51]. The increase in HDL-C resulting from CETP inhibition in rabbits is generally accompanied by a decrease in LDL-C, although in one study the anti-atherogenic effects of inhibition of CETP were apparent even when the increase in HDL-C was not accompanied by changes in other lipoprotein fractions [51].

Thus, there is robust evidence from animal studies that HDL-raising interventions are anti-atherogenic.

HDL INCREASE IN HUMAN STUDIES

Although the data from animal studies are impressive, to date they have not been supported by evidence from clinical trials designed specifically to test the hypothesis that raising the concentration of HDLs reduces cardiovascular events. However, there is mounting circumstantial evidence that this will be so.

The Lipid Research Clinics Primary Prevention Trial used cholestyramine as the lipid-modifying agent. A reduction in CHD events correlated positively with changes in LDL-C levels and negatively with changes in HDL-C. For every 1% increase in the concentration of HDL-C there was a 0.6% reduction in CHD events, which was independent of the changes in LDL-C [54].

The relationship between changes in HDL-C and CHD events in the statin trials tends to be masked by the effects of major reductions in LDL-C. However, the increase in HDL-C induced by simvastatin in the Scandinavian Simvastatin Survival Study (4S) was a significant (although weak) predictor of benefit [8], while in the AFCAPS/TexCAPS of lovastatin, the level of apoAI at one year was predictive of benefit [55]. However, the increase in HDL cholesterol induced by pravastatin in the WOSCOPS, CARE and LIPID trials did not correlate significantly with the reduction in CHD events [9, 56].

The relationship between HDL raising with statins and the progression/regression of coronary atheroma has been investigated in an analysis of data from 1455 patients in four intravascular ultrasound imaging trials [57]. Multivariate analysis showed that both the achieved level of LDL-C and the increase in concentration of HDL-C during statin treatment were significant independent predictors of coronary atheroma progression.

The results of fibrate trials have been mixed. In the Helsinki Heart Study, major CHD events were significantly reduced from 4.1% in the placebo group to 2.7% in the gemfibrozil group. In this study, a 1% increase in HDL cholesterol was associated with a 2–3% decrease in CHD events, which was independent of changes in levels of LDL cholesterol [58]. However, most of the benefit of gemfibrozil was found in subjects with an elevated level of plasma triglyceride in combination with a low level of HDL cholesterol. This was especially apparent in those who were also overweight.

In the VA-HIT study the primary endpoint (non-fatal myocardial infarction (MI) or coronary death) was significantly reduced from 21.7% in the placebo group to 17.3% in the gemfibrozil group [59]. The on-treatment HDL cholesterol level was predictive of CHD events in both the active and placebo groups. Multivariate regression analysis showed that, of all the variables examined, only the increase in HDL-C predicted benefit [60]. However, the HDL-C increase accounted for only about one-quarter of the observed benefit.

The Bezafibrate Infarction Prevention (BIP) study used bezafibrate as the active agent. In this study there was no significant effect of bezafibrate on the primary outcome (the combined incidence of non-fatal MI or death from CHD), despite an 18% increase in concentration of HDL cholesterol in those assigned bezafibrate [61]. However, *post hoc* analysis indicated a significant benefit in the subset of patients who entered the trial with an elevated level of plasma triglyceride [61]. There was also a benefit in those with other features of the metabolic syndrome [62]. Thus, while this study added support to a proposition that fibrates are effective in reducing cardiovascular risk in people with features of the metabolic syndrome, it was not possible to conclude that the benefit was secondary to the increase in concentration of HDL.

The more recently reported FIELD study using fenofibrate in people with type 2 diabetes added little to the argument, since fenofibrate treatment in this study resulted in an HDL cholesterol increase of less than 2% and a non-significant reduction in the primary endpoint of the study [63].

Studies with niacin add support to the view that increasing the concentration of HDL-C protects against cardiovascular disease. Niacin has long been used as a lipid-modifying agent. It lowers plasma triglyceride by 40–50%, lowers LDL-C by 10–15% and increases HDL-C by up to 30% [64]. When co-administered with statins, niacin not only promotes significant angiographic regression of atheromatous plaque but also reduces clinical cardiovascular events [65, 66].

The most direct evidence of a benefit of raising HDL levels in humans has been provided by studies in which humans with documented coronary atherosclerosis received infusions of rHDLs. In one study, subjects received intravenous injections of rHDLs containing apoAI$_{Milano}$ complexed with phospholipid at weekly intervals for just 5 weeks [67]. This resulted in a statistically significant reduction in the atheroma burden in the coronary arteries as assessed by intravascular ultrasound. While this study included only a small number of subjects, the result was consistent with a profound protective action of HDLs and has provided a powerful incentive to conduct further research. A comparable result has since been reported in humans receiving infusions of rHDLs containing normal apoAI [68].

EFFECTS OF RAISING HDL-C BY INHIBITING CETP IN HUMANS

CETP acts in human plasma to promote the transfer of cholesteryl esters from the protective HDL fraction to potentially pro-atherogenic particles in the VLDL/LDL fractions [69] (Figure 3.4). Drugs that inhibit CETP have been developed and tested in rabbits and humans. When such drugs are used in rabbits, the resulting increase in HDL-C is associated with a marked inhibition in the development of atherosclerosis [50, 51]. The antiatherogenic potential of inhibiting CETP in humans has been investigated in studies using torcetrapib. These studies failed to show any benefit or apparent harm of the agent.

When given to human subjects, torcetrapib increased the concentration of HDL-C by more than 50% while decreasing LDL-C by about 20%. A consistent, potentially adverse effect of torcetrapib was a small but significant increase in systolic and diastolic blood pressure by a still unknown mechanism. The human intervention trials were designed to test whether CETP inhibition translated into a reduction in cardiovascular risk over and above that achieved with effective treatment with statins.

The largest of these studies was the ILLUMINATE trial [11]. This trial included 15 000 people with manifest cardiovascular disease or type 2 diabetes. All were treated with atorvastatin at a dose necessary to reduce the LDL cholesterol level to less than 2.6 mmol/l (100 mg/dl) before being randomised in a double-blind fashion to receive torcetrapib 60 mg/day or matching placebo. The follow-up was estimated to be 4.5 years in order to achieve enough events to test the hypothesis that treatment with torcetrapib was cardioprotective. This trial was terminated early in December 2006 after a median follow-up of only 18 months because of an excess of deaths in the group assigned torcetrapib [11]. The number of deaths was 82 in the torcetrapib arm compared to 51 deaths in the control arm. This difference was statistically significant. The explanation for the excess mortality is currently not known.

Three imaging trials had been completed at around the time the ILLUMINATE trial was terminated. In all three studies, patients had been treated with atorvastatin to achieve optimal levels of LDL-C before being randomised to receive torcetrapib at a daily dose of 60 mg or matching placebo. All subjects continued on atorvastatin throughout the trial. The treatments were continued for 2 years.

One of these trials (ILLUSTRATE) [57] involved the use of intravascular ultrasound to assess coronary atheroma burden while the other two, RADIANCE 1 [11] and RADIANCE 2 [70], used ultrasound to assess the effects of torcetrapib on carotid intima-media thickness.

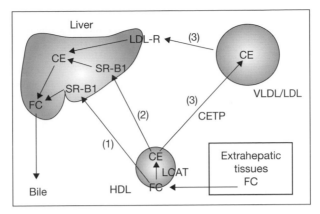

Figure 3.4 Role of cholesteryl ester transfer protein (CETP) in plasma cholesterol transport. Following incorporation of cellular free cholesterol (FC) into HDLs, it may be delivered directly to the liver in a process involving binding of HDLs to the hepatic scavenger receptor type B1 (SR-B1) (pathway 1) or it may be esterified by lecithin:cholesterol acyltransferase (LCAT) to form cholesteryl esters (CE). The HDL CE may then be delivered directly to the liver, again in a process involving binding of HDLs to hepatic SR-B1 (pathway 2), or it may first be transferred by CETP to the VLDL/LDL fraction and then delivered to the liver as a component of the LDL receptor-mediated uptake of LDLs (pathway 3) (reproduced with permission from: Barter PJ. Overview of HDL and reverse cholesterol transport. In: Packard CJ, Rader RJ (eds). *Lipids and Atherosclerosis*. Taylor & Francis, London, 2006, pp 81–92).

The ILLUSTRATE trial involved people with demonstrable coronary atheroma, while RADIANCE 1 and 2 involved patients with familial hypercholesterolaemia and mixed hyperlipidaemia, respectively. The results of all three trials were essentially the same, with no evidence that addition of torcetrapib to atorvastatin provided any benefits over and above those of atorvastatin alone. But, nor was there any evidence of harm.

The future of CETP inhibition as an anti-atherogenic strategy depends on understanding the mechanism responsible for the harm caused by torcetrapib and whether or not it can be shown that this was an off-target pharmacological effect unrelated to CETP inhibition. If this can be established, other CETP inhibitors that do not share such off-target pharmacological effects will warrant further investigation.

CONCLUSIONS

There is overwhelming epidemiological evidence of an inverse relationship between the risk of cardiovascular events and the plasma concentration of HDL-C. The fact that HDLs possess a number of properties with anti-atherogenic potential is consistent with the proposition that HDLs protect against cardiovascular disease. This proposition is further supported by numerous animal studies in which HDL-raising interventions have been shown to inhibit the development of (or even reverse) atherosclerosis. The challenge ahead is to demonstrate that raising the plasma HDL concentration also inhibits the development of atherosclerosis and reduces cardiovascular events in humans. Studies designed to address this issue are awaited with great interest.

REFERENCES

1. Gordon T, Castelli WP, Hjortland MC, Kannel WB, Dawber TR. High density lipoprotein as a protective factor against coronary heart disease. The Framingham Study. *Am J Med* 1977; 62: 707–714.

2. Enger SC, Hjermann I, Foss OP *et al*. High density lipoprotein cholesterol and myocardial infarction or sudden coronary death: a prospective case-control study in middle-aged men of the Oslo study. *Artery* 1979; 5:170–181.

3. Miller NE, Thelle DS, Forde OH, Mjos OD. The Tromso heart-study. High-density lipoprotein and coronary heart-disease: a prospective case-control study. *Lancet* 1977; 1:965–968.

4. Miller M, Seidler A, Kwiterovich PO, Pearson TA. Long-term predictors of subsequent cardiovascular events with coronary artery disease and 'desirable' levels of plasma total cholesterol. *Circulation* 1992; 86:1165–1170.

5. Pekkanen J, Linn S, Heiss G *et al*. Ten-year mortality from cardiovascular disease in relation to cholesterol level among men with and without preexisting cardiovascular disease. *N Engl J Med* 1990; 322:1700–1707.

6. Gordon DJ, Probstfield JL, Garrison RJ *et al*. High-density lipoprotein cholesterol and cardiovascular disease. Four prospective American studies. *Circulation* 1989; 79:8–15.

7. Baigent C, Keech A, Kearney PM *et al*. Efficacy and safety of cholesterol-lowering treatment: prospective meta-analysis of data from 90 056 participants in 14 randomised trials of statins. *Lancet* 2005; 366:1267–1278.

8. Pedersen TR, Olsson AG, Faergeman O *et al*. Lipoprotein changes and reduction in the incidence of major coronary heart disease events in the Scandinavian Simvastatin Survival Study (4S). *Circulation* 1998; 97:1453–1460.

9. Sacks FM, Tonkin AM, Shepherd J *et al*. Effect of pravastatin on coronary disease events in subgroups defined by coronary risk factors: the Prospective Pravastatin Pooling Project. *Circulation* 2000; 102:1893–1900.

10. Simes RJ, Marschner IC, Hunt D *et al*. Relationship between lipid levels and clinical outcomes in the Long-term Intervention with Pravastatin in Ischemic Disease (LIPID) Trial: to what extent is the reduction in coronary events with pravastatin explained by on-study lipid levels? *Circulation* 2002; 105:1162–1169.

11. Barter P, Gotto AM, LaRosa JC *et al*. HDL cholesterol, very low levels of LDL cholesterol, and cardiovascular events. *N Engl J Med* 2007; 357:1301–1310.

12. Duffy D, Rader DJ. Emerging therapies targeting high-density lipoprotein metabolism and reverse cholesterol transport. *Circulation* 2006; 113:1140–1150.

13. Levine DM, Parker TS, Donnelly TM, Walsh A, Rubin AL. In vivo protection against endotoxin by plasma high density lipoprotein. *Proc Natl Acad Sci USA* 1993; 90:12040–12044.

14. Seetharam D, Mineo C, Gormley AK *et al*. High-density lipoprotein promotes endothelial cell migration and reendothelialization via scavenger receptor-B type I. *Circ Res* 2006; 98:63–72.

15. Tso C, Martinic G, Fan WH, Rogers C, Rye KA, Barter PJ. High-density lipoproteins enhance progenitor-mediated endothelium repair in mice. *Arterioscler Thromb Vasc Biol* 2006; 26:1144–1149.

16. Sugatani J, Miwa M, Komiyama Y, Ito S. High-density lipoprotein inhibits the synthesis of platelet-activating factor in human vascular endothelial cells. *J Lipid Mediat Cell Signal* 1996; 13:73–88.

17. Mineo C, Deguchi H, Griffin JH, Shaul PW. Endothelial and antithrombotic actions of HDL. *Circ Res* 2006; 98:1352–1364.

18. Bisoendial RJ, Hovingh GK, Levels JH *et al*. Restoration of endothelial function by increasing high-density lipoprotein in subjects with isolated low high-density lipoprotein. *Circulation* 2003; 107:2944–2948.

19. Rye KA, Barter PJ. Formation and metabolism of prebeta-migrating, lipid-poor apolipoprotein A-I. *Arterioscler Thromb Vasc Biol* 2004; 24:421–428.

20. Yancey PG, Bortnick AE, Kellner-Weibel G, de la Llera-Moya M, Phillips MC, Rothblat GH. Importance of different pathways of cellular cholesterol efflux. *Arterioscler Thromb Vasc Biol* 2003; 23:712–719.

21. Yokoyama S. ABCA1 and biogenesis of HDL. *J Atheroscler Thromb* 2006; 13:1–15.

22. Wang N, Lan D, Chen W, Matsuura F, Tall AR. ATP-binding cassette transporters G1 and G4 mediate cellular cholesterol efflux to high-density lipoproteins. *Proc Natl Acad Sci USA* 2004; 101:9774–9779.

23. Nakamura K, Kennedy MA, Baldan A, Bojanic DD, Lyons K, Edwards PA. Expression and regulation of multiple murine ATP-binding cassette transporter G1 mRNAs/isoforms that stimulate cellular cholesterol efflux to high density lipoprotein. *J Biol Chem* 2004; 279:45980–45989.

24. Mackness MI, Durrington PN, Mackness B. The role of paraoxonase 1 activity in cardiovascular disease: potential for therapeutic intervention. *Am J Cardiovasc Drugs* 2004; 4:211–217.

25. Mackness MI, Durrington PN. HDL, its enzymes and its potential to influence lipid peroxidation. *Atherosclerosis* 1995; 115:243–253.

26. Garner B, Witting PK, Waldeck AR, Christison JK, Raftery M, Stocker R. Oxidation of high density lipoproteins. I. Formation of methionine sulfoxide in apolipoproteins AI and AII is an early event that accompanies lipid peroxidation and can be enhanced by alpha-tocopherol. *J Biol Chem* 1998; 273:6080–6087.

27. Navab M, Imes SS, Hama SY *et al*. Monocyte transmigration induced by modification of low density lipoprotein in cocultures of human aortic wall cells is due to induction of monocyte chemotactic protein 1 synthesis and is abolished by high density lipoprotein. *J Clin Invest* 1991; 88:2039–2046.

28. Cockerill GW, Rye KA, Gamble JR, Vadas MA, Barter PJ. High-density lipoproteins inhibit cytokine-induced expression of endothelial cell adhesion molecules. *Arterioscler Thromb Vasc Biol* 1995; 15:1987–1994.

29. Xia P, Vadas MA, Rye KA, Barter PJ, Gamble JR. High density lipoproteins (HDL) interrupt the sphingosine kinase signaling pathway. A possible mechanism for protection against atherosclerosis by HDL. *J Biol Chem* 1999; 274:33143–33147.

30. Baker PW, Rye KA, Gamble JR, Vadas MA, Barter PJ. Ability of reconstituted high density lipoproteins to inhibit cytokine-induced expression of vascular cell adhesion molecule-1 in human umbilical vein endothelial cells. *J Lipid Res* 1999; 40:345–353.

31. Baker PW, Rye KA, Gamble JR, Vadas MA, Barter PJ. Phospholipid composition of reconstituted high density lipoproteins influences their ability to inhibit endothelial cell adhesion molecule expression. *J Lipid Res* 2000; 41:1261–1267.

32. Dimayuga P, Zhu J, Oguchi S *et al*. Reconstituted HDL containing human apolipoprotein A-1 reduces VCAM-1 expression and neointima formation following periadventitial cuff-induced carotid injury in apoE null mice. *Biochem Biophys Res Commun* 1999; 264:465–468.

33. Nicholls SJ, Cutri B, Worthley SG *et al*. Impact of short-term administration of high-density lipoproteins and atorvastatin on atherosclerosis in rabbits. *Arterioscler Thromb Vasc Biol* 2005; 25:2416–2421.

34. Cockerill GW, Huehns TY, Weerasinghe A *et al*. Elevation of plasma high-density lipoprotein concentration reduces interleukin-1-induced expression of E-selectin in an in vivo model of acute inflammation. *Circulation* 2001; 103:108–112.

35. Nicholls SJ, Dusting GJ, Cutri B *et al*. Reconstituted high-density lipoproteins inhibit the acute pro-oxidant and proinflammatory vascular changes induced by a periarterial collar in normocholesterolemic rabbits. *Circulation* 2005; 111:1543–1550.

36. Puranik R, Bao S, Nobecourt E *et al*. Low dose apolipoprotein A-I rescues carotid arteries from inflammation in vivo. *Atherosclerosis* 2008; 196:240–247.

37. Spieker LE, Sudano I, Hurlimann D *et al*. High-density lipoprotein restores endothelial function in hypercholesterolemic men. *Circulation* 2002; 105:1399–1402.

38. Sumi M, Sata M, Miura S *et al*. Reconstituted high-density lipoprotein stimulates differentiation of endothelial progenitor cells and enhances ischemia-induced angiogenesis. *Arterioscler Thromb Vasc Biol* 2007; 27:813–818.

39. Rye KA, Clay MA, Barter PJ. Remodelling of high density lipoproteins by plasma factors. *Atherosclerosis* 1999; 145:227–238.

40. Warden CH, Hedrick CC, Qiao JH, Castellani LW, Lusis AJ. Atherosclerosis in transgenic mice overexpressing apolipoprotein A-II. *Science* 1993; 261:469–472.

41. Amouyel P, Isorez D, Bard JM *et al*. Parental history of early myocardial infarction is associated with decreased levels of lipoparticle AI in adolescents. *Arterioscler Thromb* 1993; 13:1640–1644.

42. Tailleux A, Bouly M, Luc G *et al*. Decreased susceptibility to diet-induced atherosclerosis in human apolipoprotein A-II transgenic mice. *Arterioscler Thromb Vasc Biol* 2000; 20:2453–2458.

43. Miller NE. Associations of high-density lipoprotein subclasses and apolipoproteins with ischemic heart disease and coronary atherosclerosis. *Am Heart J* 1987; 113:589–597.

44. van der Steeg WA, Holme I, Boekholdt SM *et al*. High-density lipoprotein cholesterol, high-density lipoprotein particle size, and apolipoprotein A-I: significance for cardiovascular risk: the IDEAL and EPIC-Norfolk studies. *J Am Coll Cardiol* 2008; 51:634–642.

45. Badimon JJ, Badimon L, Fuster V. Regression of atherosclerotic lesions by high density lipoprotein plasma fraction in the cholesterol-fed rabbit. *J Clin Invest* 1990; 85:1234–1241.

46. Chiesa G, Monteggia E, Marchesi M *et al*. Recombinant apolipoprotein A-I(Milano) infusion into rabbit carotid artery rapidly removes lipid from fatty streaks. *Circ Res* 2002; 90:974–980.

47. Duverger N, Kruth H, Emmanuel F *et al*. Inhibition of atherosclerosis development in cholesterol-fed human apolipoprotein A-I-transgenic rabbits. *Circulation* 1996; 94:713–717.

48. Rubin EM, Krauss RM, Spangler EA, Verstuyft JG, Clift SM. Inhibition of early atherogenesis in transgenic mice by human apolipoprotein AI. *Nature* 1991; 353:265–267.

49. Plump AS, Scott CJ, Breslow JL. Human apolipoprotein A-I gene expression increases high density lipoprotein and suppresses atherosclerosis in the apolipoprotein E-deficient mouse. *Proc Natl Acad Sci USA* 1994; 91:9607–9611.

50. Okamoto H, Yonemori F, Wakitani K, Minowa T, Maeda K, Shinkai H. A cholesteryl ester transfer protein inhibitor attenuates atherosclerosis in rabbits. *Nature* 2000; 406:203–207.

51. Morehouse LA, Sugarman ED, Bourassa PA *et al*. Inhibition of CETP activity by torcetrapib reduces susceptibility to diet-induced atherosclerosis in New Zealand White rabbits. *J Lipid Res* 2007; 48:1263–1272.

52. Sugano M, Makino N, Sawada S *et al*. Effect of antisense oligonucleotides against cholesteryl ester transfer protein on the development of atherosclerosis in cholesterol-fed rabbits. *J Biol Chem* 1998; 273:5033–5036.

53. Rittershaus CW, Miller DP, Thomas LJ *et al*. Vaccine-induced antibodies inhibit CETP activity in vivo and reduce aortic lesions in a rabbit model of atherosclerosis. *Arterioscler Thromb Vasc Biol* 2000; 20:2106–2112.

54. The Lipid Research Clinics Coronary Primary Prevention Trial results. I. Reduction in incidence of coronary heart disease. *JAMA* 1984; 251:351–364.

55. Gotto AM Jr, Whitney E, Stein EA *et al*. Relation between baseline and on-treatment lipid parameters and first acute major coronary events in the Air Force/Texas Coronary Atherosclerosis Prevention Study (AFCAPS/TexCAPS). *Circulation* 2000; 101:477–484.

56. Influence of pravastatin and plasma lipids on clinical events in the West of Scotland Coronary Prevention Study (WOSCOPS). *Circulation* 1998; 97:1440–1445.

57. Nicholls SJ, Tuzcu EM, Sipahi I *et al*. Statins, high-density lipoprotein cholesterol, and regression of coronary atherosclerosis. *JAMA* 2007; 297:499–508.

58. Manninen V, Tenkanen L, Koskinen P *et al*. Joint effects of serum triglyceride and LDL cholesterol and HDL cholesterol concentrations on coronary heart disease risk in the Helsinki Heart Study. Implications for treatment. *Circulation* 1992; 85:37–45.

59. Rubins HB, Robins SJ, Collins D *et al*. Gemfibrozil for the secondary prevention of coronary heart disease in men with low levels of high-density lipoprotein cholesterol. Veterans Affairs High-Density Lipoprotein Cholesterol Intervention Trial Study Group. *N Engl J Med* 1999; 341:410–418.

60. Robins SJ, Collins D, Wittes JT *et al*. Relation of gemfibrozil treatment and lipid levels with major coronary events: VA-HIT: a randomized controlled trial. *JAMA* 2001; 285:1585–1591.

61. Secondary prevention by raising HDL cholesterol and reducing triglycerides in patients with coronary artery disease: the Bezafibrate Infarction Prevention (BIP) study. *Circulation* 2000; 102:21–27.

62. Tenenbaum A, Motro M, Fisman EZ, Tanne D, Boyko V, Behar S. Bezafibrate for the secondary prevention of myocardial infarction in patients with metabolic syndrome. *Arch Intern Med* 2005; 165:1154–1160.

63. Keech A, Simes RJ, Barter P *et al*. Effects of long-term fenofibrate therapy on cardiovascular events in 9795 people with type 2 diabetes mellitus (the FIELD study): randomised controlled trial. *Lancet* 2005; 366:1849–1861.

64. Carlson LA. Niaspan, the prolonged release preparation of nicotinic acid (niacin), the broad-spectrum lipid drug. *Int J Clin Pract* 2004; 58:706–713.

65. Brown G, Albers JJ, Fisher LD *et al*. Regression of coronary artery disease as a result of intensive lipid-lowering therapy in men with high levels of apolipoprotein B. *N Engl J Med* 1990; 323:1289–1298.

66. Brown BG, Zhao XQ, Chait A *et al*. Simvastatin and niacin, antioxidant vitamins, or the combination for the prevention of coronary disease. *N Engl J Med* 2001; 345:1583–1592.

67. Nissen SE, Tsunoda T, Tuzcu EM *et al*. Effect of recombinant ApoA-I Milano on coronary atherosclerosis in patients with acute coronary syndromes: a randomized controlled trial. *JAMA* 2003; 290:2292–2300.

68. Tardif JC, Gregoire J, L'Allier PL *et al*. Effects of reconstituted high-density lipoprotein infusions on coronary atherosclerosis: a randomized controlled trial. *JAMA* 2007; 297:1675–1682.

69. Barter PJ, Hopkins GJ, Calvert GD. Transfers and exchanges of esterified cholesterol between plasma lipoproteins. *Biochem J* 1982; 208:1–7.
70. Bots ML, Visseren FL, Evans GW *et al.* Torcetrapib and carotid intima-media thickness in mixed dyslipidaemia (RADIANCE 2 study): a randomised, double-blind trial. *Lancet* 2007; 370:153–160.
71. Ashby DT, Rye KA, Clay MA, Vadas MA, Gamble JR, Barter PJ. Factors influencing the ability of HDL to inhibit expression of vascular cell adhesion molecule-1 in endothelial cells. *Arterioscler Thromb Vasc Biol* 1998; 18:1450–1455.

4

Apolipoprotein B in the therapy of atherogenic dyslipoproteinaemias

A. D. Sniderman

INTRODUCTION

The more precisely we understand the biological processes that characterise us, the more exactly we can describe them, and often, although not always, the more effectively we can manipulate them. Vascular disease has become the numerically most important cause of death worldwide and the plasma lipoproteins are the single most important determinant of the likelihood this will occur [1]. The net impact of the plasma lipoproteins on the arterial walls of any individual depends on the balance of the pro-atherogenic lipoproteins – the apoliprotein (apoB) lipoproteins: chylomicrons, very low-density lipoprotein (VLDL), LDL and lipoprotein (a) (Lp(a)) – and the anti-atherogenic lipoproteins – high-density lipoprotein (HDL) or the apoAI lipoproteins. However, because we know much less about how the anti-atherogenic lipoprotein fractions achieve their beneficial effects than we need to and because we have the ability to powerfully lower the plasma levels of the atherogenic lipoproteins, the focus here will be on apoB lipoprotein.

Each of the atherogenic lipoproteins contains one molecule of apoB. Therefore plasma apoB measures total atherogenic particle number [2]. Not only do we understand in considerable detail the processes responsible for abnormal elevation of plasma apoB, and therefore elevation of atherogenic risk [3], we also have multiple proven potent therapies to reduce the plasma apoB lipoprotein level. However, for the greatest possible success, therapies should be used in the most effective manner. For this, we must understand which marker of atherogenic risk – LDL cholesterol (LDL-C), non-HDL-C or apoB lipoprotein – is the most accurate index of the adequacy of LDL-lowering therapy.

LDL-C has been the conventional target of therapy but considerable evidence indicates that apoB is better suited for this purpose. Indeed, the American Diabetes Association and the American College of Cardiology have just issued a joint consensus statement recommending that apoB be utilised in clinical practice to determine whether LDL-lowering therapy has fully succeeded [4]. These two groups have called for a major change in clinical lipidology practice. Accordingly, the objective of this chapter is to demonstrate why apoB is a more accurate index of the risk of vascular disease and the adequacy of LDL-lowering therapy than either of the conventional cholesterol indices – LDL-C or non-HDL-C.

Allan D. Sniderman, MD, Edwards Professor of Cardiology, McGill University, Montreal, Quebec, Canada

Table 4.2 Studies in which apoB or LDL P are superior to non-HDL-C

Study	Study type	n	Gender	Clinical status	Positive parameter
AMORIS [12]	P	175 553	M + F	Asymptomatic	apoB
Leiden Heart Study [34]	CT	848	M + F		
AFCAPS/TexCAPS [18]	CT	3301	M + F	Asymptomatic	apoB
LIPID [19]	CT	4502	M + F	CAD	apoB
Casale Monferrato Study [21]	P	1565		Type II diabetes	
Health Professionals Follow-up Study [16]	NCC	266/532	M	Asymptomatic	apoB
NHANES [22]	XS	9500	M + F	Asymptomatic	apoB
The Chinese Heart Study [25]	P	3586	M + F	Asymptomatic	apoB
Framingham Offspring Study [29]	P	3066	M + F	Asymptomatic	LDL P
Carotid IMT [35]		723	M	Asymptomatic	

CT = clinical trial; NCC = nested case–control; P = prospective; XS = cross-sectional.

characterised by accumulation of massive numbers of chylomicron and VLDL remnants compared to normal. This results in marked hypertriglyceridaemia but also in disproportionately high cholesterol levels. Because VLDL particles cannot be processed normally to LDL particles, plasma apoB is typically normal, reflecting a much higher than normal VLDL apoB and a low normal LDL apoB. In this specific circumstance, apoB is misleading with respect to risk and inappropriate as a target of therapy. ApoB does add value in that if measured along with TC and triglycerides (TG), the diagnosis of type III hyperlipoproteinaemia can be made from routine laboratory tests, something that was previously not possible. In our own study of 38 cases of type III hyperlipoproteinaemia, all had a TC/apoB ratio >6.2 and a TG/apo(a) ratio of <10.0 [31].

ARGUMENTS FOR ApoB OVER NON-HDL-C

1. *ApoB more accurately identifies the key pathophysiological event responsible for atherogenesis*: trapping of apoB lipoprotein particles within the arterial wall is the key step in atherogenesis. The primary determinant of whether this will occur is the concentration – i.e., the number – of atherogenic apoB particles in the plasma. Atherosclerosis is not simply the accumulation of cholesterol within the arterial wall. Trapping of the apoB particle leads to oxidation of all its components, which results in the unregulated uptake of these partially degraded particles into macrophages and the unleashing of a complex series of inflammatory responses within the wall. Some of these lead to healing or at least 'walling off' by fibrous tissue of the area of injury, while others lead to further local cellular or tissue injury. Cholesterol is not the only 'poison' in the particle; the phospholipids, apoB and triglyceride present can all be oxidised and contribute to injury.
2. *A high correlation between non-HDL-C and apoB does not establish clinical equivalence.* The Adult Treatment Panel III (ATPIII) concluded that non-HDL-C and apoB were clinical equivalents because they were highly correlated [32]. This conclusion is not valid. Correlation relates the rate of change in one variable to the rate of change in another. Correlation is an important test of similarity. However, concordance must also be taken

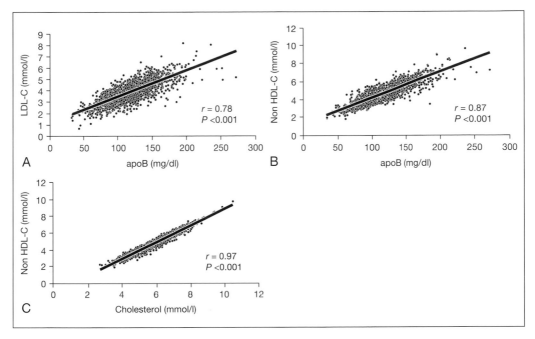

Figure 4.4 The figure illustrates the difference between correlation – the rate of change of one parameter vs. another – compared to concordance – the range of values of one parameter vs. another. (A) plots LDL-C against apoB (moderately correlated and moderately concordant); (B) plots non-HDL-C against apoB (highly correlated and moderately concordant); (C) plots non-HDL-C against TC (highly correlated and highly concordant).

into account and correlation alone is not sufficient to establish that two diagnostic measures are clinical equivalents. Concordance refers to the range of values found for one variable at any specific concentration of the other. Two measures may be highly correlated and may also be highly concordant. However, not all variables that are highly correlated are also highly concordant.

TC, LDL-C, non-HDL-C and apoB are all highly correlated but they are not all highly concordant. Figure 4.4(A) demonstrates that LDL-C and apoB are moderately correlated and moderately concordant [33]. Thus, for any particular value of one variable, there is a considerable range of values for the others. This means that apoB and LDL-C are not equivalent markers of risk in individuals and this discordance is consistent with the findings from epidemiological studies that apoB is superior to LDL-C as a marker of the risk of future vascular events. Figure 4.4(B) demonstrates that the correlation between apoB and non-HDL-C is higher than that between LDL-C and apoB. Nevertheless, apoB and non-HDL-C are only moderately concordant. This means that any specific value of non-HDL-C is associated with a wide range of values for apoB. The consequence is that, for individual cases, this will frequently lead to substantial errors in the classification of risk.

Moreover, we have shown that even though there is a high overall correlation between non-HDL-C and apoB, this differs significantly amongst normal individuals and the different forms of hyperlipidaemia [34]. As would be expected, the correlation is higher in normotriglyceridaemic subjects than those with hypertriglyceridaemia, although the relation is not the same in all hypertriglyceridaemic subjects. Correlation is higher in combined hyperlipidaemia than in simple hypertriglyceridaemia and much lower in familial dysbetalipoproteinaemia. With so many different relationships, the imprecision of correlation is apparent. The apoB that is calculated to be equivalent to non-HDL-C will vary depending on which relationship it is derived from.

By contrast, as shown in Figure 4.4(C), TC and non-HDL-C are both highly correlated and highly concordant. They are, for practical purposes, interchangeable, yet no proponent for non-HDL-C has suggested that we move back to TC.

3. *The balance of epidemiological evidence favours apoB/LDL P over non-HDL-C.* As shown in Table 4.2, a number of studies have shown that apoB and non-HDL-C are of equivalent value in identifying the risk of vascular disease. On the other hand, none have shown that non-HDL-C is superior. In contrast, a substantial number of studies listed in Table 4.2 have shown that apoB is superior to non-HDL-C in identification of the risk of vascular events in asymptomatic individuals, for quantitation of residual risk in those on LDL-lowering therapy and for better correlation with non-invasive measures of vascular disease.

4. *ApoB is the best marker of the adequacy of LDL-lowering therapy*: The American Diabetes Association and the American College of Cardiology have published a joint consensus statement on Lipoprotein Management in Patients with Cardiometabolic Risk [4]. They have recommended that apoB be used in routine clinical practice as the best test of the adequacy of LDL-lowering therapy. They also recommended that when cholesterol targets have been reached apoB should be measured to ensure that maximal LDL-lowering therapy has been achieved. The targets are shown in Table 4.3.

Among the critical elements in reaching this judgment were the multiple studies that demonstrated that apoB/LDL P are more accurate predictors than the cholesterol markers for the risk of future coronary events [10–29], as well as the studies that demonstrated apoB/LDL P to be better predictors for the risk of future coronary events while on statin or fibrate therapy (Table 4.2) [18, 19, 34–37].

Despite the fact that statins are the backbone of LDL-lowering therapy, until recently, little attention has been paid to the differential effects of LDL-lowering therapy on the three atherogenic indices: TC, non-HDL-C, and apoB. The most complete analysis is detailed elsewhere [38]. In brief, the results from 11 studies of LDL lowering, including 17 335 high-risk patients in total, were combined and analysed. These studies include all the statins at their commonly used doses. Data concerning combination therapy of a statin with ezetimibe were also analysed.

The average on-treatment levels of LDL-C, non-HDL-C, and apoB were 2.5 mmol/l (99.2 mg/dl), 3.3 mmol/l (127 mg/dl), and 2.6 mmol/l (101.6 mg/dl) respectively. The average decreases produced by LDL-lowering therapy in LDL-C, non-HDL-C and apoB are shown in Figure 4.5. These differ: LDL-C was reduced the most, by 42.1%, non-HDL-C significantly less by 39.6%; and apoB was reduced least, by 33.1%. Put differently, the decrease in apoB was only 79% of the decrease in LDL-C and non-HDL-C, respectively. Statins or statins combined with ezetimibe, therefore, reduce LDL-C and non-HDL-C more than they reduce apoB or LDL P. This means that decreases in LDL-C and non-HDL-C achieved with LDL-lowering therapy overestimate the decreases in atherogenic particle number achieved with LDL-lowering therapy and overestimate the success of therapy.

To compare LDL-C, non-HDL-C and apoB directly as therapeutic targets, absolute values must be expressed in terms of deviance from the norm. The straightforward way to do this is to express each in terms of percentile of the population. A 50th percentile value of a marker for a population means that 49% of that population have a value lower than this while 50% have a value that is higher. The absolute levels listed as targets of LDL-C, non-HDL-C and apoB for high risk in Table 4.3 all correspond to the 20th percentile of the population, whereas the absolute levels for very high-risk patients correspond to the 10th percentile of the North American population. If there was no discordance between LDL-C and apoB, or between

Table 4.3 ADA/ACC consensus targets – lipoprotein therapy

	Goals		
	LDL cholesterol (mg/dl)	*Non-HDL cholesterol (mg/dl)*	*apoB (mg/dl)*
Highest-risk patients, including those with 1) known CVD or 2) diabetes plus one or more additional major CVD risk factor	<70	<100	<80
High-risk patients, including those with 1) no diabetes or known clinical CVD but two or more additional major CVD risk factors or 2) diabetes but no other major CVD risk factors	<100	<130	<90

Other major risk factors (beyond dyslipoproteinaemia) include smoking, hypertension and family history of premature CAD.

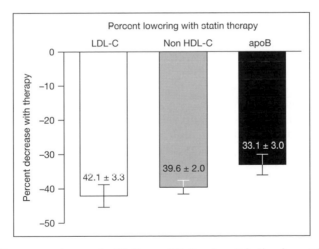

Figure 4.5 Plots of the average decrease in LDL-C, non-HDL-C and apoB in the eleven trials of LDL-lowering therapy (with permission from [39]).

non-HDL-C and apoB, then all three would be of equivalent clinical value in all patients and all three would be reached simultaneously with LDL-lowering therapy.

Figure 4.6 demonstrates the actual percentile values achieved in the eleven studies that were reviewed. LDL-C was decreased to the 21st percentile of the population. By contrast, non-HDL-C was decreased only to the 29th percentile whereas apoB was decreased substantially less to the 55th percentile. Thus, in large numbers of high-risk patients, LDL-C was reduced to target level whereas apoB was decreased only to the average level of the population leaving considerable room for further therapy. Virtually identical results were

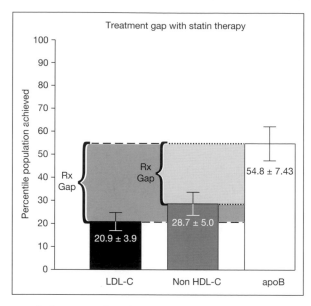

Figure 4.6 The average population percentiles of LDL-C, non-HDL-C and apoB achieved in the eleven trials of LDL-lowering therapy. The treatment gap that results is also illustrated (with permission from [39]).

obtained when studies using LDL P were reviewed. Therefore, relying on LDL-C or non-HDL-C frequently results in a treatment 'gap'.

Why is there such a substantial treatment gap if either LDL-C or non-HDL-C are used as targets for therapy? First, the studies that were analysed all deal with the high-risk classes of patients: those with coronary disease, those with high risk of coronary disease and those with diabetes or the metabolic syndrome. These are the groups of patients in whom increased numbers of small dense, cholesterol-depleted LDL are common. Thus, before therapy, if compared on population percentiles, apoB will be higher than LDL-C and non-HDL-C. Consequently, even if statins resulted in the same drop in these measures, apoB would remain farther from an ideal level than the other two because it was lowered from a higher starting point. However, there is a second explanation. As illustrated in Figure 4.5, the relative lowering from the initial values produced by statins are not the same for the three major atherogenic parameters. Statins reduce LDL-C more than non-HDL-C and they lower non-HDL-C more than apoB. The net effect of starting at a higher level and being reduced less produces a substantial gap between the population percentile achieved for apoB versus those achieved for LDL-C and non-HDL-C.

Since LDL-C drops substantially more than apoB or LDL P and since cholesteryl ester is the major core lipid in LDL, this suggests that LDL size should decrease with statin therapy, which does not occur. How can this apparent discrepancy be explained? Figure 4.7 displays the composition of LDL particles in terms of cholesterol molecules per particle versus plasma triglycerides and LDL-C. Particle size is also included. These data were derived from the Framingham Offspring Study [29]. At any concentration of LDL-C, as plasma triglycerides increase, LDL particle size decreases due to a decrease in the number of cholesterol particles per cell. This is the well-known relationship between plasma triglycerides, LDL-C/apoB ratio, and LDL size. However, the same data demonstrate what happens when LDL-C is reduced without significant change in plasma triglycerides. In this case, the number of cholesterol molecules per LDL particle is reduced but there is no change in LDL particle size.

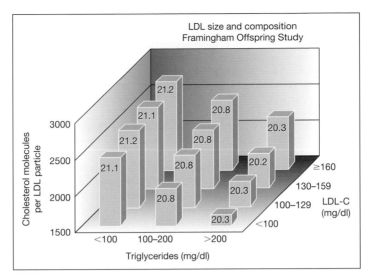

Figure 4.7 The relationships (from [39]) amongst the amount of cholesterol and triglyceride per LDL particle for different values of LDL-C and plasma triglyceride.

This is, in fact, what occurs with statin therapy. Statins lower cholesterol much more than triglycerides. Therefore statin therapy produces a triglyceride-enriched, cholesterol-diminished VLDL particle. The increase in VLDL core triglyceride accentuates TG exchange into the LDL particle, resulting in a relatively TG-enriched LDL particle compared to the pre-treatment LDL particle. Thus, particle size is maintained while core cholesteryl ester is reduced.

CONCLUSIONS

We do not know in any detail the precise sequence of events that initiates a clinical cardiovascular event and we cannot identify with any accuracy those who will be the imminent victims. We do know that trapping of an apoB particle within the arterial wall is the cardinal event that initiates and propagates the atherosclerotic process within the arterial wall. We know also that lowering the number of apoB particles within plasma is the single most powerful therapy to reduce injury to the vascular wall and to decrease the number of clinical events. The data summarized in this chapter demonstrate that both LDL-C and non-HDL-C are imperfect surrogates for apoB. Given that coronary disease is the commonest cause of death worldwide, given that apoB can be measured accurately and inexpensively on non-fasting samples, and given that the superiority of apoB has been acknowledged by the American College of Cardiology, the American Diabetes Association and the American Association of Clinical Chemistry, it is time to introduce apoB into routine clinical practice.

REFERENCES

1. Yusuf S, Hawken S, Ounpuu S *et al*. Effect of potentially modifiable risk factors associated with myocardial infarction in 52 countries (the INTERHEART study): case-control study. *Lancet* 2004; 364:937–952.
2. Sniderman AD, Furberg CD, Keech A *et al*. Apolipoproteins versus lipids as indices of coronary risk and as targets for statin therapy treatment. *Lancet* 2003; 361:777–780.

3. Barter PJ, Ballantyne CM, Carmena R *et al*. ApoB versus cholesterol in estimating cardiovascular risk and in guiding therapy: report of the thirty-person/ten-country panel. *J Intern Med* 2006; 259:247–258.

4. Brunzell JD, Davidson M, Furberg C *et al*. Lipoprotein management in patients with cardiometabolic risk. Consensus statement from the American Diabetes Association and the American College of Cardiology Foundation. *Diabetes Care* 2008; 31:811–822.

5. Jungner I, Sniderman AD, Furberg C, Aastveit AH, Holme I, Walldius G. Does low-density lipoprotein size add to atherogenic particle number in predicting the risk of fatal myocardial infarction? *Am J Cardiol* 2006; 97:943–946.

6. El Harchaoui K, Van der Steeg WA, Stroes ESG *et al*. Value of low-density lipoprotein paticle number and size as predictors of coronary artery disease in apparently healthy men and women. *J Am Coll Cardiol* 2007; 49:547–553.

7. Mora S, Szklo M, Otvos JD *et al*. LDL particle subclasses, LDL particle size, and carotid atherosclerosis in the Multi-Ethnic Study of Atherosclerosis (MESA). *Atherosclerosis* 2007; 192:211–217.

8. Pepe MS, James H, Longton G, Leisenring W, Newcomb P. Limitation of the odds ratio in gauging the performance of a diagnostic, prognostic or screening marker. *Am J Epidemiol* 2004; 159:882–890.

9. Sniderman AD, Furberg CD. Age as a modifiable risk factor for cardiovascular disease. *Lancet* 2008; 371:1547–1549.

10. Lamarche B, Moorjani S, Lupien PJ *et al*. Apoprotein A-1 and B levels and the risk of ischemic heart disease during a 5 year follow-up of men in the Québec Cardiovascular Study. *Circulation* 1996; 94:273–278.

11. Moss AJ, Goldstein RE, Marder VJ *et al*. Thrombogenic factors and recurrent coronary events. *Circulation* 1999; 99:2517–2522.

12. Walldius G, Jungner I, Holme I, Aastveit AH, Kolar W, Steiner E. High apolipoprotein B, low apolipoprotein A-1, and improvement in the prediction of fatal myocardial infarction (AMORIS study): a prospective study. *Lancet* 2001; 358:2026–2033.

13. Talmud PJ, Hawe E, Miller GJ, Humphries SE. Non-fasting apolipoprotein B and triglyceride levels as a useful predictor of coronary heart disease risk in middle-aged UK men. *Arterioscler Thromb Vasc Biol* 2002; 22:1918–1923.

14. Shai I, Rimm EB, Hankinson SE *et al*. Multivariate assessment of lipid parameters as predictors of coronary heart disease among postmenopausal women. Potential implications for clinical guidelines. *Circulation* 2004; 110:2824–2830.

15. Jiang R, Schulze MB, Li T *et al*. Non-HDL cholesterol and apolipoprotein B predict cardiovascular disease events among men with type 2 diabetes. *Diabetes Care* 2004; 27:1991–1997.

16. Pischon T, Girman CJ, Sacks FM, Rifai N, Stampfer MJ, Rimm EB. Non-high-density lipoprotein cholesterol and apolipoprotein B in the prediction of coronary heart disease in men. *Circulation* 2005; 112:3375–3383.

17. Pedersen TR, Olsson AG, Faergeman O *et al*. Lipoprotein changes and reduction in the incidence of major coronary heart disease events in the Scandinavian Simvastatin Survival Study (4S). *Circulation* 1998; 97:1453–1460.

18. Gotto AM, Whitney E, Stein EA, Shapiro DR, Clearfield M, Weis S. Relation between baseline and on-treatment lipid parameters and first acute major coronary events in the Air Force/Texas Coronary Atherosclerosis Prevention Study (AFCAPS/TexCAPS). *Circulation* 2000; 101:477–484.

19. Simes RJ, Marschner IC, Hunt D *et al*. Relationship between lipid levels and clinical outcomes in the long-term intervention with pravastatin in the ischemic disease (LIPID) trial. To what extent is the reduction in coronary events with pravastatin explained by on-study lipid levels? *Circulation* 2002; 105:1162–1169.

20. St-Pierre A, Cantin B, Dagenais GR *et al*. Low-density lipoprotein subfractions and the long-term risk of ischemic heart disease in men: 13-year follow-up data from the Quebec Cardiovascular Study. *Arterioscler Thromb Vasc Biol* 2005; 25:553–559.

21. Bruno G, Merletti F, Biggeri A *et al*. Effect of age on the association of non-high-density-lipoprotein cholesterol and apolipoprotein B with cardiovascular mortality in a Mediterranean population with type 2 diabetes: the Casale Monferrato Study. *Diabetologia* 2006; 49:937–944.

22. Hsia SH, Pan D, Berookim P, Lee M. A population-based, cross-sectional comparison of lipid-related indexes for symptoms of atherosclerotic disease. *Am J Cardiol* 2006; 98:1047–1052.

23. Benn M, Nordestgaard BG, Jensen GB, Tybjaerg-Hansen A. Improving prediction of ischemic cardiovascular disease in the general population using apolipoprotein B: the Copenhagen City Heart Study. *Arterioscler Thromb Vasc Biol* 2007; 27:661–670.

24. Ridker PM, Rifai N, Cook NR, Bradwin G, Buring JE. Non-HDL cholesterol, apolipoproteins A-1 and B100, standard lipid measures, lipid ratios, and CRP as risk factors for cardiovascular disease in women. *JAMA* 2005; 294:326–333.

25. Chien KL, Hsu HC, Su TC, Chen MF, Lee YT, Hu FB. Apolipoprotein B and non-high density lipoprotein cholesterol and the risk of coronary heart disease in Chinese. *J Lipid Res* 2007; 48:2499–2505.

26. Ingelsson E, Schaefer EJ, Contois JH *et al*. Clinical utility of different lipid measures for prediction of coronary heart disease in men and women. *JAMA* 2007; 298:776–785.

27. Blake GJ, Otvos JD, Rifai N, Ridker PM. Low-density lipoprotein particle concentration and size as determined by nuclear magnetic resonance spectroscopy as predictors of cardiovascular disease in women. *Circulation* 2002; 106:1930–1937.

28. Kuller L, Arnold A, Tracy R *et al*. Nuclear magnetic resonance spectroscopy of lipoproteins and risk of coronary heart disease in the cardiovascular health study. *Arterioscler Thromb Vasc Biol* 2002; 22:1175–1180.

29. Cromwell WC, Otvos JD, Keyes MJ *et al*. LDL particle number and risk of future cardiovascular disease in the Framingham Offspring Study – implications for LDL management. *J Clin Lipidology* 2007; 1:583–592.

30. Marcovina S, Packard CJ. Measurement and meaning of apolipoprotein AI and apolipoprotein B plasma levels. *J Intern Med* 2006; 259:437–446.

31. Sniderman A, Tremblay A, Bergeron J, Gagne C, Couture P. Diagnosis of type III hyperlipoproteinemia from plasma total cholesterol, triglyceride, and apolipoprotein B. *J Clin Lipidology* 2007; 1:256–263.

32. Adult Treatment Panel III. Executive Summary of The Third Report of The National Cholesterol Education Program (NCEP) Expert Panel on Detection, Evaluation, and Treatment of High Blood Cholesterol in Adults. *JAMA* 2001; 285:2486–2497.

33. Sniderman AD, St-Pierre A, Cantin B, Dagenais GR, Déprés J-P, Lamarche B. Concordance/discordance between plasma apolipoprotein B levels and the cholesterol indexes of atherosclerotic risk. *Am J Cardiol* 2003; 91:1173–1177.

34. Roeters van Lennep JE, Westerveld HT, Roeters van Lennep HWO, Zwinderman AH, Erkelens DW, van der Wall EE. Apolipoprotein concentrations during treatment and recurrent coronary artery disease events. *Arterioscler Thromb Vasc Biol* 2000; 20:2408–2413.

35. Ruotolo G, Ericsson CG, Tettamanti C *et al*. Treatment effects on serum lipoprotein lipids, apolipoproteins and low density lipoprotein particle size and relationships of lipoprotein variables to progression of coronary artery disease in the Bezafibrate Coronary Atherosclerosis Intervention Trial (BECAIT). *J Am Coll Cardiol* 1998; 32:1648–1656.

36. Vakkilainen J, Steiner G, Ansquer JC *et al*. Relationships between low-density lipoprotein particle size, plasma lipoproteins, and progression of coronary artery disease in the Diabetes Atherosclerosis Intervention Study (DAIS). *Circulation* 2003; 107:1733–1737.

37. Otvos JD, Collins D, Freedman DS *et al*. Low-density lipoprotein and high-density lipoprotein particle subclasses predict coronary events and are favorably changed by gemfibrozil therapy in the Veterans Affairs High-Density Lipoprotein Intervention Trial. *Circulation* 2006; 113:1553–1555.

38. Sniderman AD. Differential response of cholesterol and particle measures of atherogenic lipoproteins to LDL lowering therapy: Implications for clinical practice. *J Clin Lipidology* 2008 (in press).

39. Cromwell WC, Otvos JD, Keyes MJ *et al*. LDL particle number and risk of future cardiovascular disease in the Framingham Offspring Study – implications for LDL management. *J Clin Lipidol* 2007; 1:583–592.

5

Management of coronary heart disease patients

K. K. Ray, C. P. Cannon

INTRODUCTION

A combination of lifestyle change, improved primary prevention and better acute care for patients with acute coronary syndromes (ACS) has contributed to the decline in mortality from coronary heart disease (CHD) [1–4]. However, the incidence of non-fatal coronary events is increasing due in part to the increased prevalence of obesity, diabetes in middle age and smoking in younger people. As mortality declines and non-fatal events increase, the prevalence of CHD in our populations is set to rise. For instance, in a country such as the UK (approximate population 60 million), the prevalence of CHD is estimated at approximately 900 000 and in countries such as the USA, the prevalence is even higher with 12 million people affected (American Heart Association [AHA] Heart and Stroke Facts 2008). Observational studies indicate that a continuous positive relationship exists between blood cholesterol concentrations and CHD risk, suggesting that there is no lower threshold for lowering cholesterol [5]. A decade of trials with statins has demonstrated that cholesterol reduction, and in particular reduction of low-density lipoprotein cholesterol (LDL-C), is central to the long-term management of individuals with CHD for preventing both fatal and non-fatal events. These same drugs also reduce risk of cardiovascular events in individuals initially free from cardiovascular disease (CVD) but who may be at increased risk of CVD because they have multiple risk factors [6, 7], or have comorbid conditions such as diabetes that are considered a CHD risk equivalent [8]. Hence, in routine clinical practice, cholesterol reduction aimed principally at lowering LDL-C is considered the standard of care [9].

CHD AND ABSOLUTE RISK

Typically, individuals with CHD have cholesterol levels that are only very slightly higher than individuals without CHD (Figure 5.1(A)). However, the absolute risk of recurrent events is much higher among those with vascular disease (Figure 5.1(B)). As recurrent vascular events, such as admission with ACS, ischaemic stroke, need for revascularisation and heart failure, occur more commonly among those with CHD, any treatment used for secondary prevention in CHD patients will produce greater absolute benefits in this high-risk population, with smaller numbers needed to treat (NNT), and will hence be more cost-

Kausik K. Ray, BSc, MBChB, MRCP, MD, MPhil, FACC, FESC, Honorary Consultant Cardiologist, Department of Public Health and Primary Care, University of Cambridge; Department of Cardiology, Addenbrooke's Hospital, Cambridge, UK

Christopher P. Cannon, MD, Senior Investigator, TIMI Study Group, Cardiovascular Division, Brigham and Women's Hospital; Associate Professor of Medicine, Harvard Medical School, Boston, Massuchsetts, USA

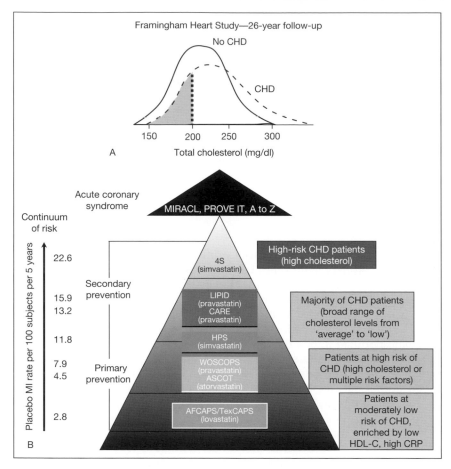

Figure 5.1 (A) Distribution of cholesterol levels among those with and without CHD. (B) Continuum of increasing risk from primary to stable CHD and ACS (with permission from Castelli WP. *Atherosclerosis* 1996; 124(suppl):S1–S9. ©1996 Elsevier Science). CHD = coronary heart disease; CRP = C reactive protein; HDL-C = high-density lipoprotein cholesterol; MI = myocardial infarction.

effective than if the same treatment is applied to a lower-risk primary prevention population (Figure 5.2).

STABLE CHD

The Heart Protection Study (HPS), which included both people with diabetes and individuals with stable CHD or a prior history of stroke or peripheral vascular disease, demonstrated that subjects with an LDL-C <2.56 mmol/l benefited proportionally as much from simvastatin 40 mg as subjects with higher cholesterol levels [10]. The Cholesterol Treatment Trialists (CTT) collaboration provided a prospective meta-analysis of data from 90 056 individuals of primary and secondary prevention. Weighted estimates were obtained of effects on different clinical outcomes as a function of the reduction in LDL-C. During half a million person-years of observation, there were significant (*P* <0.001) absolute risk reductions (ARR) in CHD mortality (1%), need for coronary revascularisation (1.8%), stroke (0.7%), and the incidence of any major vascular event (3.7%) for each 1 mmol/l reduction in LDL-C versus

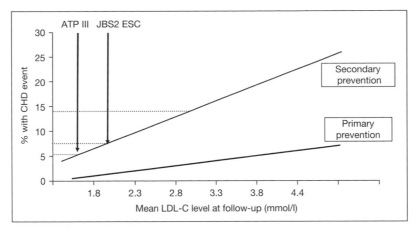

Figure 5.2 Event rates in primary and secondary prevention in relation to on-treatment LDL-C (with permission from [23]).

placebo over about 4–5 years [11]. The proportional benefit was similar across groups and related to the absolute difference in LDL-C and the duration of therapy. The greatest ARR was observed among those at highest risk, reinforcing the health economic benefit of long-term statin therapy among such individuals.

INTENSIVE STATIN THERAPY IN PATIENTS WITH STABLE CHD

Against a background in which standard of care included routine use of statin therapy , the TNT [12] and IDEAL [13] trials were designed to determine whether further LDL-C reduction with more intensive statin therapy was beneficial in subjects with stable CHD and whether this was safe over longer periods of time than previously investigated.

TNT

TNT was a double-blind, randomised trial comparing standard versus intensive therapy (10 mg vs. 80 mg atorvastatin). The study population and the overall results are shown in Table 5.1. Greater reduction in LDL-C among those randomised to intensive therapy resulted in a 2.2% ARR in major vascular events (Table 5.1) largely due to significant reductions in non-fatal myocardial infarction (MI) (hazard ratio [HR] 0.78; 95% confidence interval [CI] 0.66–0.93) and fatal or non-fatal stroke (HR 0.75; 95% CI 0.59–0.96). Overall intensive therapy was safe with no excess risk of major adverse effects. Among the 5584 patients with metabolic syndrome, intensive therapy attenuated the high risk of major cardiovascular events, the 5-year ARR being 3.5% [14].

IDEAL

IDEAL was an open-label trial in patients with a history of MI recruited months to years after this event. They were randomised to treatment with simvastatin 20 mg/40 mg or atorvastatin 80 mg. Approximately 70% of patients were on statin therapy prior to enrolment, including about half previously enrolled in the 4S trial (Table 5.1). Unlike TNT, the primary endpoint in IDEAL was the same as that in the previous 4S; a composite of CHD death, resuscitated cardiac arrest and non-fatal MI, and thus did not include stroke (a TNT endpoint) or revascularisation (a PROVE IT endpoint). The primary endpoint occurred less

Table 5.1 Summary of lipid-lowering trials of intensive versus standard statin therapy

Trial	Population	n	Run-in phase	Duration (yrs)	Regimen	Baseline LDL-C mg/dl (mmol/l)	Achieved LDL-C mg/dl (mmol/l)	Primary endpoint	HR (95% CI)	ARR
TNT	Stable CHD	10 001	Yes	4.9	10 mg atorvastatin	152 (3.9)	98 (2.6)*	Time to major CV event (CHD death, non-fatal MI, resuscitated cardiac arrest, fatal or non-fatal stroke)	0.78 (0.69–0.89)	2.2%
					80 mg atorvastatin	152 (3.9)	77 (2.0)			
IDEAL	Stable CHD	8888	No	4.8	20/40 mg simvastatin	121.4 (3.15)	104 (2.69)	Coronary death, non-fatal MI or resuscitated cardiac arrest	0.89 (0.78–1.01)	1.1%
					80 mg atorvastatin	121.6 (3.15)	82 (2.12)			
PROVE IT – TIMI 22	Post-ACS	4162	No	2	40 mg pravastatin	106 (2.74)	95 (2.46)	Death from any cause, MI, unstable angina requiring rehospitalisation, revascularisation (at least 30 days after randomisation), and stroke	0.84 (0.73–0.96)	3.9%
					80 mg atorvastatin	106 (2.74)	62 (1.60)			
A to Z	Post-ACS	4497	No	2	placebo/ 20 mg simvastatin	113 (2.93)	1 mo: 122 (3.16) 8 mo: 77 (1.99) on sim. 20 mg	Composite of CV death, non-fatal MI, re-admission for ACS and stroke	0.89 (0.76–1.04)	2.3%
					simvastatin (40/80 mg)	113 (2.93)	1 mo: 68 (1.76) on 40 mg 8 mo: 63 (1.63) on 80 mg			

*Mean LDL-C following 8-week open-label run-in phase.
LDL-C is reported as means for TNT and IDEAL, medians for PROVE IT-TIMI 22 and A to Z.
ACS = acute coronary syndromes; CHD = coronary heart disease; CV = cardiovascular; MI = myocardial infarction.

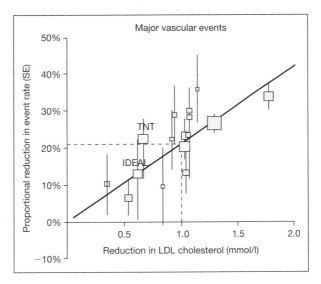

Figure 5.3 The log-linear relationship between absolute LDL reduction and proportional reduction in CHD (adapted with permission from [11]).

frequently with intensive therapy, although the difference was not statistically significant (Table 5.1). In contrast, major cardiovascular events and any CHD event were significantly reduced (ARR 1.7% and 3.6%, respectively) in those assigned intensive treatment.

IMPLICATIONS FOR CLINICAL CARE

Some observers have questioned the importance of TNT and IDEAL citing that the benefit of intensive therapy in these trials was driven by 'soft' endpoints such as recurrent MI, revascularisation or stroke when compared, for instance, to the landmark 4S trial in which the primary endpoint of total mortality was reduced in the statin group versus placebo [15]. However, the 4S trial recruited patients in the 1980s and CHD management has since improved dramatically with greater use of additional cardioprotective medications and revascularisation. Thus, modern trials and their reported benefits are simply not comparable to the early statin trials. Furthermore, atherosclerosis is a chronic disease and even the smaller absolute benefits of intensive therapy observed in TNT and IDEAL over 5 years are likely to translate into greater reductions in the number of major adverse cardiovascular events over a patient's lifetime, providing significant benefits for individuals and healthcare systems.

In summary, the results of recent trials of more intensive LDL-C reduction are consistent with the earlier placebo-controlled trials and continue to reinforce the premise that lowering LDL-C further among those with established vascular disease reduces clinical events (Figure 5.3).

ACUTE CORONARY SYNDROMES

The early statin trials (4S [15], CARE [16] and LIPID [17]) excluded patients within the first 3–6 months following ACS. Therefore, until recently, there was no evidence that statins reduced adverse events within 6 months of hospital discharge. ACS is characterised by a high rate of recurrent events, particularly within the first 6 weeks after the index event

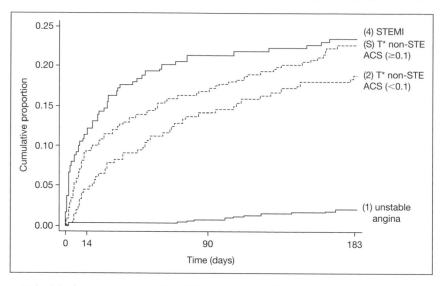

Figure 5.4 Early risk of recurrent events after different types of ACS (with permission from Ray KK, Sheridan PJ, Bolton J *et al.* Management and outcomes of acute coronary syndrome with minimal myocardial necrosis: analysis of a large prospective registry from a non-interventional centre. *Int J Clin Pract* 2006; 60:383–390)

(Figure 5.4) and evidence that statins reduce early events is therefore essential to guide the use of appropriate statin regimens during this time.

MIRACL

The MIRACL trial provided the first evidence that, compared to placebo, high-dose statin therapy with atorvastatin 80 mg initiated within 96 hours of ACS reduced adverse clinical events [18]. In the atorvastatin group, mean LDL-C level declined from 3.2 mmol/l to1.9 mmol/l. The primary endpoint event, defined as death, non-fatal acute MI, cardiac arrest with resuscitation, or recurrent symptomatic myocardial ischaemia with objective evidence and requiring emergency rehospitalisation, occurred in 14.8% of those assigned atorvastatin and in 17.4% of the placebo group (HR 0.84; 95% CI 0.70–1.00). The overall benefit was driven by a lower risk of symptomatic recurrent ischaemia (6.2% vs. 8.4%; HR 0.74; 95% CI 0.57–0.95). In contrast, the PACT trial that compared pravastatin 20–40 mg versus placebo in >3000 patients failed to demonstrate a clinically beneficial effect at 30 days [19]. The PROVE IT-TIMI 22 and the A to Z trials were subsequently designed to better understand how the timing and intensity of statin therapy following an ACS affect clinical outcomes using active comparators.

PROVE IT-TIMI 22

PROVE IT compared pravastatin 40 mg daily with atorvastatin 80 mg daily in patients with ACS hospitalised within the preceding 10 days (Table 5.1) [20]. As expected, LDL-C was lower with intensive therapy (approximate difference 0.8 mmol/l or 31 mg/dl). After 2 years there was a 3.9% ARR and a 16% relative risk reduction (RRR) in the primary endpoint in favour of intensive therapy (*P* = 0.005). There were no significant differences in major side-effects between treatments. Thus, among patients who had recently had an ACS, an intensive lipid-lowering statin regimen provided greater protection against death or major CV events than did standard therapy.

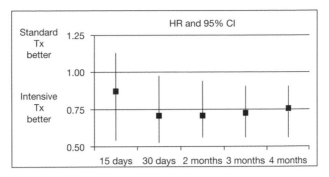

Figure 5.5 Early benefit of intensive vs. standard therapy after ACS. Clinical benefit appears at day 15 and significant by day 30.

A TO Z

This trial compared early initiation of an intensive statin regimen in ACS patients with delayed initiation of a less intensive regimen [21]. Patients received simvastatin 40 mg for 1 month followed by 80 mg thereafter versus placebo for 4 months followed by 20 mg of simvastatin (Table 5.1). Intensive therapy with simvastatin 40/80 mg reduced the risk of the primary composite endpoint by 2.3% but this was not significant [14]. Myopathy (creatine kinase >10 times the upper limit of normal [ULN] with muscle symptoms) occurred in nine patients (0.4%) receiving simvastatin 80 mg and in one patient receiving placebo ($P = 0.02$) with no cases reported at other doses.

IDEAL – RECENT MI SUBSET

The IDEAL trial included 999 patients with an MI in the preceding 2 months who were randomised to simvastatin 20/40 mg versus atorvastatin 80 mg (Pederson T, European Society of Cardiology, 2006). LDL-C differences between intensive and standard therapy were similar to the overall trial with LDL-C levels of approximately 2.1 mmol/l versus 2.6 mmol/l. This was a randomised *post hoc* comparison, and in this subgroup, followed for over 5 years, intensive therapy was associated with a significant 34% RRR in major coronary events (95% CI 0.46–0.95), a 46% reduction in non-fatal MI (95% CI 0.35–0.82), a 21% reduction in any major cardiovascular event (95% CI 0.65–0.96) and a 18% reduction in death or any vascular event (95% CI 0.67–0.99). Importantly in this high-risk population, the risk of death or any vascular event was approximately 60% in patients treated with simvastatin 20/40 mg which was reduced by approximately 10% in absolute terms by intensive therapy (ARR of 2% per year). Therefore, intensive therapy with atorvastatin 80 mg in two separate trials initiated after ACS reduced clinical events over 2 and 5 years compared to standard doses of either pravastatin or simvastatin.

EARLY BENEFITS OF INTENSIVE STATIN THERAPY IN ACS

Early statin trials in stable CHD suggested that the benefits of statin therapy appeared only after 1–2 years [15, 16], potentially questioning the clinical utility of prescribing statins in the early period after ACS. The MIRACL trial demonstrated the benefit of intensive therapy over placebo at 4 months [18]. However, it was not clear if this early benefit would be observed against an active comparator. The PROVE IT-TIMI 22 investigators assessed the risk of death, MI or rehospitalisation for ACS within 30 days of ACS [22]. The composite endpoint was reduced by 4.3% over 2 years ($P = 0.0002$) with benefits in favour of intensive therapy observed as early as 15 days after randomisation (Figure 5.5). At 30 days, the ARR for the composite endpoint was 1.2% and, importantly, this benefit was observed on a background of evidence-based therapy, with use of aspirin in >92% of patients, angiotensin converting enzyme (ACE)/angiotensin receptor blocker (ARB) and β-blockers in 85% of patients, and coronary angioplasty and stenting in approximately 70% of patients. The ARRs observed at 30 days are comparable to those observed with angioplasty and anticoagulants over a similar short time-frame. This rapid benefit coincided with a rapid reduction in C-reactive protein (CRP), independent of effects on LDL-C (1.6 mg/l vs. 2.3 mg/l intensive vs. standard therapy; P <0.0001). Commencing 6 months after ACS to the end of the study, the ARR for composite endpoints was 3.5% in favour of intensive therapy, suggesting that intensive therapy should be continued long-term and not down-titrated. Unless done on the grounds of safety or tolerance, the down-titration of statins raises levels of cholesterol in patients and should be avoided as it iatrogenically increases clinical risk akin to an increase in blood pressure [22, 23].

ROLE OF REDUCING INFLAMMATION

The PROVE IT-TIMI 22 and A to Z trials compared intensive and standard statin therapy after ACS, with apparently disparate results. There were notable differences between the trials in geographical location and use of percutaneous coronary intervention [24]. PROVE IT-TIMI 22 demonstrated that high dose statin therapy lowered LDL-C and CRP at 30 days and was associated with a reduction in cardiovascular events. In contrast, the A to Z trial showed a greater difference in LDL-C between intensive vs. moderate statin regimens but no difference in CRP at 30 days and no statistically significant early benefit was observed [21]. After 4 months the benefit of intensive vs. standard dose statin therapy was identical in PROVE IT and A to Z. Although some caution is necessary in interpreting these findings, reducing inflammation might be more important than lipid lowering in ACS patients with respect to early clinical benefits. The MIRACL trial also demonstrated an early clinical benefit and a greater reduction in CRP within the first 4 months after ACS with intensive statin therapy [25], with early clinical benefits that appeared unrelated to LDL-C [19]. In summary, those regimens which reduce early events after ACS may be those which particularly lower LDL-C and CRP early ACS (Table 5.2). Therefore reducing inflammation may be of relevance in preventing early recurrent events among those with ACS [26].

META-ANALYSES OF INTENSIVE VS. STANDARD THERAPY

RISK OF CHD DEATH, MI OR ANY MAJOR CV EVENT

The TNT [12], IDEAL [13], PROVE IT [20], and A to Z [21] trials used different endpoints to assess clinical benefit and were each underpowered to assess the composite of CHD death or non-fatal MI, which was the primary or major secondary endpoint in many of the initial statin trials. A literature based meta-analysis of these four trials provides information on 27 548 patients and roughly 120 000 years of patient follow-up and gives further evidence for the potential benefits of more intensive statin therapy over standard therapy [27]. The average pooled baseline LDL-C in the four trials was 3.3 mmol/l, which was reduced with standard therapy to an average of 2.59 mmol/l. Intensive therapy further lowered LDL-C to 1.92 mmol/l, representing a relative difference in LDL-C of 25.7% (absolute difference of 0.67 mmol/l) between the treatment groups [27]. This additional LDL-C reduction was associated with an ARR of 1.4% for CHD death or MI (OR 0.84; 95% CI 0.77–0.91; P = 0.00003) (Table 5.3). Similarly, there was an ARR of 3.4% in the risk of any major cardiovascular event (odds ratio [OR] = 0.84; 95% CI 0.80–0.89; P <0.0000001). There was a favourable trend towards reduction in CHD death (OR = 0.88; 95% CI 0.78–1.0; P = 0.054) and no excess in non-CV mortality (OR = 1.03; 95% CI 0.88–1.2; P = 0.73) [27].

Table 5.2 Differences in LDL-C, CRP and outcomes early after ACS in A to Z, MIRACL and PROVE IT–TIMI 22 (adapted with permission from Nissen SE. High-dose statins in acute coronary syndromes: not just lipid levels. *JAMA* 2004; 292:1365)

	A to Z	*MIRACL*	*PROVE IT*
Number of patients randomized	4497	3086	4162
Early* LDL achieved on treatment, mmol/l	1.6	1.85	1.6
Early* LDL cholesterol differential, mmol/l	1.6	1.6	0.85
CRP differential, %	17	34	38
Early event reduction, %	0*	16*	18†

*Measured 120 days after randomization.
†Measured 90 days after randomization.
ACS = acute coronary syndromes; CRP = C-reactive protein; LDL-C = low-density lipoprotein cholesterol

Table 5.3 Clinical benefits of intensive therapy vs. standard therapy from meta-analyses of TNT, IDEAL, A to Z and PROVE IT–TIMI 22

Endpoint	*ARR*	*NNT*	*OR*	*95% CI*
Coronary death or non-fatal MI	1.4	71	0.84	0.77–0.91
Coronary death or any cardiovascular event	3.4			
	0.5	29	0.84	0.80–0.89
Stroke		200	0.82	0.71–0.96
Mortality*	1.1	91	0.75	0.61–0.93

NNTs are based on average around 3.5 years.
*Mortality is based solely on ACS patients over 2 years.
ARR = absolute risk reduction; CI = confidence interval; MI = myocardial infarction; NNT = number needed to treat; OR = odds ratio.

ALL-CAUSE MORTALITY

Although intensive statin therapy was shown to reduce major adverse cardiovascular events, its effect on all-cause mortality remained unclear. A comparative meta-analysis of six trials, encompassing 110 271 patient-years was conducted to determine whether intensive therapy reduces all-cause mortality compared with moderate therapy in patients with recent ACS or stable CHD [27, 28]. In patients with recent ACS, intensive therapy reduced all-cause mortality from 4.6% to 3.5% over 2 years, representing an ARR of 1.1% and a 25% RRR (OR = 0.75; 95% CI 0.61–0.93) (Table 5.3) [29]. However, intensive statin therapy had no significant effect on all-cause mortality in patients with stable CHD after 4.7 years of follow-up (OR = 0.99; 95% CI 0.89–1.11) (Table 5.3) [29].

IMPLICATIONS FOR CLINICAL CARE

These meta-analyses demonstrate that beyond standard therapy, additional intensive LDL-C reduction provides further reduction in risk of non-fatal cardiovascular events among

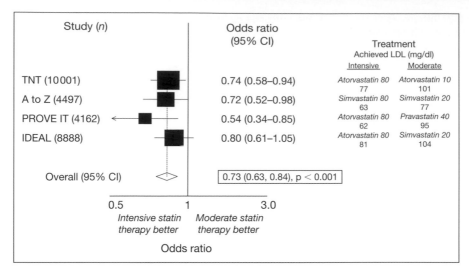

Figure 5.6 Meta-analysis of hospitalisation for heart failure with intensive vs. standard dose statin therapy (with permission from [30]).

patients with stable CHD. In patients with stable CHD, perhaps because of the extensive use of β-blockers, ACE inhibitors, aspirin and coronary revascularisation as background therapy at this time, no significant reduction in all-cause mortality was observed. This contrasts to the early (placebo-controlled) statin trials such as 4S, LIPID and even the HPS. The demonstration of a reduction in all-cause mortality today in stable patients would require some 30–40 000 to be enrolled in the trial. SEARCH, a trial of simvastatin 20 mg vs. 80 mg is nearing completion. The addition of 12 000 patients in this to the 19 000 patients in TNT and IDEAL will provide further information on all-cause mortality. Non-fatal events contribute to the health burden of CHD and even modest benefits observed over 5 years might translate into larger benefits over a patient's lifetime. Additionally, as compared with moderate therapy, intensive statin therapy reduces all-cause mortality in patients with recent ACS and should be considered a standard of care in this context.

HEART FAILURE

A separate analysis of the TNT, IDEAL, PROVE IT-TIMI 22 and A to Z trials comparing intensive versus moderate statin therapy demonstrated a significant 27% reduction in the odds of hospitalisation for heart failure (HF) (OR = 0.73; 95% CI 0.63–0.84) (Figure 5.6) [27]. Considering only the 4162 patients enrolled in PROVE IT-TIMI 22, intensive therapy was associated with a significant absolute reduction in hospitalisation for HF of 1.5% (HR 0.55; 95% CI 0.35–0.85) [27]. In the PROVE IT-TIMI 22 and TNT studies the clinical benefit of reduction in HF was mostly apparent in those individuals with pre-existing evidence of left ventricular dysfunction [30, 31]. Specifically among those with a B-type natriuretic peptide (BNP) >80 pg/ml the ARR was 4.7% with intensive therapy, the HR being 0.32 (95% CI 0.13–0.8; $P = 0.014$) [30]. Among those patients with a prior history of HF, the ARR was 6.7%, reflecting a HR of 0.59 (95% CI; $P = 0.008$) [31]. In contrast, no significant benefit was observed in patients with BNP <80 pg/ml [30] or without a prior history of HF [31]. The present data should be considered in light of the CORONA study, which recruited heart failure patients of ischaemic aetiology (including 60% with prior MI) [32]. The primary endpoint of CV death, MI or non-fatal stroke was not reduced despite achieving major reductions in LDL-C (average 1.96 mmol/l) and CRP (2.1 mg/l) with rosuvastatin 10 mg (HR 0.92; 95% CI 0.83–1.02) compared to placebo, nor were there fewer hospitalisations for heart failure (HR 0.91; 95% CI 0.82–1.02). Possible explanations for differences in trial results may include more advanced disease in patients enrolled in CORONA, a high rate of arrhythmic death (an event unlikely to be influenced by statins) and other differences in the patient populations.

IMPLICATIONS FOR CLINICAL CARE

There are currently no convincing data to support the routine use of standard doses of statins in the management of patients with heart failure. However, among those with stable CHD or ACS with evidence of significant left ventricular dysfunction, intensive statin therapy significantly reduces hospitalisation for heart failure with a low NNT. While it is not immediately clear what role lowering LDL-C plays in reducing risk of HF, the results may reflect beneficial effects of high-dose statin therapy beyond LDL-C reduction (i.e. a pleiotropic effect) [26].

SAFETY AND EFFICACY OF INTENSIVE THERAPY AND LOW LDL-C

Statins are given for life and usually only discontinued if side-effects develop. In standard doses they are remarkably safe [33]. Risks of side-effects primarily relate to the use of concomitant medications, in particular fibrates which may be metabolised through the same cytochrome P450 pathways [33]. In order to optimise patient outcomes, clinicians should be aware of specific patient characteristics, such as advancing age, gender, body mass index, or glomerular filtration rate, which predict muscle and hepatic statin toxicity [34]. Risks of myopathy are of the order of 0.016% for standard doses of statins and rise with increasing doses [33, 34]. Increases in liver enzymes are also dose-dependent but improve with discontinuation of therapy or down-titration of the statin dose and do not appear to result in hepatitis [33, 34].

Among nearly 2000 subjects receiving atorvastatin 80 mg in the PROVE IT trial, about 90% had a LDL-C <2.56 mmol/l at month 4 [35]. Muscle side-effects were at the expected low rate (2–3%) and unrelated to LDL-C levels, with no episode of rhabdomyolysis observed. Similar results were observed for liver-related side-effects with no relationship between achieved LDL-C and the frequency of either liver enzyme elevations or discontinuation for abnormal liver enzyme levels. There was no significant association between the achieved LDL-C and adverse opthalmological events, suicide, trauma, total strokes, or intracranial haemorrhage. Compared to the reference group (LDL-C 2.05–2.56 mmol/l) the hazard of death, MI, stroke, recurrent ischaemia and coronary revascularisation was lower among patients with an LDL-C between 1.03–1.54 mmol/l (HR 0.76; 95% CI 0.50–0.92) and lowest among those with an LDL-C ≤1.03 mmol/l (HR 0.61; 95% CI 0.40–0.91). Thus, when treating patients with intensive statin therapy after an ACS, there was no relationship between achieved LDL-C levels and the risk of adverse side-effects over a 2-year period. However, the rates of cardiovascular events in those achieving lower LDL-C levels decreased progressively according to the level of LDL-C.

The TNT trial observed identical findings in patients with stable CHD [36]. Subjects in the lowest quintile of on-treatment LDL-C (<1.64 mmol/l) had the lowest incidence of the primary endpoint with a gradation of increasing risk across quintiles of LDL-C. Of note, TNT provided safety data on 1836 patients over 5 years who achieved LDL-C levels <1.8 mmol/l, with no excess risk of side-effects compared with higher achieved LDL-C levels [37]. These results suggest that further LDL lowering beyond current guidelines could translate into additional clinical benefit. Ongoing trials are examining this.

IMPLICATIONS FOR CLINICAL CARE

The analyses conducted in the PROVE IT and TNT trials suggest that patients with CHD who are receiving statin therapy should not have their dose down-titrated if a very low LDL-C is observed. However, as these treatments are lifelong, patients receiving high doses of statins should be counselled to be vigilant if additional medications not routinely considered as causing myopathy are coprescribed in the future. These include macrolide antibiotics, antifungals, retroviral agents and amiodarone, which act on the CYP3A4 system.

COSTS OF MORE INTENSIVE TREATMENT

The current guidelines recommending lower LDL-C targets among patients with CHD have major implications for healthcare. Simvastatin 40 mg which costs, for instance, £1.39/month in the UK, reduces total cholesterol by approximately 30–35%, but is unlikely to enable patients to reach their LDL-C goal (European Society of Cardiology [ESC] goal of <2 mmol/l, American College of Cardiology/American Heart Association [ACC/AHA] goal <1.8 mmol/l) if starting cholesterols are >6 mmol/l. Therefore, advocating lower targets will result in greater use of non-generic statins at higher doses such as atorvastatin 40 or 80 mg and rosuvastatin 20 or 40 mg. Given the greater absolute benefit achieved in secondary prevention for any given level of cholesterol reduction, a rational option in patients with stable CHD is to advocate generic therapy in the first instance. Risks of high-dose simvastatin appear to be significantly greater than for other equipotent agents, hence, among patients not at goal with generic statins, high-dose non-generic treatments with appropriate safety data should be considered.

In stable CHD patients, a high-dose statin strategy would yield a gain of 0.10 quality-adjusted life years (QALYs) and is sensitive to model assumptions about statin efficacy [37]. The daily cost difference between a high- and conventional-dose statin would need to be <$1.70, $2.65, and $3.55 (US) to yield incremental cost-effective ratios below $50 000, $100 000 and $150 000 per QALY. In ACS patients, a high-dose versus conventional-dose statin strategy resulted in a gain of 0.35 QALYs. In threshold analyses, a high-dose statin strategy consistently yielded incremental cost-effective ratios below $30 000 per QALY even under conservative model assumptions [37].

IMPLICATIONS FOR CLINICAL CARE

High-dose statin therapy is potentially highly cost-effective in patients with ACS. In patients with stable CHD, however, the cost-effectiveness of high-dose statin therapy is highly sensitive to model assumptions about statin efficacy and cost. Routine use of high-dose statins can be supported on health economic grounds in patients with ACS, but the case is less clear for patients with stable CHD.

RESIDUAL RISK – THE ROLE OF TRIGLYCERIDES AND HDL

There is compelling epidemiological data which suggest that a high triglyceride (TG) concentration [38] and a low high-density lipoprotein cholesterol level (HDL-C) [39] are each independently associated with increased CV risk. Most statins have modest effects on TG levels (approximately 10% reduction) although the newer and more potent statins atorvastatin and rosuvastatin are somewhat more powerful with respect to TG (approximately 30% reduction) even when used at low doses. Similarly, all statins very weakly increase HDL-C by approximately 5–12% (i.e. absolute increase 0.05–0.12 mmol/l), although there are data to suggest that the more potent statins rosuvastatin and atorvastatin more favourably alter HDL subclass compared to others [40, 41]. As the magnitude of CHD risk reduction using statin therapy compared to placebo ranges between 25% and 35%, one potential

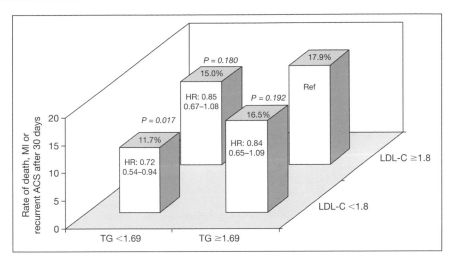

Figure 5.7 Event rate and adjusted hazard of death, MI and recurrent ACS between 30 days and 2 years of follow-up with achieved LDL-C and TG adjusted for age, sex, low HDL-C, smoking, hypertension, obesity, diabetes, prior statin therapy, prior ACS, PVD. ACS = acute coronary syndromes; HR = hazard ratio; HDL-C = high-density lipoprotein cholesterol; LDL-C = low-density lipoprotein cholesterol; MI = myocardial infarction; PVD = peripheral vascular disease; TG = triglyceride.

impediment limiting further reduction in CHD events despite low on-treatment LDL-C is residual elevation in serum TG levels or a low HDL-C.

TRIGLYCERIDES

Recently, observational data from the PROVE IT-TIMI 22 trial suggested that at every level of achieved LDL-C, the risk of recurrent CHD events was reduced by about 15% over 2 years among patients who additionally achieve a TG <1.69 mmol/l [42]. Importantly, even among patients who achieve an on-treatment LDL-C <1.8mmol/l, the risk of recurrent events was lower if TG levels were <1.69 mmol/l (Figure 5.7). These data support the concept that strategies which lower both LDL-C and TG may reduce cardiovascular risk further than strategies which reduce LDL-C alone. In the PROVE IT-TIMI 22 study, 56.1% of patients allocated atorvastatin 80 mg reached an LDL-C <1.8 mmol/l and a TG <1.69 mmol/l compared with only 12% assigned pravastatin 40 mg. This may have contributed to the clinical benefit of intensive statin therapy observed in this trial. However, even intensive statin therapy failed to achieve a dual goal of low LDL-C and TG, suggesting that combination therapy with perhaps a combination of a statin and a fibrate may be of benefit in reducing this residual risk. Such a strategy is being investigated in the ACCORD trial which is comparing statin alone versus statin plus fibrate in high-risk diabetic patients.

HDL-C

In the TNT trial, the achieved LDL-C levels in the intensive- and standard-dose statin regimens were approximately 2 and 2.6 mmol/l, respectively. The TNT trialists conducted an observational study to assess the relevance of HDL-C levels and risk of events using month 3 on-treatment data [43]. Compared to subjects with a HDL-C <0.97 mmol/l (quintile 1), the risk of recurrent events was lower across increasing quintiles of HDL-C, with the lowest risk (HR 0.75; 95% CI 0.60–0.95) observed among those with a HDL-C >1.41 mmol/l (quintile 5) (Figure 5.8(A)). These trends were consistently observed across all categories of achieved LDL-C (<1.8 mmol/l, 1.8–2.56 mmol/l and >2.56 mmol/l) (Figure 5.8(B)). In all,

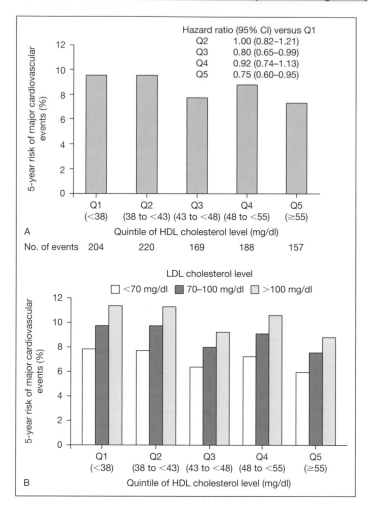

Figure 5.8 (A) Relationship between quintiles of HDL-C and risk in the TNT trial. (B) Relationship between quintiles of HDL-C at different levels of achieved LDL-C in the TNT trial.

2661 subjects achieved an LDL-C <1.8 mmol/l. Among these low LDL-C subjects, those with HDL-C in the highest quintile had a lower risk of major cardiovascular events than subjects in the lowest quintile of HDL-C (HR 0.61; 95% CI 0.38–0.97). These data and prior studies suggest that treatments which raise HDL-C may further reduce CHD risk. HDL-C raising therapy has been limited by what may be off-target toxicity observed with the cholesteryl ester transfer protein (CETP) inhibitor torcetrapib [44]. However, two large trials in 4000 and 20 000 patients (AIM-HIGH and HPS II-THRIVE, respectively in patients after ACS and with stable CHD) are currently underway to assess the incremental benefit of HDL-C raising using nicotinic acid derivates which raise HDL-C by an average 25–30% via ABCA1 and apoAI-mediated pathways on a background of statin therapy.

OTHER AGENTS

Meta-regression studies have suggested that less potent methods for reducing LDL-C or total cholesterol should also produce clinical benefit [45]. Studies with agents such as bile acid sequestrants, fibrates and ileal bypass have suggested that reductions in clinical events may be observed. However the totality of data for benefit of these agents is weaker than for statins [46] and these agents may take longer to demonstrate a clinical benefit. Therefore, statins remain the first-line treatment for CHD. Newer agents such as ezetemibe which block intestinal absorption of cholesterol lower cholesterol by an additional 20% when added to a statin. There are as yet no outcome data with this agent and the recent ENHANCE trial [47] suggested that there were no demonstrable changes in carotid artery intima-media thickness (cIMT) despite 20% lower LDL-C levels with ezetemibe 10 mg plus simvastatin 80 mg versus simvastatin 80 mg. Similar differences in LDL-C using statins have shown differences in both cIMT and clinical outcome [20, 48]. Thus, at present, ezetemibe is best reserved for additional therapy among patients intolerant of high-dose statins. However, a clinical outcomes study is ongoing at present (IMPROVE IT).

CONCLUSIONS

Data from recent high- versus moderate-dose statin trials are consistent with earlier trials and support a 'lower is better' strategy for LDL-C reduction in CHD, with greatest absolute benefit observed among those with greatest absolute risk. This greater effectiveness must also be balanced by acquisition costs. Given the lower risk in stable CHD patients, a balanced approach is to aim for lower LDL-C targets initially with generic statins such as simvastatin 40 mg but using more potent high-dose regimens if these goals are not met. However in high-risk ACS patients, early intensive therapy is required rather than slower up-titration with the weight of evidence at this time favouring high-dose atorvastatin. The absolute benefit observed from statin therapy is related chiefly to the absolute risk of cardiovascular events, reinforcing the need to consider long-term intensive therapy among those individuals at high risk of any type of major vascular event. Overall, the available safety data provide good evidence that very low levels of LDL-C are not harmful and that further reductions in the risk of major CHD events are achieved with reductions in LDL-C well below current goals. Future studies such as IMPROVE IT are prospectively evaluating these hypotheses.

REFERENCES

1. Unal B, Critchley JA, Capewell S. Explaining the decline in coronary heart disease mortality in England and Wales between 1981 and 2000. *Circulation* 2004; 109:1101–1107.
2. Hardoon SL, Whincup PH, Lennon LT, Wannamethee SG, Capewell S, Morris RW. How much of the recent decline in the incidence of myocardial infarction in British men can be explained by changes in cardiovascular risk factors? Evidence from a prospective population-based study. *Circulation* 2008; 117:598–604.
3. Ford ES, Capewell S. Coronary heart disease mortality among young adults in the U.S. from 1980 through 2002: concealed leveling of mortality rates. *J Am Coll Cardiol* 2007; 50:2128–2132.
4. Ford ES, Ajani UA, Croft JB *et al*. Explaining the decrease in U.S. deaths from coronary disease, 1980–2000. *N Engl J Med* 2007; 356:2388–2398.
5. Law MR, Wald NJ. Risk factor thresholds: their existence under scrutiny. *Br Med J* 2002; 324:1570–1576.
6. Shepherd J, Cobbe SM, Ford I *et al*. Prevention of coronary heart disease with pravastatin in men with hypercholesterolemia. West of Scotland Coronary Prevention Study Group. *N Engl J Med* 1995; 333:1301–1307.
7. Sever PS, Dahlof B, Poulter NR *et al*. Prevention of coronary and stroke events with atorvastatin in hypertensive patients who have average or lower-than-average cholesterol concentrations, in the Anglo-Scandinavian Cardiac Outcomes Trial–Lipid Lowering Arm (ASCOT-LLA): a multicentre randomised controlled trial. *Lancet* 2003; 361:1149–1158.
8. Colhoun HM, Betteridge DJ, Durrington PN *et al*. Primary prevention of cardiovascular disease with atorvastatin in type 2 diabetes in the Collaborative Atorvastatin Diabetes Study (CARDS): multicentre randomised placebo-controlled trial. *Lancet* 2004; 364:685–696.

9. Grundy SM, Cleeman JI, Merz CN *et al*. Implications of recent clinical trials for the National Cholesterol Education Program Adult Treatment Panel III guidelines. *Circulation* 2004; 110:227–239.

10. MRC/BHF Heart Protection Study of cholesterol lowering with simvastatin in 20 536 high-risk individuals: a randomised placebo-controlled trial. *Lancet* 2002; 360:7–22.

11. Baigent C, Keech A, Kearney PM *et al*. Efficacy and safety of cholesterol-lowering treatment: prospective meta-analysis of data from 90 056 participants in 14 randomised trials of statins. *Lancet* 2005; 366:1267–1278.

12. LaRosa JC, Grundy SM, Waters DD *et al*. Intensive lipid lowering with atorvastatin in patients with stable coronary disease. *N Engl J Med* 2005; 352:1425–1435.

13. Pedersen TR, Faergeman O, Kastelein JJ *et al*. High-dose atorvastatin vs. usual-dose simvastatin for secondary prevention after myocardial infarction: the IDEAL study: a randomized controlled trial. *JAMA* 2005; 294:2437–2445.

14. Deedwania P, Barter P, Carmena R *et al*. Reduction of low-density lipoprotein cholesterol in patients with coronary heart disease and metabolic syndrome: analysis of the Treating to New Targets study. *Lancet* 2006; 368:919–928.

15. Randomised trial of cholesterol lowering in 4444 patients with coronary heart disease: the Scandinavian Simvastatin Survival Study (4S). *Lancet* 1994; 344:1383–1389.

16. Sacks FM, Pfeffer MA, Moye LA *et al*. The effect of pravastatin on coronary events after myocardial infarction in patients with average cholesterol levels. Cholesterol and Recurrent Events Trial investigators. *N Engl J Med* 1996; 335:1001–1009.

17. Prevention of cardiovascular events and death with pravastatin in patients with coronary heart disease and a broad range of initial cholesterol levels. The Long-Term Intervention with Pravastatin in Ischaemic Disease (LIPID) Study Group. *N Engl J Med* 1998; 339:1349–1357.

18. Schwartz GG, Olsson AG, Ezekowitz MD *et al*. Effects of atorvastatin on early recurrent ischemic events in acute coronary syndromes: the MIRACL study: a randomized controlled trial. *JAMA* 2001; 285:1711–1718.

19. Olsson AG, Schwartz GG, Szarek M *et al*. High-density lipoprotein, but not low-density lipoprotein cholesterol levels influence short-term prognosis after acute coronary syndrome: results from the MIRACL trial. *Eur Heart J* 2005; 26:890–896.

20. Cannon CP, Braunwald E, McCabe CH *et al*. Intensive versus moderate lipid lowering with statins after acute coronary syndromes. *N Engl J Med* 2004; 350:1495–1504.

21. De Lemos JA, Blazing MA, Wiviott SD *et al*. Early intensive vs. a delayed conservative simvastatin strategy in patients with acute coronary syndromes: phase Z of the A to Z trial. *JAMA* 2004; 292:1307–1316.

22. Ray KK, Cannon CP, McCabe CH *et al*. Early and late benefits of high-dose atorvastatin in patients with acute coronary syndromes: results from the PROVE IT-TIMI 22 trial. *J Am Coll Cardiol* 2005; 46:1405–1410.

23. Ray KK, Schofield PM. Secondary prevention for coronary heart disease in the United Kingdom, low-density lipoprotein cholesterol goals and statin switching – an expression of concern. *Int J Clin Pract* 2007; 61:1608–1611.

24. Wiviott SD, de Lemos JA, Cannon CP *et al*. A tale of two trials: a comparison of the post-acute coronary syndrome lipid-lowering trials A to Z and PROVE IT-TIMI 22. *Circulation* 2006; 113:1406–1414.

25. Kinlay S, Schwartz GG, Olsson AG *et al*. High-dose atorvastatin enhances the decline in inflammatory markers in patients with acute coronary syndromes in the MIRACL study. *Circulation* 2003; 108:1560–1566.

26. Ray KK, Cannon CP. The potential relevance of the multiple lipid-independent (pleiotropic) effects of statins in the management of acute coronary syndromes. *J Am Coll Cardiol* 2005; 46:1425–1433.

27. Cannon CP, Steinberg BA, Murphy SA, Mega JL, Braunwald E. Meta-analysis of cardiovascular outcomes trials comparing intensive versus moderate statin therapy. *J Am Coll Cardiol* 2006; 48:438–445.

28. Murphy SA, Cannon CP, Wiviott SD *et al*. Effect of intensive lipid-lowering therapy on mortality after acute coronary syndrome (a patient-level analysis of the Aggrastat to Zocor and Pravastatin or Atorvastatin Evaluation and Infection Therapy-Thrombolysis in Myocardial Infarction 22 trials). *Am J Cardiol* 2007; 100:1047–1051.

29. Afilalo J, Majdan AA, Eisenberg MJ. Intensive statin therapy in acute coronary syndromes and stable coronary heart disease: a comparative meta-analysis of randomised controlled trials. *Heart 2007*; 93:914–921.
30. Scirica BM, Morrow DA, Cannon CP *et al*. Intensive statin therapy and the risk of hospitalization for heart failure after an acute coronary syndrome in the PROVE IT-TIMI 22 study. *J Am Coll Cardiol* 2006; 47:2326–2331.
31. Khush KK, Waters DD, Bittner V *et al*. Effect of high-dose atorvastatin on hospitalizations for heart failure: subgroup analysis of the Treating to New Targets (TNT) study. *Circulation* 2007; 115:576–583.
32. Kjekshus J, Apetrei E, Barrios V *et al*. Rosuvastatin in Older Patients with Systolic Heart Failure. *N Engl J Med* 2007; 357:2248–2261.
33. Armitage J. The safety of statins in clinical practice. *Lancet* 2007; 370:1781–1790.
34. Davidson MH, Robinson JG. Safety of aggressive lipid management. *J Am Coll Cardiol* 2007; 49:1753–1762.
35. Wiviott SD, Cannon CP, Morrow DA, Ray KK, Pfeffer MA, Braunwald E. Can low-density lipoprotein be too low? The safety and efficacy of achieving very low low-density lipoprotein with intensive statin therapy: a PROVE IT-TIMI 22 substudy. *J Am Coll Cardiol* 2005; 46:1411–1416.
36. Chan PS, Nallamothu BK, Gurm HS, Hayward RA, Vijan S. Incremental benefit and cost-effectiveness of high-dose statin therapy in high-risk patients with coronary artery disease. *Circulation* 2007; 115:2398–2409.
37. LaRosa JC, Grundy SM, Kastelein JJ, Kostis JB, Greten H. Safety and efficacy of Atorvastatin-induced very low-density lipoprotein cholesterol levels in Patients with coronary heart disease (a post hoc analysis of the treating to new targets [TNT] study). *Am J Cardiol* 2007; 100:747–752.
38. Sarwar N, Danesh J, Eiriksdottir G *et al*. Triglycerides and the risk of coronary heart disease: 10,158 incident cases among 262,525 participants in 29 Western prospective studies. *Circulation* 2007; 115:450–458.
39. Gordon DJ, Probstfield JL, Garrison RJ *et al*. High-density lipoprotein cholesterol and cardiovascular disease. Four prospective American studies. *Circulation* 1989; 79:8–15.
40. Asztalos BF, Cupples LA, Demissie S *et al*. High-density lipoprotein subpopulation profile and coronary heart disease prevalence in male participants of the Framingham Offspring Study. *Arterioscler Thromb Vasc Biol* 2004; 24:2181–2187.
41. Asztalos BF, Horvath KV, McNamara JR, Roheim PS, Rubinstein JJ, Schaefer EJ. Comparing the effects of five different statins on the HDL subpopulation profiles of coronary heart disease patients. *Atherosclerosis* 2002; 164:361–369.
42. Miller M, Cannon CP, Murphy SA, Qin J, Ray KK, Braunwald E. Impact of triglyceride levels beyond low-density lipoprotein cholesterol after acute coronary syndrome in the PROVE IT-TIMI 22 trial. *J Am Coll Cardiol* 2008; 51:724–730.
43. Barter P, Gotto AM, LaRosa JC *et al*. HDL cholesterol, very low levels of LDL cholesterol, and cardiovascular events. *N Engl J Med* 2007; 357:1301–1310.
44. Barter PJ, Caulfield M, Eriksson M *et al*. Effects of torcetrapib in patients at high risk for coronary events. *N Engl J Med* 2007; 357:2109–2122.
45. Robinson JG, Smith B, Maheshwari N, Schrott H. Pleiotropic effects of statins: benefit beyond cholesterol reduction? A meta-regression analysis. *J Am Coll Cardiol* 2005; 46:1855–1862.
46. Keech A, Simes RJ, Barter P *et al*. Effects of long-term fenofibrate therapy on cardiovascular events in 9795 people with type 2 diabetes mellitus (the FIELD study): randomised controlled trial. *Lancet* 2005; 366:1849–1861.
47. Kastelein JJ, Akdim F, Stroes ES *et al*; ENHANCE Investigators. Simvastatin with or without ezetimibe in familial hypercholesterolemia. *N Engl J Med* 2008; 358:1431–1443. Erratum in *N Engl J Med* 2008; 358:1977.
48. Taylor AJ, Kent SM, Flaherty PJ, Coyle LC, Markwood TT, Vernalis MN. ARBITER: Arterial Biology for the Investigation of the Treatment Effects of Reducing Cholesterol: a randomized trial comparing the effects of atorvastatin and pravastatin on carotid intima medial thickness. *Circulation* 2002; 106:2055–2060.

6

Stroke and transient ischaemic attack prevention

P. Amarenco, P. Lavallée, M. Mazighi, J. Labreuche

INTRODUCTION

It is estimated that stroke affects about 10 million people worldwide every year. Ischaemic stroke is more frequent than myocardial infarction (MI) in Asia and there is now evidence that ischaemic stroke has also become more frequent in Europe as well [1]. This has prompted considerable interest in both the primary and secondary prevention of stroke which is set to continue in future decades. The occurrence of stroke increases with age, particularly affecting the older elderly, a population who are also at a higher risk of developing coronary heart disease (CHD). Regardless of stroke subtype, the prevalence of coronary atherosclerosis in patients with stroke is about 75% [2]. After a first stroke, the 5-year risk of having another stroke is 20% and the 5-year risk of MI is 10% [3], which qualifies stroke as a CHD risk equivalent (i.e. a 10-year risk of MI of 20%).

High blood pressure is the most important risk factor for stroke [4] and by controlling blood pressure, the risk of first-ever or recurrent stroke can be reduced by 40% [5]. Epidemiological and observational studies have not shown a clear association between cholesterol levels and all causes of stroke [6]. Nonetheless, large, long-term statin trials in patients with established CHD or at high risk of developing CHD have shown that statins decrease stroke incidence [7]. This is consistent with other epidemiological studies that have shown a positive and continuous relationship between cholesterol levels and the risk of ischaemic stroke, and possibly an increased risk of haemorrhagic stroke at low cholesterol levels [8].

STATINS IN THE PREVENTION OF STROKE IN HIGH-RISK PATIENTS

Statin trials have included more than 90 000 patients to determine the effect of statins on the incidence of major cardiovascular events in patients at a high risk of vascular events [9]. In these trials, stroke was a secondary endpoint. The relative risk reduction for stroke was 21% (odds ratio [OR] 0.79; confidence interval [CI] 0.73–0.85) with no heterogeneity between trials [8]. Fatal strokes were reduced, but not significantly, by 9% (OR 0.91; CI 0.76–1.10). The

Pierre Amarenco, MD, Professor of Neurology, INSERM U-698 and Paris-Diderot University, Department of Neurology and Stroke Center, Bichat University Hospital, Paris, France

Philippa Lavallée, MD, Associate Professor of Neurology, INSERM U-698 and Paris-Diderot University, Department of Neurology and Stroke Center, Bichat University Hospital, Paris, France

Mikael Mazighi, MD, PhD, Assistant Professor of Neurology, INSERM U-698 and Paris-Diderot University, Department of Neurology and Stroke Center, Bichat University Hospital, Paris, France

Julien Labreuche, BS, Biostatistician, INSERM U-698 and Paris-Diderot University, Department of Neurology and Stroke Center, Bichat University Hospital, Paris, France

extent of the effect of statins was closely associated with the magnitude of low-density lipo-protein cholesterol (LDL-C) reduction. It was estimated that LDL-C reduction explained 34–80% of the observed benefit, consistent with other, possibly pleiotropic, effects. Each 10% reduction in LDL-C was estimated to reduce the risk of all strokes by 13.2% (95% CI 4.8–20.6) and carotid intima-media thickness (cIMT) by 0.73% per year (95% CI 0.27–1.19). This meta-analysis showed that statins may reduce the incidence of all strokes, and this effect was mainly driven by the extent of the between-group LDL-C reduction.

The meta-analysis of the Cholesterol Treatment Trialists (CTT) collaboration, using data from 90 000 individuals, came to the same conclusion [9]. This study showed a reduction in fatal and non-fatal stroke (hazard ratio [HR] 0.83; 95% CI 0.78–0.88; P <0.0001) and indicated that statin therapy could reduce the 5-year incidence of major coronary events, coronary revascularisation and stroke by about one-fifth per 1 mmol/l reduction in LDL-C, largely irrespective of the initial lipid profile or other presenting characteristics, and with a good overall safety profile with no increased incidence of haemorrhagic stroke or cancer [9].

Recent studies such as the Treat to New Target (TNT) trial have confirmed that more aggressive cholesterol lowering with statins reduced the risk of first-ever stroke in patients with coronary artery disease. Benefits of aggressive treatment have also been seen in other high-risk populations, such as in diabetic patients (the Heart Protection Study [HPS] and Collaborative AtoRvastatin Diabetes Study [CARDS] trials), and hypertensives (the Anglo-Scandinavian Cardiac Outcomes Trial [ASCOT] trial), and even in patients with a normal baseline blood cholesterol level, all of which supports the case for a global cardiovascular risk-based treatment strategy [10–12].

STATINS IN SECONDARY STROKE PREVENTION

Until recently, statins have not been shown to prevent recurrent stroke in patients with prior stroke and additional studies in patients representative of the typical stroke population were required to investigate this further. In the HPS, the risk of recurrent stroke of all types was 10.3% in those assigned simvastatin and 10.4% in the placebo group, with significant hetero-geneity (P = 0.002) within the group with no prior cerebrovascular disease at randomisation, and there were 21 (1.3%) haemorrhagic strokes in those assigned simvastatin compared with 11 (0.7%) in the placebo group (P = 0.03) [13]. The main explanations for this neutral effect were the fact that the study was not powered for this comparison and that the patients had their qualifying stroke on average 4.3 months prior to randomisation, at a time when the risk of recurrent stroke has naturally decreased to its lowest level. This contrasts with the risk of MI, which increases continually over time after a stroke or transient ischaemic attach (TIA).

STROKE PREVENTION BY AGGRESSIVE REDUCTION IN CHOLESTEROL LEVELS (SPARCL) STUDY

The SPARCL study focussed only on stroke patients. This unique, large, randomised, placebo-controlled trial evaluated atorvastatin 80 mg/day in patients with previous stroke or TIA [14].

In this trial, 4731 patients with stroke or TIA within 1–6 months of study entry and LDL-C levels of 2.6–4.9 mmol/l (100–190 mg/dl) without known coronary heart disease were randomly assigned to double-blind treatment with atorvastatin 80 mg/day or placebo. The primary endpoint was occurrence of first fatal or non-fatal stroke.

Mean LDL-C over the course of the trial was 73 mg/dl on atorvastatin, and 129 mg/dl in those assigned placebo. After 4.9 years median follow-up, a fatal or non-fatal stroke occurred in 265 patients (11.2%) in the atorvastatin arm and 311 patients (13.1%) in those given placebo (5-year absolute risk reduction 2.2%; adjusted HR 0.84; 95% CI 0.71–0.99; P = 0.03;). Two hundred and eighteen ischaemic and 55 haemorrhagic strokes occurred with atorvastatin, and 274 ischaemic and 33 haemorrhagic strokes with placebo. The absolute 5-year risk

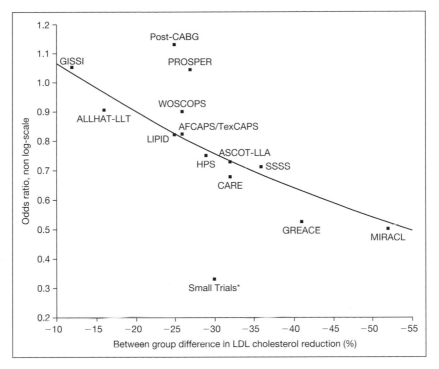

Figure 6.1 Stroke risk reduction according to LDL cholesterol reduction (%) in statin trials.

reduction in major cardiovascular events was 3.5% (HR 0.80; 95% CI 0.69–0.92; *P* = 0.002). All-cause mortality was unchanged (216 deaths in the atorvastatin arm versus 211 deaths in the placebo arm; *P* = 0.98). The rates of serious adverse events such as muscle pain, myopathy and rhabdomyolysis were similar in both treatment groups.

This trial therefore showed that in patients with recent stroke or TIA without known CHD, 5-year treatment with atorvastatin 80 mg/day reduced the incidence of stroke and cardiovascular events (Figure 6.1).

SPARCL SUBANALYSES

Who benefited most?
This result was obtained despite relatively poor adherence to the allocated randomised treatment, particularly in the placebo group. On average, 25% of patients assigned placebo were prescribed a commercially available statin outside the trial. In a *post hoc* analysis, LDL-C reduction was therefore chosen as the best marker for adherence to the allocated treatment, with the hypothesis that patients with no change or an increase in LDL-C (compared to baseline) were not on a statin or were adhering to the allocated placebo treatment regimen, while the group with a >50% LDL-C reduction from baseline were likely to be adhering to treatment with atorvastatin 80 mg/day. Based on 55 045 blinded LDL-C measurements (with an average of 11.6 measurements per patient performed during follow-up), the percentage change in LDL-C from baseline was classified – *post hoc* – as either no change, <50% reduction or ≥50% reduction. Compared to the group with no change or an increase in LDL-C, the group with the most profound LDL-C lowering (>50% from baseline) had a 31% relative risk reduction in stroke and no increase in intracerebral haemorrhage [15].

Haemorrhagic stroke

Another *post hoc* analysis [16] showed that haemorrhagic stroke was more frequent in those treated with atorvastatin, in those with a haemorrhagic stroke as their qualifying event, in men and with increasing age. Those with stage 2 hypertension at the last visit prior to the haemorrhagic stroke during follow-up were also at increased risk. Treatment did not disproportionately affect the haemorrhagic stroke risk associated with these other factors. There was no relationship between the risk of haemorrhagic stroke and baseline LDL cholesterol level or recent LDL cholesterol level in treated patients.

Although the 1409 patients with small vessel disease had a risk of haemorrhagic stroke over the course of the trial that was similar to other ischaemic stroke subgroups, the 708 patients with small vessel disease randomised to atorvastatin were at higher risk of haemorrhagic stroke. The published multivariate analysis [16] did not identify the small vessel disease subgroup as an independent predictor of haemorrhagic stroke. Thus, there was no heterogeneity due to treatment in this subgroup. Data not collected in SPARCL, such as imaging data (e.g. extent of leukoaraiosis, cerebral microbleeding, multilacunae), might have confounded or explained some of the significant associations found. The patients with small vessel disease had a higher baseline systolic and diastolic blood pressure than other ischaemic stroke subgroups. They also had an absolute event rate of recurrent stroke and rate of major cardiovascular events similar to patients with large vessel disease (14.3% and 15.9%, respectively). This similarity between both subgroups was unexpected, although it was consistent with recent autopsy data showing that patients with small vessel disease (with no history of CHD) had coronary plaques in 79% of cases and coronary stenosis >50 % in 37% of cases as compared to 77% and 33% of cases respectively in atherothrombotic strokes and those with no history of symptomatic CHD [17]. Data from the SPARCL trial clearly show that patients with small vessel disease had a long-term risk of major cardiovascular events similar to other ischaemic stroke subtypes. They therefore require the same intensive preventive strategies, including statin therapy. Indeed, the effect of atorvastatin on major cardiovascular events in SPARCL was as great in those with small vessel disease as in those with large vessel disease.

TARGET LDL CHOLESTEROL

The same time-varying analysis of SPARCL showed that achieving LDL-C levels of 1.8 mmol/l (<70 mg/dl) as compared to 2.6 mmol/l (>100 mg/dl) was followed by a 28% relative risk reduction in stroke [15]. This result was obtained *post hoc* and should therefore be considered to be hypothesis-generating. A next step would be to demonstrate in patients with stroke and/or TIA that low LDL-C target levels of 1.8 mmol/l (<70 mg/dl) are associated with a lower incidence of recurrent stroke or other major vascular events than the currently recommended LDL-C target after a stroke of 2.6 mmol/l (<100 mg/dl).

Recent trials have shown that intense LDL-C lowering reduces the risk of major cardiovascular events to a greater degree than standard therapy [10, 18–20]. The PROVE-IT trial randomised 4162 patients with recent acute coronary syndromes to either pravastatin 40 mg/day or atorvastatin 80 mg/day, with an achieved average on-treatment LDL-C of 95 mg/dl and 62 mg/dl respectively [18]. The TNT study randomised 10 001 patients with stable CHD to atorvastatin 80 mg/day or atorvastatin 10 mg/day, achieving an average on-treatment LDL-C of 77 mg/dl and 101 mg/dl respectively [10]. The IDEAL trial randomised patients with CHD to either simvastatin 20–40 mg/day or atorvastatin 80 mg/day, achieving an average on-treatment LDL-C of 100 mg/dl and 80 mg/dl respectively [19].

Finally, the ALLIANCE trial randomised 2442 CHD patients to atorvastatin titrated to a LDL-C target of <70 mg/dl (median dose of atorvastatin 41 mg/day) or 'usual care', achiev-

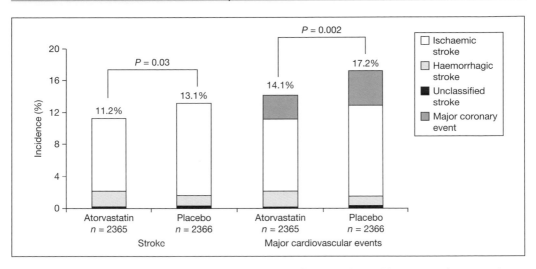

Figure 6.2 Net benefit of treatment with atorvastatin 80 mg/day in patients with recent stroke or transient ischaemic attack (analysis of incidence of haemorrhagic stroke was *post hoc*) in the SPARCL trial. Left panel: primary endpoint stroke fatal or non-fatal; right panel: secondary endpoint major cardiovascular events (stroke fatal or non-fatal and major coronary events).

Study	Intensive arm n/N	Conventional arm n/N	OR 95% CI	Weight %	OR (fixed) (95% CI)
A to Z	28/2265	35/2232		8.48	0.79 (0.48–1.30)
ALLIANCE	35/1217	39/1225		9.19	0.90 (0.57–1.43)
PROVE IT	21/2099	19/2063		4.62	1.09 (0.58–2.03)
IDEAL	151/4439	174/4449		40.89	0.87 (0.69–1.08)
TNT	117/4995	155/5006		36.82	0.75 (0.59–0.96)
Overall: $P = 0.01$ Heterogeneity: $I^2 = 0\%$, $P = 0.80$				100.00	0.83 (0.72–0.96)

0.1   0.2   0.5   1   2   5   10

Log-scale

Figure 6.3 Meta-analysis of five statin trials that evaluated the effect of intensive lipid-lowering therapy vs. standard statin therapy: fatal and non-fatal stroke incidence.

ing an average on-treatment LDL-C of 95 mg/dl and 110 mg/dl, respectively [20]. The crude meta-analysis of these trials ($n = 25\ 409$) shows that, compared to standard statin therapy, intensive statin therapy reduced the risk of stroke by 17% (95% CI 3.0–28.0) with no heterogeneity between trials (Figure 6.2). Seven hundred and thirteen patients had a stroke and the incidence of stroke in the intensive arms was 2.54% ($n = 324/12\ 750$) compared to 3.04% ($n = 387/12\ 743$) in the conventional arm (OR 0.83; 95% CI 0.72–0.97; $P = 0.02$]). These results are shown in Figure 6.3. For major cardiovascular events (stroke, MI and vascular death), the same crude meta-analysis found a relative risk reduction of 21% with no heterogeneity between trials (Figure 6.4); 2857 patients had such an event and the incidence of major cardiovascular events in the intensive arm was 10.05% ($n = 1282/12\ 750$) compared to 12.36% ($n = 1575/12\ 743$) in the conventional arm (OR 0.79; 95% CI 0.73–0.86; $P <0.0001$).

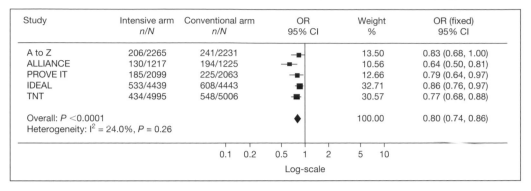

Study	Intensive arm n/N	Conventional arm n/N	OR 95% CI	Weight %	OR (fixed) 95% CI
A to Z	206/2265	241/2231		13.50	0.83 (0.68, 1.00)
ALLIANCE	130/1217	194/1225		10.56	0.64 (0.50, 0.81)
PROVE IT	185/2099	225/2063		12.66	0.79 (0.64, 0.97)
IDEAL	533/4439	608/4443		32.71	0.86 (0.76, 0.97)
TNT	434/4995	548/5006		30.57	0.77 (0.68, 0.88)
Overall: $P < 0.0001$ Heterogeneity: $I^2 = 24.0\%$, $P = 0.26$				100.00	0.80 (0.74, 0.86)

0.1   0.2   0.5   1   2   5   10

Log-scale

Figure 6.4 Meta-analysis of five statin trials that evaluated the effect of intensive lipid-lowering therapy vs. 'standard' statin therapy: major cardiovascular events (including stroke, myocardial infarction and vascular death).

The results of this meta-analysis, together with the *post hoc* analysis of the SPARCL trial mentioned above, reinforce the case for an evaluation of the two LDL-C-lowering strategies (achieved LDL-C <70 mg/dl vs. a standard dose of statin) in the secondary prevention of stroke.

MECHANISMS OF BENEFIT

Table 6.1 shows the potential mechanisms by which statins may reduce stroke risk. The importance of LDL-C lowering in particular and the reduction in progression of carotid atherosclerosis is clear. However, other potential mechanisms exist. Among these, the pleiotropic effects of statins include upregulating endothelial localised nitric oxide (NO) synthase, plaque stabilisation by a decrease in the effects of inflammatory cytokines and matrix metalloproteinases, decreased tissue factor expression and other thrombotic mechanisms, and an effect on the oxidised LDL receptor. Neuroprotection may be mediated by effects both upstream (the ischaemic penumbra) and downstream (the cerebral infarct).

FUTURE PERSPECTIVES

Current recommendations use target LDL-C levels together with associated risk factors or disease (e.g. diabetes, carotid stenosis) or clinical events (e.g. myocardial infarction) to drive the prescription of statins. The results obtained in the SPARCL study should now be implemented and included in guidelines and recommendations to spread the prescription of statins following stroke or TIA. This may also improve the adherence of patients to treatments. SPARCL secondary analyses showing that LDL-C levels less than 70 mg/dl may be associated with 2-fold greater risk reduction than that observed in the intention-to-treat analysis may also inform such recommendations. However, target LDL-C levels in secondary stroke prevention should currently be considered to be hypothesis-generating from *post hoc* analyses rather than evidence-based. A personal recommendation after a stroke or a TIA would be to 'prescribe a statin', particularly atorvastatin 80 mg/day.

A randomised, controlled trial should evaluate whether achieving a LDL-C level <70 mg/dl is superior to a standard dose of statin (LDL around 100–110 mg/dl) in the secondary prevention of stroke. Other directions should include an evaluation of combination therapy (e.g. statin plus ezetimibe, statin plus HDL-raising drugs), of the primary preven-

Table 6.1 Potential mechanisms whereby statins may reduce the risk of stroke

Evidence-based
LDL-C lowering
Reduction of carotid atherosclerosis progression (IMT studies)
Putative (not demonstrated)
Reduction of myocardial infarction and mural thrombus in the left ventricle (and subsequent thrombo-embolic complication)
Plaque stabilisation
Antiinflammatory effect
Antithrombotic properties
Blood pressure-lowering effect
Improvement of endothelial dysfunction
Neuroprotective effect (upregulation of nitric oxide) with increased cerebral blood flow

tion of stroke and TIA as well as other cardiovascular events in patients at intermediate risk, and of the benefit versus risk of peroxisome proliferator-activated receptor (PPAR) agonists such as fibrates, alone or in combination with statins.

CONCLUSIONS

Previous randomised controlled trials have shown that statins may reduce the risk of stroke in high-risk patients (those with established vascular disease or multiple risk factors). Recent evidence from the SPARCL trial has further established that statins can reduce recurrent strokes. In this study, when compared to placebo, those patients with a recent stroke or TIA who were randomised to atorvastatin 80 mg/day had a significant 16% relative risk reduction of stroke and a 35% reduction in major coronary events. This was obtained despite 25% of those patients assigned to receive placebo being prescribed a commercially available statin outside the trial. A *post hoc* analysis used blinded LDL-C measurements (taken at study visits during the trial) as a marker of adherence to lipid-lowering therapy. Compared to the group with no change or an increase in LDL-C (the group adherent to placebo or not taking a statin), the group with >50% reduction in LDL-C had a statistically significant 31% reduction in stroke.

The meta-analysis of trials that evaluated intensive LDL-C lowering ($n = 29\,906$ patients) showed that, compared to 'standard' statin therapy, intensive therapy reduced the risk of stroke by 17% (95% CI 4–28%; $P = 0.01$) with no heterogeneity between trials, and the risk of major cardiovascular events (stroke, MI and vascular death) by 20% (95% CI 14–26%; $P < 0.0001$) with no heterogeneity between trials. Current recommendations use target LDL-C levels together with associated risk factors or disease (e.g. diabetes) or clinical events (e.g. MI) to drive the prescription of statins. The results obtained in SPARCL should now be implemented and included in guidelines and recommendations that are appropriate to the general prescription of statins following stroke or TIA. Measures are also necessary to improve the adherence of patients to treatment. SPARCL secondary analyses, which showed that LDL-C levels less than 70 mg/dl may be associated with 2-fold greater risk reduction than that observed in the intention-to-treat analysis may help develop recommendations. However, target LDL-C levels in secondary stroke prevention are currently hypothesis-generating from *post hoc* analysis rather than evidence-based.

A next step is to define whether achieving a LDL-C <70 mg/dl is better than a standard dose of statin (to achieve an LDL-C of approximately 100–110 mg/dl) in the secondary prevention of stroke. Other future directions include the evaluation of combination therapy (statin plus ezetimide, statin plus HDL-raising drugs), of the primary prevention of stroke and TIA as well as other cardiovascular events in subjects at intermediate risk and of the benefits and risks of PPAR agonists such as fibrates, alone or in combination with statins.

Statins are effective in reducing both first-ever and recurrent stroke, and this effect appears to be driven by the extent of LDL-C lowering. Statins are among the most effective drugs in reducing the risk of stroke in a population of patients at high vascular risk, as well as the risk of major coronary events. In the secondary prevention of stroke, statins clearly reduced the risk of major coronary events and, in the SPARCL trial, atorvastatin reduced the risk of recurrent stroke.

Disclosure

Pierre Amarenco has received honoraria for educational symposia and advisory boards as well as research grants from Pfizer.

REFERENCES

1. Rothwell PM, Coull AJ, Silver LE *et al*. Population-based study of event-rate, incidence, case fatality, and mortality for all acute vascular events in all arterial territories (Oxford Vascular Study). *Lancet* 2005; 366:1773–1783.
2. Gongora-Rivera F, Labreuche J *et al*. The prevalence of coronary atherosclerosis in patients with stroke. *Stroke* 2007; 38:1203–1210.
3. Dhamoon MS, Sciacca RR, Rundek T, Sacco RL, Elkind MS. Recurrent stroke and cardiac risks after first ischemic stroke: the Northern Manhattan Study. *Neurology* 2006; 66:641–646.
4. Sacco RL, Benjamin EJ, Broderick JP *et al*. American Heart Association Prevention Conference. IV. Prevention and Rehabilitation of Stroke. *Risk Factors Stroke* 1997; 28:1507–1517.
5. MacMahon S. Blood pressure and the prevention of stroke. *J Hypertens* 1996; 14:39–46.
6. Amarenco P, Lavallée P, Touboul P-J. Stroke prevention, blood cholesterol, and statins. *Lancet Neurol* 2004; 3:271–278.
7. Amarenco P, Labreuche J, Lavallée P, Touboul P-J. Statins in stroke prevention and carotid atherosclerosis: systematic review and up-to-date meta-analysis. *Stroke* 2004; 35:2902–2909.
8. Asia Pacific Cohort Studies Collaboration. Joint effects of systolic blood pressure and serum cholesterol on cardiovascular disease in the Asia Pacific Region. *Circulation* 2005; 112:3384–3390.
9. Baigent C, Keech A, Kearney PM *et al*. Efficacy and safety of cholesterol-lowering treatment: prospective meta-analysis of data from 90 056 participants in 14 randomised trials of statins. *Lancet* 2005; 366:1267–1278.
10. LaRosa JC, Grundy SM, Waters DD *et al*. For the Treating to New Target (TNT) Investigators. Intensive lipid lowering with atorvastatin in patients with stable coronary disease. *N Engl J Med* 2005; 352:1425–1435.
11. Colhoun HM, Betteridge DJ, Durrington PN *et al*. Primary prevention of cardiovascular disease with atorvastatin in type 2 diabetes in the Collaborative Atorvastatin Diabetes Study (CARDS): multicentre randomised placebo-controlled trial. *Lancet* 2004; 364:685–696.
12. Sever PS, Dahlof B, Poulter NR *et al*. Prevention of coronary and stroke events with atorvastatin in hypertensive patients who have average or lower-than-average cholesterol concentrations, in the Anglo-Scandinavian Cardiac Outcomes Trial – Lipid Lowering Arm (ASCOT-LLA): a multicentre randomised controlled trial. *Lancet* 2003; 361:1149–1158.
13. Heart Protection Study Collaborative Group. MRC/BHF Heart Protection Study of cholesterol-lowering with simvastatin in 5963 people with diabetes: a randomised placebo-controlled trial. *Lancet* 2003; 361:2005–2016.
14. Amarenco P, Bogousslavsky J, Callahan A 3rd *et al*., for the SPARCL investigators. High-dose atorvastatin after stroke or transient ischemic attack. *N Engl J Med* 2006; 355:549–555.
15. Amarenco P, Goldstein LB, Szarek M *et al*., for the SPARCL Investigators. Effects of intense LDL-C reduction in patients with stroke or transient ischemic attack: the Stroke Prevention by Aggressive Reduction in Cholesterol Levels (SPARCL) trial. *Stroke* 2007; 38:3198–3204.
16. Goldstein LB, Amarenco P, Szarek M *et al*. Hemorrhagic stroke in the Stroke Prevention by Aggressive Reduction in Cholesterol Levels Study. *Neurology* 2008; 70:2364–2370.

17. Gongora-Rivera F, Labreuche J, Jaramilo A, Steg PG, Hauw J-J, Amarenco P. The prevalence of coronary atherosclerosis in patients with stroke. *Stroke* 2007; 38:1203–1210.

18. Cannon CP, Braunwald E, McCabe CH *et al*. Pravastatin or Atorvastatin Evaluation and Infection Therapy-Thrombolysis in Myocardial Infarction 22 Investigators. Intensive versus moderate lipid lowering with statins after acute coronary syndromes. *N Engl J Med* 2004; 350:1495–1504.

19. Pedersen TR, Faergeman O, Kastelein JJ *et al*. High-dose atorvastatin versus usual-dose simvastatin for secondary prevention after myocardial infarction. The IDEAL study: a randomized controlled trial. *JAMA* 2005; 294:2437–2445.

20. Koren MJ, Hunninghake DB, on behalf of the ALLIANCE investigators. Clinical outcomes in managed-care patients with coronary heart disease treated aggressively in lipid-lowering disease management clinics: The ALLIANCE Study. *J Am Coll Cardiol* 2004; 44:1772–1779.

7

Diabetes and the metabolic syndrome

A. J. Cameron, J. Shaw, P. Zimmet

INTRODUCTION

Type 2 diabetes and its counterpart, the metabolic syndrome, have been increasing in prevalence worldwide at least since the second half of the twentieth century, and appear set to continue apace well into the new century [1]. Diabetes is now one of the most common non-communicable diseases globally, and the fourth or fifth leading cause of death in most developed countries [1]. The global prevalence of diabetes was estimated to be 5.9% in 2007, representing almost a quarter of a billion people, about 90% of whom had type 2 diabetes. It is predicted that this number will approach 400 million, or 7.1%, by 2025 (Table 7.1) [1]. Strikingly, some 80% of those with diabetes in 2007 live in developing countries [1], despite type 2 diabetes often being perceived as a Western condition.

The threat to healthcare systems, health financing and individual health and wellbeing that these two conditions represent in both developed and developing nations has been recently recognised in a United Nations resolution on diabetes. This made diabetes only

Table 7.1 Global projections for the number of people with diabetes (20–79 years), 2007 to 2025 (adapted with permission from the *Diabetes Atlas*, 3rd edition, 2006, International Diabetes Federation)

Region	Number with diabetes (millions)		
	2007	*2025*	*% increase*
Africa	10.4	18.7	80%
Eastern Mediterranean and Middle East	24.5	44.5	81%
Europe	53.2	64.1	21%
North America	28.3	40.5	43%
South and Central America	16.2	32.7	102%
South-East Asia	46.5	80.3	73%
Western Pacific	67	99.4	48%
World	246	380	55%

Adrian J. Cameron, BSc(Hons), MPH, Grad Dip Int Hlth, Epidemiologist, Baker IDI Heart and Diabetes Institute, Department of Clinical Diabetes and Epidemiology, Melbourne, Australia

Jonathan Shaw, MD, MRCP(UK), FRACP, Associate Director / Consultant Physician, Baker IDI Heart and Diabetes Institute, Department of Clinical Diabetes and Epidemiology, Melbourne, Australia

Paul Zimmet, MD, PhD, FRACP, FRCN, FTSE, Hon Causa Doctoris (Complutense, Spain), Director Emeritus and Director, International Research, Baker IDI Heart and Diabetes Institute, Department of Clinical Diabetes and Epidemiology, Melbourne, Australia

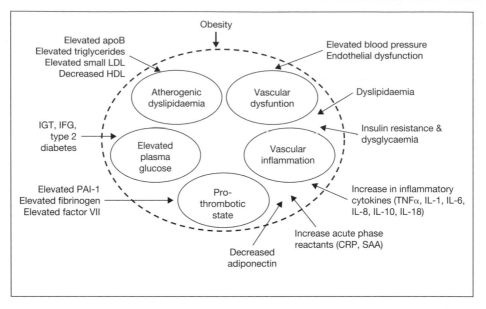

Figure 7.1 Components of the metabolic syndrome (adapted with permission from [8]). apoB = apolipoproten B; CRP = C-reactive protein; IFG = impaired fasting glucose; IGT = impaired glucose tolerance; IL = interleukin; PAI-1 = plasminogen activator inhibitor-1; SAA = serum amyloid A; TNFα = tumour necrosis factor-alpha.

the second disease after acquired immune deficiency syndrome (AIDS) to be so recognised. This dubious honour was the result of a diabetes epidemic that began with modernisation and a Western lifestyle and is set to escalate as this lifestyle is adopted globally.

Considerable evidence now exists linking diabetes with an increased risk of cardiovascular disease (CVD). Various estimates suggest that between one-half and two-thirds of deaths among people with diabetes are due to cardiovascular causes such as ischaemic heart disease and stroke [2–4]. Compared to those without diabetes, the risk of coronary artery disease (CAD), stroke and peripheral arterial disease is two to four times higher in the diabetic population, more particularly among women, and many now see diabetes as having a risk equivalent to that associated with previously diagnosed coronary heart disease (CHD) [5–7].

The metabolic syndrome and type 2 diabetes are closely linked, with the clustering of the abnormalities that make up the metabolic syndrome constituting a major risk for diabetes and both being significant risk factors for atherosclerotic CVD. While the increase in the risk of CVD among those with diabetes and the metabolic syndrome is multifactorial, much of the excess risk can be attributed to dyslipidaemia. The metabolic syndrome is made up of a number of core components, including obesity, atherogenic dyslipidaemia, elevated blood pressure, elevated plasma glucose and prothrombotic and pro-inflammatory states [8]. Each of these components has several markers or constituents (Figure 7.1).

'SYNDROME X' AND THE METABOLIC SYNDROME

Insulin resistance – the inability of normal levels of insulin to elicit an insulin-mediated response from fat, muscle and liver cells – has been recognised to be a precursor of hyperglycaemia and diabetes since as early as the 1930s. In his Banting lecture of 1988 [9], Reaven outlined the other negative consequences of insulin resistance, which included an increased likelihood of glucose intolerance, high plasma triglyceride and low HDL cholesterol (HDL-C) concentrations, and elevated blood pressure, labelling this 'syndrome X' and effectively giving birth to the concept that was later to become the metabolic syndrome. Since these abnormalities each increase the risk of CVD, the most common cause of death in people with diabetes, it was acknowledged that, by association, insulin resistance must also have close links with the development of CVD. The term 'syndrome X' was coined in an attempt to explain why insulin resistance might be associated with CVD as well as diabetes and its precursors. It has since emerged that numerous other CVD risk factors that can exist with or without hyperglycaemia (in addition to those identified as part of syndrome X) can also develop as a result of insulin resistance, and indeed, that obesity is likely to be the major underlying cause of the syndrome.

DEFINITIONS OF THE METABOLIC SYNDROME

With the increasing awareness and acknowledgement of Reaven's syndrome X throughout the late 1980s and early 1990s, a clear need arose for a clinical and research tool that would identify those individuals who did not have clinically diagnosed diabetes, but who were nevertheless at increased risk of CVD and diabetes by virtue of their having components of syndrome X. Since the World Health Organization included a clinical definition of what is now commonly known as the 'metabolic syndrome' in their publication on the Definition, Diagnosis and Classification of Diabetes Mellitus and its Complications in 1998, alternative definitions have been proposed [10–13]. While syndrome X, as described by Reaven [9] and Himsworth [14] before him, was focused on the consequences of insulin resistance and the physiological process surrounding this, the goal of clinical definitions of the metabolic syndrome has been to *identify* those individuals who have the characteristic clustering of abnormalities associated with insulin resistance. All have included overweight or obesity, which is recognised not as a consequence, but rather as a cause, of insulin resistance. Indeed, evidence has now emerged that visceral obesity and not insulin resistance may actually be the cause of the metabolic syndrome. The importance of obesity is highlighted in the most recent definition of the metabolic syndrome published by the International Diabetes Federation (IDF), which includes central adiposity as a prerequisite, with any two of the four consequences originally included in syndrome X (hyperglycaemia, a high plasma triglyceride and low HDL-C concentration, and elevated blood pressure) [11]. More recently identified factors that could be thought of as part of the metabolic syndrome include obesity-induced low-grade inflammation, microalbuminuria, elevated levels of leptin, decreased adiponectin levels and endothelial dysfunction [15 19]. A summary of clinical definitions of the metabolic syndrome is found in Table 7.2.

USES OF THE METABOLIC SYNDROME

Debate has surrounded not only the exact composition of a clinical metabolic syndrome definition but also the cut-points to define abnormality in the various components, and the purpose. A popular argument for the clinical utility of the metabolic syndrome is its ability to predict future diabetes and CVD. Since insulin resistance is not the only avenue to the development of CVD or diabetes, and there are several other potent CVD risk factors not included in the definition of the metabolic syndrome (e.g. LDL cholesterol LDL-C, small dense LDL particle concentration and smoking), a strong argument can be put that as a predictor of CVD in the clinical setting it is preferable to use dedicated CVD risk constructs such as the Framingham risk algorithms [20, 21], rather than the metabolic syndrome.

Table 7.2 Definitions of the metabolic syndrome

	WHO 1999[10]	EGIR 1999[13]	ATPIII 2005[85]	IDF 2005[11]
Compulsory requirement	Diabetes or impaired glucose regulation (IFG or IGT) or insulin resistance*	Insulin resistance (defined as hyperinsulinaemia–top 25% of fasting insulin values among the non-diabetic population)	None	Central obesity: waist circumference (ethnicity specific)†‡
	Plus two or more of the following:	**Plus two or more of the following:**	**Three or more of the following:**	**Plus any two of the following:**
Obesity	Men: waist:hip ratio >0.9	Men: waist circumference ≥94 cm	Men: waist circumference >102 cm§	
	Women: waist:hip ratio >0.85 *and/or* BMI > 30 kg/m²	Women: waist circumference ≥80 cm	Women: waist circumference >88 cm	
Triglycerides	Triglycerides ≥1.7 mmol/l (150 mg/dl) *and/or* HDL Men:	Triglycerides >2.0 mmol/l (178 mg/dl) or treatment *and/or* HDL <1.0 mmol/l (39 mg/dl) or treatment	≥1.7 mmol/l (150 mg/dl)	≥1.7 mmol/l (150 mg/dl) or specific treatment for this abnormality
HDL cholesterol	<0.9 mmol/l (35 mg/dl); Women: <1.0 mmol/l (39 mg/dl)		Men: <1.03 mmol/l (40 mg/dl) Women: ≥1.29 mmol/l (50 mg/dl)	Men: <1.03 mmol/l (40 mg/dl) Women: ≥1.29 mmol/l (50 mg/dl) or specific treatment for this abnormality
Fasting plasma glucose		≥6.1 mmol/l (110 mg/dl) but non-diabetic	≥5.6 mmol/l (100 mg/dl)**	≥5.6 mmol/l (100 mg/dl) or previously diagnosed type 2 diabetes ‖#
Blood pressure	≥140/90 mmHg	≥140/90 mmHg or medication	≥130/85 mmHg	≥130/85 mmHg or treatment of previously diagnosed hypertension
Microalbuminuria	Urinary albumin excretion rate ≥ 20 µg/min or albumin:creatinine ratio ≥30 mg/g			

*Insulin sensitivity measured under hyperinsulinaemic euglycaemic conditions, glucose uptake below lowest quartile for background population under investigation.

†Europids Male ≥94 cm; Female ≥80 cm. South Asians, Chinese, Japanese Male ≥90 cm; Female ≥80 cm. Ethnic South and Central Americans – use South Asian recommendations until more specific data are available. Sub-Saharan Africans and people from the Eastern Mediterranean and Middle East – use Europid data until more specific data are available.

‡If body mass index is >30 kg/m² then central obesity can be assumed, and waist circumference does not need to be measured.

§Some male patients can develop multiple metabolic risk factors when the waist circumference is only marginally increased, e.g. 94–102 cm (37–39 in). Such patients may have a strong genetic contribution to insulin resistance. They should benefit from changes in life habits, similarly to men with categorical increases in waist circumference.

‖In clinical practice, impaired glucose tolerance is also acceptable, but all reports of the prevalence of the metabolic syndrome should use only the fasting plasma glucose and presence of previously diagnosed diabetes to assess this criterion. Prevalences also incorporating the 2-h glucose results can be added as supplementary findings.

#If >5.6 mmol/l or 100 mg/dl, oral glucose tolerance test is strongly recommended but is not necessary to define presence of the syndrome.

** The 2001 ATPIII definition identified fasting plasma glucose of ≥6.1 mmol/l (110 mg/dl) as elevated. This was modified in 2004 to be ≥5.6 mmol/l (100 mg/dl) in the American Diabetes Association updated definition of impaired fasting glucose (IFG) and this modified version was therefore included in the 2005 updated ATPIII criteria.

Diabetes risk algorithms are not routinely used in clinical practice and the metabolic syndrome is acknowledged to have strong associations with incident diabetes because of the presence in the definition of several important diabetes risk factors (obesity, dysglycaemia and insulin resistance). Despite this, there are several important diabetes risk factors not included in definitions of the metabolic syndrome (age, physical activity/inactivity, diet), and several studies have shown that the metabolic syndrome is inferior to published risk algorithms, as well as to simple measurement of fasting or 2-hour post load glucose level [22, 23].

Prediction of either incident CVD or diabetes was not, however, the sole rationale for construction of a clinical definition of the metabolic syndrome. Valuable additional roles include:

1. Placing an emphasis on the interaction between, and importance of, multiple modifiable diabetes and CVD risk factors.
2. Explaining to patients why they are developing multiple chronic diseases.
3. Ensuring that tackling the components of the metabolic syndrome (using proven lifestyle approaches or pharmacotherapy) will prevent or delay the onset of not only diabetes and CVD, but also other conditions associated with a modern Western lifestyle.
4. Providing further information regarding the options for drug therapy for the clinician, including treatments for elevated cholesterol and blood pressure, glucose control and aspirin prophylaxis [24].

The plethora of epidemiological, metabolic and genetic studies resulting from the introduction of clinical and research definitions of the metabolic syndrome has led to a heightened understanding of its prevalence, aetiology and pathogenesis. The metabolic syndrome has also been a catalyst for the development and discovery of new drugs or combinations of existing drugs that will simultaneously modify multiple risk factors [8, 24].

However, despite its frequent application in epidemiological research and the considerable and often passionate discussion surrounding the syndrome in medical and scientific literature [25], many questions relating to the public health utility of its definitions remain unanswered [26, 27].

AETIOLOGY OF THE METABOLIC SYNDROME

Both insulin resistance and abdominal obesity have been advanced as likely causes for the clustering of abnormalities seen in the metabolic syndrome. However, its pathogenesis is likely to be complex and multifactorial, with considerable heterogeneity seen in the number and composition of the constituent abnormalities [11]. Factor analysis has been extensively utilised in an attempt to explore the nature of the clustering that is characteristic of the syndrome. Earlier reports varied in the number of factors identified and the nature of their clustering [28]. However, a common finding was the presence of three or four factors, representing insulin/glucose, obesity, lipid and blood pressure components. This was seen by some as evidence that no single underlying factor unified the components of the syndrome, but later studies specifically testing the hypothesis that a single factor united all of these sub-factors, provided good support for the single factor model [28, 29]. An explanation for the apparent disparity in these results is the nature of the earlier analyses, with multiple variables representing each of the four components often included in the models. This ensured that these variables clustered, despite the fact that each component could also cluster together as a 'second order' factor in a model including only single variables representing each component [30]. If a single unifying factor can indeed explain the frequent clustering of abnormalities, its identity has remained elusive.

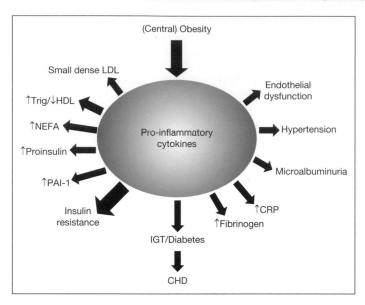

Figure 7.2 An inflammation-centred paradigm of the metabolic syndrome (adapted with permission from [33]). CHD = coronary heart disease; CRP = C-reactive protein; IGT = impaired glucose tolerance; NEFT = non-esterified fatty acid; PAI-1 = plasminogen activator inhibitor-1; Trig = triglycerides.

Despite major advances in the understanding of the relationship between obesity and insulin resistance and their role in type 2 diabetes and cardiovascular disease, the physiological mechanisms that link them and whether one or the other is the unifying feature of the metabolic syndrome, are both far from clear [9, 31, 32]. The recent discovery of novel factors such as inflammatory cytokines and endothelial dysfunction that are associated with components of the metabolic syndrome has led to the hypothesis of a causal pathway based on inflammation (Figure 7.2). Since the inflammatory process is thought to result from an increase in adipose tissue, obesity remains the preceding condition, with components linked through their association with pro-inflammatory cytokines [33]. Further critique of this model will undoubtedly include new studies of the role of inflammation and endothelial dysfunction in the deterioration seen in various components of the metabolic syndrome.

The difficulty in elucidating the relationships between the components of the metabolic syndrome results from multiple challenges, including the complexity of a condition that involves multiple interrelated disorders; the uncertainty as to how most conveniently and accurately to measure insulin resistance in particular, but also other components (including anthropometric measures); and the fact that environmental and genetic factors are usually not accounted for in most analyses [33]. It is likely that the issue of causation will only be resolved through a combination of approaches, including epidemiology, human and animal genetic studies, and analysis of the physiological and biochemical processes involved at the cellular, organ, individual and population levels.

There is only limited and unconvincing evidence to suggest that the metabolic syndrome, at least using published definitions, identifies risk for fatal and non-fatal CVD and diabetes over and above that identified by its component parts or established risk factors [22, 34, 35]. However, if this was shown definitively, an argument could be made that treatment of lipid parameters should be particularly aggressive among those with abnormal lipid levels as well as a diagnosis of the syndrome.

DYSLIPIDAEMIA IN PEOPLE WITH DIABETES AND THE METABOLIC SYNDROME

The typical features of dyslipidaemia in people with diabetes and the metabolic syndrome include both quantitative and qualitative changes in the lipid profile. Quantitative changes commonly observed include an increase in elevated circulating levels of triglycerides and a decrease in HDL-C and its major structural protein, apolipoprotein AI (apoAI). Qualitative changes to the size and density of lipid particles resulting in a preponderance of small dense LDL particles, and increase in levels of apolipoprotein B (apoB), are also typical and very common in diabetes and the metabolic syndrome [36].

Various lipid subfractions exist, which are divided into three main types:

1. Very low-density lipoprotein (VLDL).
2. Low-density lipoprotein (LDL).
3. High-density lipoprotein (HDL).

Of these subtypes, the size and density of LDL particles have attracted the most attention in basic, clinical and population research, with several lines of evidence implicating particularly small, dense LDLs, rather than large buoyant LDL particles, in the aetiology of CHD [37]. Small, dense LDL particles have a low content of cholesterol at their core, while their triglyceride content is either similar to or greater than that of larger particles [38, 39]. Their atherogenic effect is thought to result from the extended amount of time they are able to spend in plasma (because of reduced postprandial clearance) as well as enhanced oxidisability, arterial proteoglycan binding and permeability through the endothelial wall [40]. The formation of small, dense LDLs takes place through multiple metabolic pathways, including the removal of lipids from larger LDL particles by hepatic lipase, remodelling (removal of cholesteryl esters) of LDLs by cholesteryl ester transfer protein (CETP), through secretion from the liver into plasma [37], or a combination of these. The concentration of LDL and VLDL particles in the circulation can be estimated by measurement of the number of apolipoprotein B100 (apoB100) molecules, with one apoB100 molecule present per lipoprotein particle. The top quartile of the ratio of apoB to apoAI (a surrogate for the ratio of HDL-C to LDL-C and VLDL cholesterol) was shown to increase risk for acute myocardial infarction 3.25-fold (representing 49% of the total population attributable risk) in the INTERHEART study [41].

The typical dyslipidaemic profile seen in insulin resistance and diabetes begins with an increase in the number of VLDL particles secreted by the liver. Increased VLDL production is stimulated by an increase in the amount of triglycerides (the main substrate regulating VLDL production) available to the liver. In diabetes, all three sources of hepatic triglycerides are disturbed. First, lipolysis of the stored triglycerides in insulin-resistant fat cells into their component fatty acid and glycerol parts results in an increase in free fatty acids in the circulation. Secondly, peripheral removal of triglycerides (by lipolysis) in VLDL particles and chylomicron is reduced, and thirdly, de novo hepatic lipidogenesis is increased [36].

Elevated VLDL levels in the plasma, in conjunction with CETP, result in an exchange of triglycerides and cholesterol between VLDL and both LDL and HDL particles. This leads to more LDL particles that are cholesteryl ester depleted, but triglyceride enriched. The triglyceride in these particles can then be lipolysed by either lipoprotein lipase or hepatic lipase, resulting in small, dense LDLs. However, other avenues for the generation of small, dense LDLs are likely to exist, with the observation that in individuals who are insulin-resistant or have type 2 diabetes, small, dense LDLs can be present even with relatively normal triglyceride concentrations. These other possible avenues include the increase in hepatic lipase seen in insulin resistance, which could result in the triglycerides in LDLs being hydrolysed more effectively, as well as the type of VLDL (usually larger and triglyceride enriched in people with type 2 diabetes) originally assembled by the liver and secreted into plasma [36].

Despite much research testing the hypothesis that the size and density of lipoprotein particles is important in atherogenesis, consensus has not been reached in this area. A key critique of much of the research implicating small, dense LDLs is that even though small and dense LDL particles correlate strongly with CHD and possess several properties that make them a good candidate for a pivotal atherogenic role, there is less evidence that they are important *independent* of existing, acknowledged risk factors such as overall LDL and triglyceride concentrations [37]. After adjustment for lipids (as well as other risk factors), LDL size often does not remain as an independent predictor of CVD events. Both large and small LDL subtypes have been shown to be atherogenic in metabolic studies and until evidence is produced to the contrary, any type of LDL particle should be viewed as being harmful.

TREATMENT RECOMMENDATIONS FOR DIABETIC DYSLIPIDAEMIA

Multiple prospective studies have conclusively shown that elevated LDL-C is a major risk factor for CHD. In turn, a large number of randomised controlled trials have shown that interventions to reduce LDL-C also reduce CHD events. Similar relative risk reductions are seen among those with and without diabetes [42–44]. Therefore, both the American Diabetes Association (ADA) and the (US) National Cholesterol Education Program (NCEP) Expert Panel on Detection, Evaluation, and Treatment of High Blood Cholesterol in Adults (Adult Treatment Panel III [ATP III]) have published clinical guidelines to inform physicians' judgment in the treatment of dyslipidaemia in people with diabetes [12, 45]. Both recommend reduction of LDL-C to ≤2.6 mmol/l (≤100 mg/dl) as the first target for treatment, with the ADA then recommending treatment of HDL-C and triglyceride abnormalities as secondary and tertiary targets respectively once the primary target has been met. The NCEP recommends treatment of non-HDL (VLDL) cholesterol as a secondary target. In the individual patient, the 2004 ADA statement recommends that treatment should aim for a 30–40% reduction in LDL-C level, with a recent discussion paper by the NCEP mirroring this recommendation [46].

Targets for treatment of dyslipidaemia in those with diabetes are similar to those for non-diabetic individuals with prevalent CAD, reflecting the status of diabetes as a CHD risk equivalent. Although findings are not consistent, those studies showing a similar relative risk for fatal or non-fatal heart disease (~20% over 6 years) among people with diabetes but no prior myocardial infarction (MI) and those with a prior MI but without diabetes [5–7] underline this viewpoint.

STATINS

Statins are the recommended front-line drug therapy for dyslipidaemia in people both with and without diabetes due to their powerful ability to lower LDL-C (they in fact lower all apoB-containing lipoproteins [12]). A reduction in risk for coronary and other major vascular events of roughly 20% for every 1 mmol/l reduction in LDL-C is seen [47, 48], with some of this reduction thought to be due to anti-inflammatory effects above and beyond reduction in LDL-C [49, 50], although this hypothesis is yet to be proven [51]. However, whether or not statins have anti-inflammatory effects may be somewhat academic because their clear benefits for high-risk patients are already established [8].

The Heart Protection Study, a large trial including around 6000 people with diabetes, showed that the reduction in vascular events with simvastatin was no different in those with high and low baseline LDL-C levels. The observation among those with and without diabetes that the magnitude of the reduction in relative risk was unrelated to baseline levels of LDL-C was consistent with a benefit of statins in those with diabetes, regardless of their LDL-C level. The reduction in relative risk of first major vascular event among the group

Table 7.3 Meta-analysis of effects of statin therapy on major vascular events per mmol/l lower LDL cholesterol in people with diabetes (*n* = 18 686) (adapted with permission from [48])

| Outcome | Subgroup | Events (%) | | RR (95%CI) per 1mmol/l lower LDL cholesterol |
		Treatment	Control	
Vascular death	All diabetes	604 (6.4%)	674 (7.2%)	0.87 (0.76–1.00)
Non-vascular death	All diabetes	427 (4.6%)	430 (4.6%)	0.97 (0.82–1.16)
All-cause mortality	All diabetes	1031 (11.0%)	1104 (11.9%)	0.91 (0.82–1.01)
Major coronary event	All diabetes	776 (8.3%)	979 (10.5%)	0.78 (0.69–0.87)
Coronary revascularisation	All diabetes	491 (5.2%)	627 (6.7%)	0.75 (0.64–0.88)
Stroke	All diabetes	407 (4.4%)	501 (5.4%)	0.79 (0.67–0.93)
Major vascular event	All diabetes	1465 (15.6%)	1782 (19.2%)	0.79 (0.72–0.86)
Major vascular event	Type 1 diabetes	147 (20.5%)	196 (26.2%)	0.79 (0.62–1.01)
	Type 2 diabetes	1318 (15.2%)	1586 (18.5%)	0.79 (0.72–0.87)
	Men	1082 (17.2%)	1332 (21.4%)	0.78 (0.71–0.86)
	Women	383 (12.4%)	450 (14.6%)	0.81 (0.67–0.97)
	Age ≤65 years	701 (13.1%)	898 (17.1%)	0.77 (0.68–0.87)
	Age >65 years	764 (18.9%)	884 (21.8%)	0.81 (0.67–0.97)
	Current smoker	266 (17.5%)	347 (22.5%)	0.78 (0.64–0.96)
	Non-smoker	1199 (15.2%)	1435 (18.5%)	0.79 (0.72–0.87)
	Predicted risk of vascular disease <4.5%	474 (8.4%)	631 (11.2%)	0.74 (0.64–0.85)
	Predicted risk of vascular disease 4.5–8.0%	472 (23.2%)	540 (27.3%)	0.80 (0.66–0.96)
	Predicted risk of vascular disease ≥8.0%	519 (30.5%)	611 (35.8%)	0.82 (0.70–0.95)
	LDL cholesterol ≤3.5 mmol/l	694 (13.9%)	812 (16.3%)	0.79 (0.69–0.92)
	LDL cholesterol 3.5–4.5 mmol/l	591 (17.0%)	721 (21.1%)	0.82 (0.73–0.93)
	LDL cholesterol ≥4.5 mmol/l	166 (23.0%)	216 (30.5%)	0.78 (0.63–0.96)

with diabetes and LDL <3.0 mmol/l (116 mg/dl) at baseline and no vascular disease was around one-quarter, and similar to the risk reduction among all of those with diabetes [44]. The risk reduction among those with LDL <2.6 mmol/l (100 mg/dl) was not reported. Absolute benefits will be greater in those with diabetes because of the high baseline risk. Those with both diabetes and manifest CVD, who were at very high risk of future CVD events, obtained the greatest absolute risk reduction. The NCEP recommendation for this very high-risk group is initiation of statin therapy *regardless* of pre-treatment LDL levels, with a target of a very low LDL-C (<1.8 mmol/l or 70 mg/dl) [46]. Lifestyle measures and attention to other risk factors are also imperative.

A recent meta-analysis assessed the overall relative risk reduction for a major coronary event with statin therapy and found it was very similar in those with diabetes (20%) and in non-diabetic subjects (23%) [52]. This analysis showed a similar risk reduction in primary and secondary prevention settings, and for CHD death.

Another seminal, and more recently published, meta-analysis is that by the Cholesterol Treatment Trialists' (CTT) Collaboration of 14 randomised trials, including a total of 17 220 individuals with type 2 diabetes and 1466 with type 1 diabetes [48]. This meta-analysis found that statin therapy reduced the risk of major coronary events, major vascular events, stroke and coronary revascularisation, each by around 21% per mmol/l lower LDL-C (a similar risk reduction to that reported in those without diabetes). This benefit was found not only among those with type 2 diabetes but, importantly, also in those with type 1 diabetes, was present in those with and without vascular disease, and was independent of baseline age, gender, blood pressure, smoking status, renal function, HDL-C , triglycerides or LDL-C level [48] (Table 7.3). A 9% reduction in all-cause mortality ($P = 0.02$), and a 13% reduction in vascular mortality ($P = 0.008$) were also reported in this analysis. These results support the earlier claim that statin therapy is important regardless of pre-treatment LDL-C level. The conclusions from this meta-analysis were that statin therapy should be considered for all people with diabetes, apart from those in whom there is a compelling reason not to treat with statins (e.g. pregnancy), and for those in whom there is a very low short-term absolute risk of vascular disease (as in type 1 diabetes in children), and that treatment should be considered irrespective of whether vascular disease has developed and irrespective of lipid profile [48]. Table 7.4 summarises individual statin and fibrate trials in people with diabetes and the metabolic syndrome.

OTHER PHARMACOLOGICAL THERAPIES FOR DYSLIPIDAEMIA IN DIABETES AND THE METABOLIC SYNDROME

While statins are the drugs of choice, other treatment options include fibrates, niacin, cholesterol absorption inhibitors and bile acid-binding resins.

Niacin

Niacin, or nicotinic acid, blocks the breakdown of fats in adipose tissue. Because of this effect, the level of circulating free fatty acids also decreases, resulting in a decrease in secretion of VLDLs and cholesterol by the liver. By lowering VLDL levels, niacin also increases the concentration of HDL-C.

In the Coronary Drug Project, niacin decreased the risk of recurrent fatal and non-fatal atherosclerotic CVD events and mortality both in individuals with the metabolic syndrome and type 2 diabetes and those without these conditions [53, 54]. A limitation in the use of niacin among patients with the metabolic syndrome and type 2 diabetes has been a demonstrated increase in insulin resistance and plasma glucose during therapy. Recent studies, however, have suggested that if diabetes is well controlled and glucose status monitored carefully, titration of current hypoglycaemic medication can limit any negative effects of niacin [55]. Another side-effect that limits the utility of niacin is flushing, although a long-acting formulation (niaspan) and its combination with a prostaglandin inhibitor, which minimises but does not completely eliminate flushing, are being trialled. Among patients with type 2 diabetes or the metabolic syndrome and very low levels of HDL-C that cannot be raised using lifestyle modification alone, niacin should be considered as a complementary therapy because of its uniquely powerful effect on HDL-C [36]. Current development of drug options that combine niacin with statin therapy may be useful in treating both LDL and HDL abnormalities in people with diabetic dyslipidaemia [8].

Cholesterol absorption inhibitors

Plant sterols or stanols and ezetimibe inhibit dietary cholesterol absorption in the intestine. This decreases the content of cholesterol in circulating chylomicrons, which deliver triglycerides to muscle and fat tissues, but return to the liver rich in cholesterol absorbed in the intestine. Therefore, ezetimibe reduces the flux of cholesterol from the intestine to the liver, with consequent reduction in hepatic VLDL production. To compensate for the reduction in cholesterol returning to the liver, however, the liver is stimulated to upregulate cholesterol biosynthesis.

In practice, ezetimibe is often combined with a statin to result in even greater reduction in LDL-C. Ezetimibe is also very useful in patients who cannot tolerate, or have side-effects to, statins. Ezetimibe is largely free of major side-effects and has largely replaced the use of bile acid-binding resins such as cholestyramine, colesevelam and colestipol due to their frequent undesirable side-effects such as abdominal fullness, flatulence and constipation. In addition, bile acid-binding resins can inhibit intestinal absorption of fat-soluble vitamins, warfarin, digoxin, thiazide diuretics, folic acid and even statins. They also often increase triglyceride concentration, a particular problem in those with diabetes or the metabolic syndrome [56].

Fibrates

Fibrates, or fibric acids, including gemfibrozil, fenofibrate and bezafibrate, lower triglyceride levels, transform small, dense LDL particles into larger, more buoyant particles, and raise HDL-C. In addition, fibrates also have a moderate effect on total apoB levels. Because of their specific effects on the components of atherogenic dyslipidaemia, fibrates are primarily recommended for the typical dyslipidaemia observed in the metabolic syndrome and type 2 diabetes [8]. Indeed, in trials such as the Helsinki Heart Study [57], VA-HIT [58], and BIP [59], benefits with a fibrate were particularly seen in those subjects with features of the metabolic syndrome or with diabetes. Used in combination with statins, fibrates can result in particularly favourable changes to the total lipid profile [60–62], however whether this reduces risk of CHD beyond that achieved by statins alone is yet to be determined [8].

The FIELD (Fenofibrate Intervention and Event Lowering in Diabetes) study tested the efficacy of fenofibrate alone in reducing CVD events in 9995 people with type 2 diabetes [63]. The effect on risk of all cardiovascular events with fibrates was less than anticipated, with the FIELD trial showing an 11% risk reduction in this endpoint ($P = 0.035$), but importantly no significant reduction in the primary endpoint of total CHD events (CHD mortality or non-fatal MI), or CHD mortality [63]. Another analysis of the FIELD study showed a reduction in risk of diabetic retinopathy with fenofibrate [64]. It is important to note that, perhaps because of an increase in homocysteine levels and resultant decrease in synthesis of apoA, fenofibrate resulted in only a small increase in HDL-C in FIELD. The absence of a greater effect on CVD endpoints, and the absence of effects on CHD events and CHD mortality seen in the FIELD study may also have been influenced by differential uptake of statin therapy, with the placebo group initiating therapy at roughly twice the rate of those assigned the fenofibrate (17% vs. 8%; $P < 0.0001$) [63], although the precise effects of this differential are unclear [65].

Table 7.4 CHD prevention trials using statin and fibrate therapy that include patients with diabetes.

		Medication	Diabetes patients (n)	CHD % risk reduction		P (in people with diabetes)
				Overall	Diabetes	
Statin trials	**Primary prevention**					
	AFCAPS/TexCAPS [86]	Lovastatin	155	37	43	ns
	ASCOT-LLA [87]	Atorvastatin	2532	36	16	ns
	HPS [44, 88]	Simvastatin	2912	27	33	0.0003
	CARDS [89]	Atorvastatin	2838	37	37	ns
	ASPEN [90]	Atorvastatin	1905	19	19	ns
	Secondary prevention					
	CARE [43]	Pravastatin	586	23	25	0.05
	4S [91]	Simvastatin	202	32	55	0.002
	4S extended [92]	Simvastatin	483	32	42	0.001
	LIPID [93]	Pravastatin	1077	24	19	ns
	HPS [44]	Simvastatin	1981	27	18	0.002
	TNT [94]	Atorvastatin	1501	22	25	0.026
	ASPEN [90]	Atorvastatin	505	36	36	ns
	Post-CABG [95]	Lovastatin	116	47	39	ns
	Primary/Secondary prevention					
	ALLHAT-LLS [96]	Pravastatin	3638	9	11	ns
	Meta-analysis: Type 2 diabetes					
	14 randomised trials [97]	Statins	17 220	23% per mmol/l LDL reduction	22% per mmol/l LDL reduction	<0.0001
	Meta-analysis: Type 1 diabetes					
		Statins	1466		22% per mmol/l LDL reduction	0.05

Fibrate trials				
Helsinki Heart Study [98]	Gemfibrozil	135	68% risk reduction in MI or sudden cardiac death	ns
SENDCAP [99]	Bezafibrate	164	70% reduction in definite CHD events	0.01
VA-HIT [100]	Gemfibrozil	769	32% risk reduction for composite endpoint	0.004
DAIS [101]	Fenofibrate	418	23% reduction in cardiac endpoints	ns
FIELD [63]	Fenofibrate	9795	11% reduction in coronary endpoints	ns
BIP [59]	Bezafibrate	516	2.3% reduction in MI	ns

Fibrates are generally well tolerated, however concern persists regarding the risk for muscle-related adverse events, particularly with concurrent use of gemfibrozil [60]. With fenofibrate, the risk for adverse events such as rhabdomyolysis appears to be lower than with gemfibrozil, and the FIELD trial showed that in patients with type 2 diabetes, the combination of fenofibrate and a statin was well tolerated.

DIETARY AND PHYSICAL ACTIVITY MODIFICATION

The primary goal of lipid-lowering treatment for those with type 2 diabetes and the metabolic syndrome is to prevent or delay associated CVD events. Among the first tools that should be used for this purpose is lifestyle therapy or therapeutic lifestyle change (TLC), achieved through improvement of dietary and physical activity habits. These are crucial in any patient with the metabolic syndrome or type 2 diabetes, and should be introduced early and aggressively, and continued at every stage of the clinical management of these conditions [8]. The ATPIII recommends TLC in all people with dyslipidaemia, regardless of LDL-C levels, with weight reduction, increased physical activity, reduced intake of saturated fats (<7% of total calories) and cholesterol (<200 mg/day), and increased intake of dietary factors such as plant stanols/sterols (2 g/day) and viscous (soluble) fibre (10–25 g/day). Numerous studies have shown that lipid profiles can be improved following such interventions independently of the associated weight loss [66–71].

The three large-scale randomised controlled trials examining the effect of TLC on the prevention of diabetes and the metabolic syndrome in at-risk individuals with glucose intolerance (Da Qing IGT and Diabetes Study in China, the Diabetes Prevention Program [DPP] in the USA and the Diabetes Prevention Study [DPS] in Finland) all demonstrated conclusively the preventive benefits of improvements in diet and lifestyle, with a 40–58% risk reduction in the incidence of diabetes and the metabolic syndrome [72–76].

The lifestyle intervention in the US DPP led to a reduction in the numbers of participants with small, dense, atherogenic LDL particles, a decrease in triglycerides of 0.28 mmol/l and an increase in HDL-C of 0.025 mmol/l, although there were no observable differences in either total or LDL-C levels [77]. Similarly, there was no effect on total and LDL-C in the DPS [75], possibly limiting the impact of the intervention on prevention of CVD events. A possible reason for an absence of effects on lipid levels in these trials was the modest weight loss observed.

Among people with diabetes, a meta-analysis of available trials suggested that aerobic exercise has little impact on total cholesterol, HDL-C, triglycerides or total- to HDL-C ratio [78]. A potentially important but modest reduction of 5% in LDL-C was found, and the authors noted that changes to the physical structure of the protein particle carrying cholesterol may be important independently of the conventional measures of lipid concentration [78, 79]. However, only seven studies including 220 individuals were available for this meta-analysis, suggesting that further data are required to more accurately determine the effects of exercise on the lipid profile among people with diabetes. It appears that dietary interventions may be more effective than aerobic exercise in improving lipid abnormalities. However, the evidence from observational studies of the beneficial effects of physical activity on the incidence of fatal and non-fatal CVD events [80], and its effects on other chronic diseases implies that despite limited evidence for the impact of physical activity on lipid concentrations among people with diabetes, physical activity is still recommended as a key component of TLC [81, 82]. The impact of dietary interventions is predominantly to lower total and LDL-C, while physical activity interventions target HDL-C and triglyceride levels albeit, it appears, with limited impact [83]. Even among those who require pharmacological intervention to bring lipid levels to a desirable level, concurrent TLC can bring about further benefits beyond those achieved with medication alone and should be part of any therapeutic strategy [84].

CONCLUSIONS

Type 2 diabetes is increasing in prevalence worldwide. Diabetic dyslipidaemia, characterised by increased triglyceride and decreased HDL-C concentrations and an increase in small, dense LDL-C, is an important contributor to the increased risk of morbidity and mortality related to CVD in those with both diabetes and the metabolic syndrome. Therapeutic lifestyle change as both a measure to prevent dyslipidaemia and diabetes, and introduced early and aggressively as a form of treatment for both hyperglycaemia and dyslipidaemia, should be the foundation on which other treatment for diabetic dyslipidaemia is built. Robust evidence now exists to suggest that statin therapy in people with diabetes significantly reduces the risk of major vascular events by 20% per 1 mmol/l lower LDL-C, regardless of the presence or absence of vascular disease, and irrespective of age, gender, blood pressure, LDL-C level, smoking status and renal function [48]. The Cholesterol Treatment Trialists' Collaboration meta-analysis demonstrated that similar risk reductions are also seen in those with type 1 diabetes. Therefore, statin therapy should be considered in people with diabetes irrespective of LDL-C levels and irrespective of whether they have had a previous vascular event. Although consistent evidence of an effect on CHD risk reduction does not exist for fibrates or nicotinic acid, they can be considered for use in those with low HDL-C and elevated triglyceride concentration given their specific effects on this form of dyslipidaemia. Future trials of the combined effects of statins and fibrates may help to quantify the benefits of adding fibrates to statin therapy. Due to their high risk for CVD, lipid-lowering therapy in those with diabetes and the metabolic syndrome should be aggressive, and should aim to achieve a 30–40% reduction in LDL-C levels. While glycaemic control may help lower lipid levels, this should not be seen as a substitute for specific lipid-lowering therapy in those with diabetes.

REFERENCES

1. International Diabetes Federation. *Diabetes Atlas*, 3rd edition. Brussels, 2006.
2. Barr EL, Zimmet PZ, Welborn TA *et al*. Risk of cardiovascular and all-cause mortality in individuals with diabetes mellitus, impaired fasting glucose, and impaired glucose tolerance: the Australian Diabetes, Obesity, and Lifestyle Study (AusDiab). *Circulation* 2007; 116:151–157.
3. Morrish NJ, Wang SL, Stevens LK, Fuller JH, Keen H. Mortality and causes of death in the WHO Multinational Study of Vascular Disease in Diabetes. *Diabetologia* 2001; 44:S14–S21.
4. Grundy SM, Benjamin IJ, Burke GL *et al*. Diabetes and cardiovascular disease: a statement for healthcare professionals from the American Heart Association. *Circulation* 1999; 100:1134–1146.
5. Becker A, Bos G, de Vegt F *et al*. Cardiovascular events in type 2 diabetes: comparison with nondiabetic individuals without and with prior cardiovascular disease. 10-year follow-up of the Hoorn Study. *Eur Heart J* 2003; 24:1406–1413.
6. Haffner SM, Lehto S, Rönnemaa T, Pyörälä K, Laakso M. Mortality from coronary heart disease in subjects with type 2 diabetes and in nondiabetic subjects with and without prior myocardial infarction. *N Engl J Med* 1998; 339:229–234.
7. Whiteley L, Padmanabhan S, Hole D, Isles C. Should diabetes be considered a coronary heart disease risk equivalent?: results from 25 years of follow-up in the Renfrew and Paisley survey. *Diabetes Care* 2005; 28:1588–1593.
8. Grundy SM. Drug therapy of the metabolic syndrome: minimizing the emerging crisis in polypharmacy. *Nat Rev Drug Discov* 2006; 5:295–309.
9. Reaven G. Role of insulin resistance in human disease. *Diabetes* 1988; 37:1595–1607.
10. World Health Organization. *Definition, diagnosis and classification of diabetes mellitus and its complications. Part 1: Diagnosis and classification of diabetes mellitus.* Department of Non-communicable Diseases Surveillance, World Health Organization, Geneva, 1999.
11. Alberti KG, Zimmet P, Shaw J. Metabolic syndrome – a new world-wide definition. A Consensus Statement from the International Diabetes Federation. *Diabet Med* 2006; 23:469–480.
12. Executive Summary of The Third Report of The National Cholesterol Education Program (NCEP) Expert Panel on Detection, Evaluation, And Treatment of High Blood Cholesterol In Adults (Adult Treatment Panel III). *JAMA* 2001; 285:2486–2497.

13. Balkau B, Charles MA, Drivsholm T *et al.* Frequency of the WHO metabolic syndrome in European cohorts, and an alternative definition of an insulin resistance syndrome. *Diabetes Metab* 2002; 28:364–376.

14. Himsworth H. Diabetes mellitus: its differentiation into insulin-sensitive and insulin-insensitive types. *Lancet* 1936; 1:117–120.

15. Shoelson SE, Herrero L, Naaz A. Obesity, inflammation, and insulin resistance. *Gastroenterology* 2007; 132:2169–2180.

16. Matsuzawa Y, Funahashi T, Kihara S, Shimomura I. Adiponectin and metabolic syndrome. *Arterioscler Thromb Vasc Biol* 2004; 24:29–33.

17. Snijder MB, Heine RJ, Seidell JC *et al.* Associations of adiponectin levels with incident impaired glucose metabolism and type 2 diabetes in older men and women: the Hoorn study. *Diabetes Care* 2006; 29:2498–2503.

18. Soderberg S, Zimmet P, Tuomilehto J *et al.* Leptin predicts the development of diabetes in Mauritian men, but not women: a population-based study. *Int J Obes* 2007; 31:1126–1133.

19. Hotamisligil GS. Inflammation and metabolic disorders. *Nature* 2006; 444:860–867.

20. Anderson K, Odell P, Wilson P, Kannel W. Cardiovascular disease risk profiles. *Am Heart J* 1991; 121:293–298.

21. Kannel WB, D'Agostino RB, Sullivan L, Wilson PW. Concept and usefulness of cardiovascular risk profiles. *Am Heart J* 2004; 148:16–26.

22. Cameron AJ, Zimmet PZ, Soderberg S *et al.* The metabolic syndrome as a predictor of incident diabetes mellitus in Mauritius. *Diabet Med* 2007; 24:1460–1469.

23. Stern MP, Williams K, Gonzalez-Villalpando C, Hunt KJ, Haffner SM. Does the metabolic syndrome improve identification of individuals at risk of type 2 diabetes and/or cardiovascular disease? *Diabetes Care* 2004; 27:2676–2681.

24. Grundy SM. Metabolic syndrome: a multiplex cardiovascular risk factor. *J Clin Endocrinol Metab* 2007; 92:399–404.

25. Kahn R, Buse J, Ferrannini E, Stern M. The metabolic syndrome: time for a critical appraisal: joint statement from the American Diabetes Association and the European Association for the Study of Diabetes. *Diabetes Care* 2005; 28:2289–2304.

26. Greenland P. Critical questions about the metabolic syndrome. *Circulation* 2005; 112:3675–3676.

27. Kahn R. The metabolic syndrome (emperor) wears no clothes. *Diabetes Care* 2006; 29:1693–1696.

28. Shen BJ, Todaro JF, Niaura R *et al.* Are metabolic risk factors one unified syndrome? Modeling the structure of the metabolic syndrome X. *Am J Epidemiol* 2003; 157:701–711.

29. Pladevall M, Singal B, Williams LK *et al.* A single factor underlies the metabolic syndrome: a confirmatory factor analysis. *Diabetes Care* 2006; 29:113–122.

30. McCaffery JM, Shen BJ, Todaro JF, Niaura RS. A single factor underlies the metabolic syndrome: a confirmatory factor analysis: response to Pladevall *et al.* *Diabetes Care* 2006; 29:1719–1720.

31. Grundy SM. What is the contribution of obesity to the metabolic syndrome? *Endocrinol Metab Clin North Am* 2004; 33:267–282.

32. Kahn SE, Hull RL, Utzschneider KM. Mechanisms linking obesity to insulin resistance and type 2 diabetes. *Nature* 2006; 444:840–846.

33. Yudkin JS. Insulin resistance and the metabolic syndrome – or the pitfalls of epidemiology. *Diabetologia* 2007; 50:1576–1586.

34. Sundström J, Risérus U, Byberg L, Zethelius B, Lithell H, Lind L. Clinical value of the metabolic syndrome for long term prediction of total and cardiovascular mortality: prospective, population based cohort study. *Br Med J* (Clinical Research Edn.) 2006; 332:878–882.

35. Sundström J, Vallhagen E, Risérus U *et al.* Risk associated with the metabolic syndrome versus the sum of its individual components. *Diabetes Care* 2006; 29:1673–1674.

36. Chahil TJ, Ginsberg HN. Diabetic dyslipidemia. *Endocrinol Metab Clin North Am* 2006; 35:491–510.

37. Sacks FM, Campos H. Clinical review 163: Cardiovascular endocrinology: Low-density lipoprotein size and cardiovascular disease: a reappraisal. *J Clin Endocrinol Metab* 2003; 88:4525–4532.

38. Capell WH, Zambon A, Austin MA, Brunzell JD, Hokanson JE. Compositional differences of LDL particles in normal subjects with LDL subclass phenotype A and LDL subclass phenotype B. *Arterioscler Thromb Vasc Biol* 1996; 16:1040–1046.

39. McNamara JR, Small DM, Li Z, Schaefer EJ. Differences in LDL subspecies involve alterations in lipid composition and conformational changes in apolipoprotein B. *J Lipid Res* 1996; 37:1924–1935.

40. Krauss RM. Heterogeneity of plasma low-density lipoproteins and atherosclerosis risk. *Curr Opin Lipidol* 1994; 5:339–349.

41. Yusuf S, Hawken S, Ounpuu S *et al*. Effect of potentially modifiable risk factors associated with myocardial infarction in 52 countries (the INTERHEART study): case-control study. *Lancet* 2004; 364:937–952.

42. Haffner SM, Alexander CM, Cook TJ *et al*. Reduced coronary events in simvastatin-treated patients with coronary heart disease and diabetes or impaired fasting glucose levels: subgroup analyses in the Scandinavian Simvastatin Survival Study. *Arch Intern Med* 1999; 159:2661–2667.

43. Goldberg RB, Mellies MJ, Sacks FM *et al*. Cardiovascular events and their reduction with pravastatin in diabetic and glucose-intolerant myocardial infarction survivors with average cholesterol levels: subgroup analyses in the cholesterol and recurrent events (CARE) trial. The Care Investigators. *Circulation* 1998; 98:2513–2519.

44. Collins R, Armitage J, Parish S, Sleigh P, Peto R. MRC/BHF Heart Protection Study of cholesterol-lowering with simvastatin in 5963 people with diabetes: a randomised placebo-controlled trial. *Lancet* 2003; 361:2005–2016.

45. Supplement 1. American Diabetes Association: clinical practice recommendations 2000. *Diabetes Care* 2000; 23(suppl 1):S1–S116.

46. Grundy SM, Cleeman JI, Merz CN *et al*. Implications of recent clinical trials for the National Cholesterol Education Program Adult Treatment Panel III Guidelines. *J Am Coll Cardiol* 2004; 44:720–732.

47. Baigent C, Keech A, Kearney PM *et al*. Efficacy and safety of cholesterol-lowering treatment: prospective meta-analysis of data from 90 056 participants in 14 randomised trials of statins. *Lancet* 2005; 366:1267–1278.

48. Cholesterol Treatment Trialists' (CTT) Collaborators. Efficacy of cholesterol-lowering therapy in 18 686 people with diabetes in 14 randomised trials of statins: a meta-analysis. *Lancet* 2008; 371:117–125.

49. Ridker PM. Connecting the role of C-reactive protein and statins in cardiovascular disease. *Clin Cardiol* 2003; 26(4 suppl 3):III39–III44.

50. Jialal I, Stein D, Balis D, Grundy SM, Adams-Huet B, Devaraj S. Effect of hydroxymethyl glutaryl coenzyme a reductase inhibitor therapy on high sensitive C-reactive protein levels. *Circulation* 2001; 103:1933–1935.

51. Robinson JG, Smith B, Maheshwari N, Schrott H. Pleiotropic effects of statins: benefit beyond cholesterol reduction? A meta-regression analysis. *J Am Coll Cardiol* 2005; 46:1855–1862.

52. Costa J, Borges M, David C, Vaz Carneiro A. Efficacy of lipid lowering drug treatment for diabetic and non-diabetic patients: meta-analysis of randomised controlled trials. *Br Med J* (Clinical Research Edn.) 2006; 332:1115–1124.

53. Canner PL, Furberg CD, McGovern ME. Benefits of niacin in patients with versus without the metabolic syndrome and healed myocardial infarction (from the Coronary Drug Project). *Am J Cardiol* 2006; 97:477–479.

54. Canner PL, Furberg CD, Terrin ML, McGovern ME. Benefits of niacin by glycemic status in patients with healed myocardial infarction (from the Coronary Drug Project). *Am J Cardiol* 2005; 95:254–257.

55. Meyers CD, Kashyap ML. Management of the metabolic syndrome-nicotinic acid. *Endocrinol Metab Clin North Am* 2004; 33:557–575.

56. Volkova N, Deedwania P. Dyslipidaemia in the Metabolic Syndrome. In: Krentz A, Wong N (eds). *Metabolic Syndrome and Cardiovascular Disease: Epidemiology, Assessment and Management*. Informa Healthcare, New York, 2007, pp 191–217.

57. Frick MH, Elo O, Haapa K *et al*. Helsinki Heart Study: primary-prevention trial with gemfibrozil in middle-aged men with dyslipidemia. Safety of treatment, changes in risk factors, and incidence of coronary heart disease. *N Engl J Med* 1987; 317:1237–1245.

58. Rubins HB, Robins SJ, Collins D *et al*. Gemfibrozil for the secondary prevention of coronary heart disease in men with low levels of high-density lipoprotein cholesterol. Veterans Affairs High-Density Lipoprotein Cholesterol Intervention Trial Study Group. *N Engl J Med* 1999; 341:410–418.

59. Secondary prevention by raising HDL cholesterol and reducing triglycerides in patients with coronary artery disease: the Bezafibrate Infarction Prevention (BIP) study. *Circulation* 2000; 102:21–27.

60. Keating GM, Croom KF. Fenofibrate: a review of its use in primary dyslipidaemia, the metabolic syndrome and type 2 diabetes mellitus. *Drugs* 2007; 67:121–153.

61. Vega GL, Ma PT, Cater NB et al. Effects of adding fenofibrate (200 mg/day) to simvastatin (10 mg/day) in patients with combined hyperlipidemia and metabolic syndrome. Am J Cardiol 2003; 91:956–960.

62. Grundy SM, Vega GL, Yuan Z, Battisti WP, Brady WE, Palmisano J. Effectiveness and tolerability of simvastatin plus fenofibrate for combined hyperlipidemia (the SAFARI trial). Am J Cardiol 2005; 95:462–468.

63. Keech A, Simes RJ, Barter P et al. Effects of long-term fenofibrate therapy on cardiovascular events in 9795 people with type 2 diabetes mellitus (the FIELD study): randomised controlled trial. Lancet 2005; 366:1849–1861.

64. Keech AC, Mitchell P, Summanen PA et al. Effect of fenofibrate on the need for laser treatment for diabetic retinopathy (FIELD study): a randomised controlled trial. Lancet 2007; 370:1687–1697.

65. Keech A, Simes J, Barter P, Best J, Scott R, Taskinen MR. Correction to the FIELD study report. Lancet 2006; 368:1415.

66. Kodama S, Tanaka S, Saito K et al. Effect of aerobic exercise training on serum levels of high-density lipoprotein cholesterol: a meta-analysis. Arch Intern Med 2007; 167:999–1008.

67. Prong N. Short term effects of exercise on plasma lipids and lipoprotein in humans. Sports Med 2003; 16:431–448.

68. Katzel LI, Bleecker ER, Rogus EM, Goldberg AP. Sequential effects of aerobic exercise training and weight loss on risk factors for coronary disease in healthy, obese middle-aged and older men. Metabolism 1997; 46:1441–1447.

69. Torjesen PA, Birkeland KI, Anderssen SA, Hjermann I, Holme I, Urdal P. Lifestyle changes may reverse development of the insulin resistance syndrome. The Oslo Diet and Exercise Study: a randomized trial. Diabetes Care 1997; 20:26–31.

70. Anderssen SA, Holme I, Urdal P, Hjermann I. Associations between central obesity and indexes of hemostatic, carbohydrate and lipid metabolism. Results of a 1-year intervention from the Oslo Diet and Exercise Study. Scand J Med Sci Sports 1998; 8:109–115.

71. Dengel DR, Hagberg JM, Pratley RE, Rogus EM, Goldberg AP. Improvements in blood pressure, glucose metabolism, and lipoprotein lipids after aerobic exercise plus weight loss in obese, hypertensive middle-aged men. Metabolism 1998; 47:1075–1082.

72. Knowler WC, Barrett-Connor E, Fowler SE et al. Reduction in the incidence of type 2 diabetes with lifestyle intervention or metformin. N Engl J Med 2002; 346:393–403.

73. Pan X, Li G, Hu Y et al. Effects of diet and exercise in preventing NIDDM in people with impaired glucose tolerance: The Da Qing IGT and Diabetes Study. Diabetes Care 1997; 20:537–544.

74. Orchard TJ, Temprosa M, Goldberg R et al. The effect of metformin and intensive lifestyle intervention on the metabolic syndrome: the Diabetes Prevention Program randomized trial. Ann Intern Med 2005; 142:611–619.

75. Lindström J, Louheranta A, Mannelin M et al. The Finnish Diabetes Prevention Study (DPS): Lifestyle intervention and 3-year results on diet and physical activity. Diabetes Care 2003; 26:3230–3236.

76. Tuomilehto J, Lindström J, Eriksson J et al. Prevention of type 2 diabetes mellitus by changes in lifestyle among subjects with impaired glucose tolerance. New Engl J Med 2001; 344:1343–1350.

77. Ratner R, Goldberg R, Haffner S et al. Impact of intensive lifestyle and metformin therapy on cardiovascular disease risk factors in the diabetes prevention program. Diabetes Care 2005; 28:888–894.

78. Kelley GA, Kelley KS. Effects of aerobic exercise on lipids and lipoproteins in adults with type 2 diabetes: a meta-analysis of randomized-controlled trials. Public Health 2007; 121:643–655.

79. Kraus WE, Houmard JA, Duscha BD et al. Effects of the amount and intensity of exercise on plasma lipoproteins. N Engl J Med 2002; 347:1483–1492.

80. Blair SN, Kohl HW 3rd, Barlow CE, Paffenbarger RS, Jr, Gibbons LW, Macera CA. Changes in physical fitness and all-cause mortality. A prospective study of healthy and unhealthy men. JAMA 1995; 273:1093–1098.

81. U.S. Department of Health and Human Services. Physical activity and health: a report of the Surgeon General. U.S. Department of Health and Human Services, Centers for Disease Control, National Center for Chronic Disease Prevention and Health Promotion, Atlanta, GA, 1996.

82. Warburton DE, Nicol CW, Bredin SS. Health benefits of physical activity: the evidence. Can Med Assoc J 2006; 174:801–809.

83. Varady KA, Jones PJ. Combination diet and exercise interventions for the treatment of dyslipidemia: an effective preliminary strategy to lower cholesterol levels? J Nutr 2005; 135:1829–1835.

84. Wadden TA, Berkowitz RI, Womble LG *et al.* Randomized trial of lifestyle modification and pharmacotherapy for obesity. *N Engl J Med* 2005; 353:2111–2120.

85. Grundy SM, Cleeman JI, Daniels SR *et al.* Diagnosis and management of the metabolic syndrome: an American Heart Association/National Heart, Lung, and Blood Institute Scientific Statement. *Circulation* 2005; 112:e285-e290.

86. Downs JR, Clearfield M, Weis S *et al.* Primary prevention of acute coronary events with lovastatin in men and women with average cholesterol levels: results of AFCAPS/TexCAPS. Air Force/Texas Coronary Atherosclerosis Prevention Study. *JAMA* 1998; 279:1615–1622.

87. Sever PS, Dahlof B, Poulter NR *et al.* Prevention of coronary and stroke events with atorvastatin in hypertensive patients who have average or lower-than-average cholesterol concentrations, in the Anglo-Scandinavian Cardiac Outcomes Trial–Lipid Lowering Arm (ASCOT-LLA): a multicentre randomised controlled trial. *Lancet* 2003; 361:1149–1158.

88. MRC/BHF Heart Protection Study of cholesterol lowering with simvastatin in 20 536 high-risk individuals: a randomised placebo-controlled trial. *Lancet* 2002; 360:7–22.

89. Colhoun HM, Betteridge DJ, Durrington PN *et al.* Primary prevention of cardiovascular disease with atorvastatin in type 2 diabetes in the Collaborative Atorvastatin Diabetes Study (CARDS): multicentre randomised placebo-controlled trial. *Lancet* 2004; 364:685–696.

90. Knopp RH, d'Emden M, Smilde JG, Pocock SJ. Efficacy and safety of atorvastatin in the prevention of cardiovascular end points in subjects with type 2 diabetes: the Atorvastatin Study for Prevention of Coronary Heart Disease Endpoints in non-insulin-dependent diabetes mellitus (ASPEN). *Diabetes Care* 2006; 29:1478–1485.

91. Pyörälä K, Pedersen T, Kjeksus J, Faergeman O, Olsson A. Cholesterol lowering with simvastatin improves prognosis of diabetic patients with coronary heart disease: a subgroup analysis of the Scandinavian Simvastatin Survival Study. (4S). *Diabetes Care* 1997; 20:614–620.

92. Haffner S, Alexander C, Cook T *et al.* Reduced coronary events in simvastatin-treated subjects with coronary heart disease and diabetes or impaired fasting glucose: subgroup analyses in the Scandinavian Simvastatin Survival Study (4S). *Arch Intern Med* 1999; 159:2661–2667.

93. Keech A, Colquhoun D, Best J *et al.* Secondary prevention of cardiovascular events with long-term pravastatin in patients with diabetes or impaired fasting glucose: results from the LIPID trial. *Diabetes Care* 2003; 26:2713–2721.

94. Shepherd J, Barter P, Carmena R *et al.* Effect of lowering LDL cholesterol substantially below currently recommended levels in patients with coronary heart disease and diabetes: the Treating to New Targets (TNT) study. *Diabetes Care* 2006; 29:1220–1226.

95. Hoogwerf BJ, Waness A, Cressman M *et al.* Effects of aggressive cholesterol lowering and low-dose anticoagulation on clinical and angiographic outcomes in patients with diabetes: the Post Coronary Artery Bypass Graft Trial. *Diabetes* 1999; 48:1289–1294.

96. ALLHAT Officers and Coordinators for the ALLHAT Collaborative Research Group. The Antihypertensive and Lipid-Lowering Treatment to Prevent Heart Attack Trial. Major outcomes in moderately hypercholesterolemic, hypertensive patients randomized to pravastatin vs. usual care. *JAMA* 2002; 288:2998–3007.

97. Kearney PM, Blackwell L, Armitage J *et al.* Benefits of reducing LDL Cholesterol among 18 686 patients with diabetes: meta-anlaysis of 14 randomized trials of a statin versus control. American Diabetes Association; 2006 09/06/2006; Washington, DC; 2006, p. A215.

98. Koskinen P, Manttari M, Manninen V, Huttunen JK, Heinonen OP, Frick MH. Coronary heart disease incidence in NIDDM patients in the Helsinki Heart Study. *Diabetes Care* 1992; 15:820–825.

99. Elkeles RS, Diamond JR, Poulter C *et al.* Cardiovascular outcomes in type 2 diabetes. A double-blind placebo-controlled study of bezafibrate: the St. Mary's, Ealing, Northwick Park Diabetes Cardiovascular Disease Prevention (SENDCAP) Study. *Diabetes Care* 1998; 21:641–648.

100. Rubins HB, Robins SJ, Collins D *et al.* Diabetes, plasma insulin, and cardiovascular disease: subgroup analysis from the Department of Veterans Affairs high-density lipoprotein intervention trial (VA-HIT). *Arch Intern Med* 2002; 162:2597–2604.

101. The DAIS investigators. Effect of fenofibrate on progression of coronary-artery disease in type 2 diabetes: the Diabetes Atherosclerosis Intervention Study, a randomised study. *Lancet* 2001; 357:905–910.

8

Hypertension

R. H. Grimm, Jr

INTRODUCTION

An increase in normal blood pressure (BP) above an ideal of around 115 mmHg systolic has been estimated to account for the single largest proportion (4.4%) of the global burden of disease [1]. Elevation in cholesterol (above a theoretical minimum of ~3.8 mmol/l) also ranks high among risk factors, accounting for 2.8% of the global disease burden [2]. The great importance of these two risk factors is underscored by the estimate that about two-thirds of strokes and half of cases of ischaemic heart disease (for blood pressure) and about 18% of strokes and 55% of cases of ischaemic heart disease (for cholesterol) can be attributed to risk factor levels above these theoretical minima [3].

Abnormalities in many cardiovascular risk factors largely reflect adverse lifestyle factors. Concerning blood pressure, seminal observational studies undertaken almost 40 years ago showed that in populations such as in Africa, the Amazon and rural Thailand, blood pressure did not rise above 110–115 mmHg systolic with advancing age as it did in Western societies. The populations whose blood pressure did not rise with ageing had very low dietary salt intake, high intake of fruit and vegetables, and had high levels of physical activity and low rates of overweight [4].

Forward projections to 2025 based on what are probably conservative estimates related to country, age and sex-specific population estimates, also emphasize the increasing numbers with hypertension and associated cardiovascular disease (CVD). To a large extent, this increase is related to the ageing of societies [5].

EPIDEMIOLOGY

For both blood pressure and cholesterol, the association with coronary heart disease (CHD) and stroke (ischaemic stroke for usual cholesterol) is continuous and log-linear as risk factor levels increase [6]. Such associations are seen in older as well as younger individuals. In an overview of blood pressure and mortality, including 1 million adults in 61 prospective observational studies, and 55 000 vascular events, with each decade the risk of vascular death was the same [7]. Although the proportional differences in vascular mortality related to risk factor increments are less in the elderly, the absolute difference in risk is greater with ageing.

On the other hand, most CVD events occur in those individuals with only moderate elevation rather than in those with the highest risk factor levels. For systolic blood pressure, it has been estimated that only 21% of patients with ischaemic heart disease and 28% of patients with stroke have blood pressure levels in the highest decile of the population distribution [8].

Richard H. Grimm, Jr, MD, MPH, PhD, Professor of Cardiology and Epidemiology, Department of Medicine, Division of Cardiology, University of Minnesota, Minneapolis, Minnesota, USA

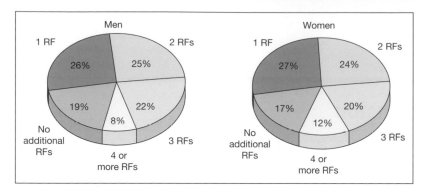

Figure 8.1 Cardiovascular risk factor clustering in association with hypertension among those aged 18–74 years in the Framingham Offspring Study: >50% of hypertension occurs in presence of two or more risk factors (adapted with permission [9]). RFs = Risk factors.

It is important to note that cardiovascular risk factors, including elevated blood pressure, tend to cluster. Accepting the limitation of the use of categorical variables, the Framingham study showed that of all those with hypertension – arbitrarily defined as having a blood pressure >140/90 mmHg or receiving treatment with antihypertensive drugs – less than 20% had this diagnosis in isolation from other risk factors that tend to accompany it. These risk factors include glucose intolerance, obesity, left ventricular hypertrophy and different manifestations of dyslipidaemia [9]. In the Framingham Offspring Study [8], clusters of more than three of these additional risk factors occurred at a rate that was about four times that expected by chance (Figure 8.1). This finding probably related to associations with abdominal adiposity and related insulin resistance.

Blood pressure and cholesterol have a less than additive effect on CVD risk due to the multifactorial causation of this condition as well as the joint action of these two risk factors. However, their joint importance is illustrated in the seminal study of over 361 000 middle-aged (35–57) males screened for eligibility for the Multiple Risk Factor Intervention Trial (MRFIT) [10] (Figure 8.2). The hazards of increasing systolic blood pressure are evident at all levels of cholesterol and *vice versa* [10, 11].

BENEFITS OF CHOLESTEROL AND BLOOD PRESSURE LOWERING

There is a wealth of evidence supporting the value of cholesterol-lowering agents, particularly statins, in a wide variety of subjects with or at risk of cardiovascular disease, many of whom had hypertension [12]. There is similar evidence to show a reduction in cardiovascular events, particularly stroke, with blood pressure-lowering therapy [13]. For both cholesterol and blood pressure lowering, the magnitude of benefit is related in a linear manner to the extent to which the risk factors are reduced.

Among the landmark studies, the Heart Protection Study (HPS) [14] in patients with vascular disease or diabetes, and PROGRESS, a secondary prevention trial in patients with previous stroke, showed that there was no difference in the proportional treatment effect observed according to baseline levels of cholesterol and blood pressure, respectively [14, 15].

CHOLESTEROL LOWERING IN PEOPLE WITH HYPERTENSION

The large-scale trials of statins have included many patients with hypertension. Subgroup analyses in hypertensive and normotensive subjects, both in primary [16] and secondary

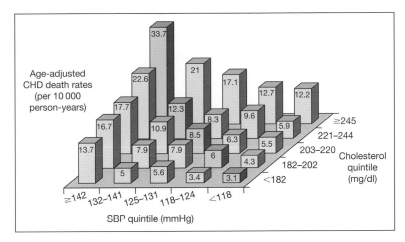

Figure 8.2 The impact of elevated systolic blood pressure and total cholesterol on CHD mortality among male subjects in the Multiple Risk Factor Intervention Trial (MRFIT) (adapted with permission from [10]).

prevention [17] of coronary heart disease have shown no heterogeneity in the proportional treatment effect of statins [16, 17].

Two large-scale trials have examined the role of cholesterol lowering (in addition to blood pressure lowering) in patients with hypertension.

ALLHAT

The Antihypertensive and Lipid-Lowering Treatment to Prevent Heart Attack Trial (ALLHAT) was undertaken in 10 355 participants (49%) in North America, men and women aged ≥55 years (mean 66 years), with low-density lipoprotein cholesterol (LDL-C) 120–185 mg/dl (100–129 mg/dl if known CHD) and triglycerides less than 350 mg/dl. A total of 35% of the subjects had type 2 diabetes [18]. They were randomised to receive either pravastatin 40 mg/day (*n* = 5170) or 'usual care' (*n* = 5185). The sample size was reduced after the trial began, but a cohort of 10 000 subjects was estimated to provide 84% power to detect a 20% difference in all-cause mortality, the primary endpoint.

The difference in LDL-C averaged over a mean follow-up period of 4.8 years was only 16.7%. In addition to drop-outs among those assigned to receive pravastatin, this almost certainly related to the fact that 32% and 29% of usual care participants with and without CHD, respectively, were placed on statins or other lipid-lowering agents by their personal physicians. All-cause mortality was 14.9% for the pravastatin group and 15.3% in those assigned to usual care (relative risk [RR] 0.99; 95% confidence interval [CI] 0.89–1.11; *P* = 0.88). Also, CHD event rates were not significantly different (9.3% for pravastatin, 10.4% for usual care: RR 0.91; 95% CI 0.79–1.04; *P* = 0.16). The power of the lipid study was greatly diminished due to the much reduced delta for change in LDL as a result of the high 'drop-in' rate.

ASCOT

The Anglo-Scandinavian Cardiac Outcomes Trial (ASCOT) [19] included 19 257 hypertensive subjects aged 40–79 years with screening and baseline blood pressure ≥160/100 mmHg if untreated or systolic blood pressure ≥140 mmHg if treated with antihypertensive drugs [20]. Participants had no previous manifestations of CHD. They were required to have three or more other risk factors for cardiovascular disease. ASCOT had utilised a Prospective Randomised Open Blinded Endpoints (PROBE) design.

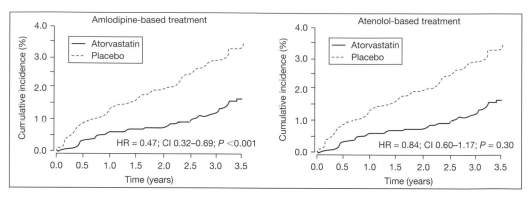

Figure 8.3 Cumulative incidence of non-fatal myocardial infarction and fatal coronary heart disease in ASCOT (with permission from [20]).

Of the total cohort, 10 305 individuals (81% men; mean age 63 years) with total cholesterol ≤6.5 mmol/l (250 mg/dl) and not taking a statin or a fibrate entered the double-blind Lipid Lowering Arm (LLA) of the study. They were randomised to receive either atorvastatin 10 mg/day or placebo. Follow-up was planned for an average of 5 years. However, the LLA of the study was terminated prematurely after a median 3.3 years follow-up. At this time, the differences in both total and LDL-C between placebo and atorvastatin-assigned patients were around 1.0 mmol/l. There were minimal changes in high-density lipoprotein cholesterol (HDL-C), and serum triglycerides fell with atorvastatin by about 0.3 mmol/l. The study terminated early because of a 36% relative risk reduction (from 3.0 to 1.9%) in the primary endpoint of non-fatal myocardial infarction including silent myocardial infarction and CHD death (hazard ratio [HR] 0.64; 95% Cl 0.50–0.83; P = 0.0005). There were also significant reductions in total cardiovascular events including coronary revascularisation, total CHD events, non-fatal myocardial infarction (excluding myocardial infarction) and CHD death. In addition, there were significant reductions in fatal and non-fatal stroke, which were among the prespecified secondary endpoints. Concerning other secondary endpoints, there was no significant reduction in all-cause cardiovascular mortality or heart failure.

There were no significant differences in the proportional treatment effect of atorvastatin in prespecified subgroups. Reductions in the primary endpoint with atorvastatin were significant and similar in those with baseline cholesterol above and below the median of 5.6 mmol/l (HR 0.65; P = 0.015 and HR 0.63; P = 0.012, respectively). *Post hoc* analyses showed benefit across the ranges of cholesterol, <5.0, 5.0–5.9, ≥6.0 mmol/l [Sever P; personal communication].

It is noteworthy that atorvastatin resulted in an early benefit on CHD events, although there was some delay before benefit on stroke, a secondary endpoint, was observed [21].

After the premature closure of the LLA of ASCOT, all subjects initially assigned placebo were offered atorvastatin. The Blood-Pressure Lowering Arm (BPLA) of the study [22] was also terminated prematurely because of a significant reduction in all-cause mortality (HR 0.89; 95% CI 0.81–0.99; P = 0.025) in those assigned amlodipine (adding perindopril as required) compared to treatment based on atenolol (and adding bendroflumethiazide as required) [22]. The primary endpoint for the BPLA was also non-fatal myocardial infarction (including silent myocardial infarction) and CHD death, where a non-significant trend to reduction in this endpoint with the amlodipine-based regimen compared with the atenolol-based regimen (unadjusted HR 0.90; 95% CI 0.79–1.02; P = 0.11) was observed (Figure 8.3).

At the time of closure of the BPLA after 5.5 years, approximately two-thirds of both initial treatment groups in the LLA (whether assigned atorvastatin or placebo) were taking statins, both groups having reached identical LDL-C levels after this further period of follow-up beyond the randomised phase of the LLA. Despite this, there was still a 36% relative risk reduction in CHD death or non-fatal myocardial infarction (P <0.0001) [20]. Such persistence of benefit despite both assigned groups having received active treatment has also been observed in other studies such as the Long-Term Intervention with Pravastatin in Ischaemic Disease (LIPID) study [23]. This observation underscores the importance of long-term maintenance of statin therapy in those with hypertension, particularly because of the increased risk with ageing.

A further prespecified analysis of ASCOT suggested there was synergy between the effects on CHD events of atorvastatin and amlodipine in the LLA and BPLA respectively (P for interaction = 0.025) [20]. The relative risk reduction in CHD events with atorvastatin was 53% (HR 0.47; 95% CI 0.32–0.69; P <0.0001) among those assigned amlodipine in the BPLA and 16% (HR 0.84; 95% CI 0.60–1.17) among those assigned atenolol (Table 8.1). It has been suggested that this could have a plausible explanation associated with the role of vascular smooth muscle cells in the development of atherosclerotic plaques. The authors have proposed that statins could promote a more differentiated vascular smooth muscle cell phenotype that restores functionality of L-type calcium channels in vascular smooth muscle cells [24]. This action could lead to plaque stabilisation, decreased release of matrix metalloproteinases and preservation of the intercellular matrix.

EFFECTS OF ANTIHYPERTENSIVE DRUGS ON LIPIDS AND LIPOPROTEINS

HISTORICAL BACKGROUND

The first publication citing a relationship of high blood pressure and vascular disease was published by Dr Richard Bright in 1836 [25]. It took six more decades before an Italian physician, Riva-Rossi, invented the pneumatic sphygmomanometer which, for the first time, provided a simple way to indirectly measure blood pressure [26]. Due to the measurement possibilities of the Rossi device, a new field of medicine – the study of hypertension – arose and with it increasing interest in the area of hypertension generally. Early in the 20th century, Anitschkow made a serendipitous observation that feeding cholesterol (in the form of milk, eggs and meat) to rabbits resulted in the development of atherosclerotic arterial atherosclerotic lesions. In so doing, he inadvertently developed the first animal model for studying atherosclerosis [27]. In the late 1940s, major epidemiological observational studies were launched, and the study cohorts were followed long term. These and similar studies confirmed the relationship of high blood pressure and blood cholesterol to atherosclerosis [28–31]. Soon, these epidemiological studies were being conducted around the world with similar results [32].

The clinical management of hypertension was very limited until 1958 when the thiazide diuretic, chlorothiazide, was introduced for general use, soon followed by hydrochlorothiazide, bendroflumethiazide and the iazide-like diuretic chlorthalidone [33]. These drugs lowered BP with significantly fewer side-effects, providing practical tools for general practitioners to lower and control many of their patients' blood pressures.

From the early 1970s to the mid 1990s, a steady progression of new classes of antihypertensive agents became available for use in clinical practice. The major new classes of antihypertensive agents included β-blockers, methyldopa, α-1 antagonists, centrally acting agents, angiotensin converting enzyme (ACE) inhibitors, calcium channel blockers, and angiotensin receptor blockers (ARBs). By 2000, it was firmly established both by observational studies and by well designed and powered clinical trials that both cholesterol (LDL)

Table 8.1 Summary of lipid and lipoprotein effects of classes of antihypertensive drugs

Drug class	Total cholesterol	LDL	HDL	TG	TC/HDL
Thiazides	↑	↑		↑↑	↑
Chlorthalidone			−		
Indapamide	5–15%	4–10%		15–25%	
Non-selective β-blocker (atenolol, propranolol)	−	↑↑	↓↓	↓	↑
		30%		−13%	30%
Cardioselective β-blockers (metoprolol)			↓	↑	↑
	−	−	5–9%	15–30%	
ISA β-blocker (oxyprenolol, pindolol)					↓
Acebutolol	−	−	−	−	
	↓	↓			↓
	8–10%	8–12%	−	−	
α-I antagonists (prazosin, doxazosin, terazosin)	↓	↓	↑	↓	↓
	4–6%	5–7%	2–5%	5–10%	
Dihydropyridine calcium blocker	−	−	−	−	−
ACE ARB (diltiazem, verapamil)	−	−	−	−	−
Methyl dopa	−	−	−	−	−
Reserpine (central)	−	−	−	−	−
Spironolactone aldosterone antagonist	−	−	−	−	−
Furosemide			↓	↑	↑
	−	−	5–10%	20–25%	
Hydralazine	↓		−	−	↓
	15–20%	−			

(−) = Neutral no to minimal effects.

and BP (especially systolic) were strong causal risk factors which, when treated, would prevent CVD to impressive – statistically and clinically significant – degrees.

Although the BP trials showed impressive lowering of stroke, heart failure and other vascular disease, the results were negative for fatal and non-fatal CHD, thus raising the possibility that the reason for the lack of CHD effects could be the result of the adverse effects of some antihypertensive drugs on blood lipids [34, 35].

In 1964, Schoenfield and Goldberger reported an increase in serum cholesterol in four of six cardiac patients treated with the diuretic bendroflumethiazide given at a dose of 5 mg/day [36]. This was a brief report prior to post-observation of individual patients serving as their own controls. The mean increase in serum cholesterol was 9.1 mg/dl. The report went largely unnoticed, but 14 years later the issue resurfaced as a result of early data from the Multiple Risk Factor Intervention Trial. MRFIT was a study of 12 866 middle-aged men who were at high risk (upper 10–15% Framingham) for a first coronary event due to a combination of increased blood pressure, elevated blood cholesterol and cigarette smoking. These men were randomised to special intervention (SI) or usual care (UC). SI men were all given dietary advice and training to lower their blood cholesterol, behavioural therapy to quit smoking and for the men with hypertension (diastolic blood pressure [DBP] >90 mmHg) pharmacologic therapy using the 'stepped care' approach. Drug therapy in the SI group was initiated with a diuretic, either hydrochlorothiazide (HCTZ) or chlorthalidone (50–100 mg daily) [37].

Early in the trial it became apparent that SI men taking diuretics were experiencing only about 50% of the lowering of the blood cholesterol on the cholesterol-lowering diet compared to the normotensives on the same diet but not taking antihypertensive drugs [38]. This result was widely noted and several other trials using diuretics examined their data and confirmed the MRFIT findings [34, 39]. Not long after the initial report, the hypothesis was once again put forward that the diuretic increase in lipids could account for the failure of previous trials to show reductions in CHD endpoints [40–43]. Another speculation was that the increase in lipids was simply a result of haemoconcentration from the plasma volume loss when taking a diuretic. As a result of these questions, an ancillary study on subjects ineligible for MRFIT was undertaken using a modified Latin square design [44–46]. This study confirmed that the effects on lipids of hydrochlorothiazide and chlorthalidone were significant with LDL increases (compared to placebo of 13–18 mg/dl and triglyceride [TG] increases of 16–21 mg/dl). These increases could not be explained by haemoconcentration but could be neutralised by giving cholesterol lowering dietary advice. Soon after the MRFIT report, numerous studies began to report the lipid effects with other classes of antihypertensive drugs, including the α-1 antagonists, finding decreases in LDL, TG and no effect or slight increases in HDL with prazosin [47, 48], non-selective and cardioselective β-blockers (propranolol, atenolol), and intrinsic sympathomimetic activity (ISA) β-blockers (acebutolol). Table 8.1 provides a summary of lipid and lipoprotein effects of the most commonly used agents in medical practice [49–52].

Thiazides and thiazide-like (chlorthalidone) increase total cholesterol and LDL cholesterol around 5–8% and triglycerides 10–20%, and have no effect on HDL-C. These lipid effects tend to be somewhat greater with higher doses (50–100 mg). The changes in lipids are less pronounced over longer treatment duration and can be neutralised with weight loss and/or a cholesterol-lowering diet [53, 54]. Another non-thiazide, indapamide, has similar effects on lipids and minimal effects on other metabolic measures. Cardioselective β-blockers, such as metoprolol, appear to only minimally affect lipids [49]. The ISA β-blockers oxyprenolol and pindolol both adversely affect the total cholesterol/HDL but the effect is minimal [55]. Acebutolol is an ISA β-blocker that stands out in the sense that in the Treatment of Mild Hypertension Study (TOMHS) it was one of the top drugs, along with chlorthalidone and amlodipine, in lowering systolic pressure. However, acebutolol's most unique finding was a reduction in LDL of about 10%, no effect on TG and HDL, and a favourable effect on the total cholesterol/HDL ratio [54].

Several reviews on the topic of antihypertensives and lipids have been published [56, 57].

CONCLUSIONS

A great deal of attention and concern about the lipid effects of antihypertensive agents were sparked by the MRFIT diuretic findings of relatively small changes on LDL and TG which dissipate over time and are countered by a weight loss cholesterol-lowering diet [44, 58]. Finally, numerous large long-term trials using diuretic-based treatment regimens with placebo and active control designs have consistently shown impressive reductions in rates of numerous cardiovascular endpoints [2, 34, 37, 59].

There remain concerns about β-blockers, especially the non-selective agents such as propranolol which was disappointing in the first Medical Research Council (MRC) study, with cardiovascular results inferior to the thiazide diuretic and similar to placebo [49]. The BHAT (β-Blocker Heart Attack Trial) outcomes also suggested that the lipid effects observed with propranolol may have influenced the trial outcomes, as was the case with the MRC study [14]. Several trials using atenolol have reported similar results, indicating that the combination of poor blood pressure lowering and the lipid effects of increases in TG and lowering of HDL are associated with atenolol [14, 22, 60, 61].

With the possible exception of non-selective β-blockers, the adverse lipid effects observed primarily with the diuretics and α-1 antagonists should be a lower priority in terms of clinical importance in the clinical management of hypertension.

REFERENCES

1. Ezzati M, Hoorn SV, Rodgers A, Lopez AD, Mathers CD, Murray CJ; Comparative Risk Assessment Collaborating Group. Estimates of global and regional potential health gains from reducing multiple major risk factors. *Lancet* 2003; 362:71–80.
2. ALLHAT Officers and Coordinators for the ALLHAT Collaborative Research. Major outcomes in high-risk hypertensive patients randomized to angiotensin-converting enzyme inhibitor or calcium channel blocker vs. diuretic: The Antihypertensive and Lipid-Lowering Treatment to Prevent Heart Attack Trial (ALLHAT). *JAMA* 2002; 288:2981–2997.
3. Murray CJL, Lauer JA, Hutubessy RC *et al*. Effectiveness and costs of interventions to lower systolic blood pressure and cholesterol: a global and regional analysis on reduction of cardiovascular-disease risk. *Lancet* 2003; 361:717–725.
4. Epstein FH, Eckoff RD. The epidemiology of high blood pressure – geographic distribution and etiological factors. In: Stamler J *et al*. *The epidemiology of hypertension*. New York: Grune & Stratton, 1967:155–163.
5. Kearney PM, Whelton M, Reynolds K, Muntner P, Whelton PK, He J. Global burden of hypertension: analysis of worldwide data. *Lancet* 2005; 365:217–223.
6. Prospective Studies Collaboration. Blood cholesterol and vascular mortality by age, sex, and blood pressure: a meta-analysis of individual data from 61 prospective studies with 55 000 vascular deaths. *Lancet* 2007; 370:1829–1839.
7. Ames RP. Serum lipid response to antihypertensives. *Drug Therapy* 1977:37.
8. Law MR, Wald NJ. Risk factor thresholds: their existence under scrutiny. *Br Med J* 2002; 324:1570–1576.
9. Kannel WB. Risk stratification in hypertension: new insights from the Framingham Study. *Am J Hypertens* 2000; 13:3S–10S.
10. Neaton JD, Blackburn H, Jacobs D *et al*. Serum cholesterol, blood pressure, cigarette smoking, and death from coronary heart disease. Overall findings and differences by age for 316,099 white men. Multiple Risk Factor Intervention Trial Research Group. *Arch Internal Med* 1992; 152:56–64.
11. Asia Pacific Cohort Studies Collaboration, Joint Effects of Systolic Blood Pressure and Serum Cholesterol on Cardiovascular Disease in the Asia Pacific Region. *Circulation* 2005; 112:3384–3390.
12. Cholesterol Treatment Trialists' Collaborators. Efficacy and safety of cholesterol-lowering treatment: prospective meta-analysis of data from 90 056 participants in 14 randomised trials of statins. *Lancet* 2005; 366:1267–1278.
13. Blood Pressure Lowering Treatment Trialists' Collaboration. Effects of different blood-pressure-lowering regimens on major cardiovascular events: results of prospectively-designed overviews of randomised trials. *Lancet* 2003; 362:1527–1535.
14. Heart Protection Study Collaborative Group. MRC/BHF Heart Protection Study of cholesterol lowering with simvastatin in 20 536 high-risk individuals: a randomised placebo-controlled trial. *Lancet* 2002; 360:7–22.
15. Progress Collaborative Group. Randomised trial of a perindopril based blood-pressure-lowering regimen among 6105 individuals with previous stroke or transient ischaemic attack. *Lancet* 2001; 358:1033–1041.

16. Downs JR, Clearfield M, Weis S *et al.* for the AFCAPS/TexCAPS Research Group. Primary prevention of acute coronary events with lovastatin in men and women with average cholesterol levels: results of AFCAPS/TexCAPS. *JAMA* 1998; 279:1615–1622.
17. Long-Term Intervention with Pravastatin Group in Ischaemic Disease (LIPID) Study Group. Prevention of cardiovascular events and death with pravastatin in patients with coronary heart disease and a broad range of initial cholesterol levels. *N Engl J Med* 1998; 339:1349–1357.
18. ALLHAT Officers and Coordinators for the ALLHAT Collaborative Research Group. Major outcomes in moderately hypercholesterolemic, hypertensive patients randomised to pravastatin vs. usual care. *JAMA* 2002; 288:2998–3007.
19. Sever PS, Dahlöf B, Poulter NR *et al.*; ASCOT Investigators. Prevention of coronary and stroke events with atorvastatin in hypertensive patients who have average or lower-than-average cholesterol concentration, in the Anglo-Scandinavian Cardiac Outcomes Trial - Lipid Lowering Arm (ASCOT-LLA): a multicentre randomised controlled trial. *Lancet* 2003; 361:1149–1158.
20. Sever P, Dahlöf B, Poulter N *et al.*; ASCOT Steering Committee Members. Potential synergy between lipid-lowering and blood-pressure-lowering in the Anglo-Scandinavian Cardiac Outcomes Trial. *Eur Heart J* 2006; 27:2982–2988.
21. Sever PS, Poulter NR, Dahlöf B, Wedel H; Anglo-Scandinavian Cardiac Outcomes Trial Investigators. Different time course for prevention of coronary and stroke events by atorvastatin in the Anglo-Scandinavian Cardiac Outcomes Trial - Lipid Lowering Arm (ASCOT-LLA). *Am J Cardiol* 2005; 96(suppl):39F–44F.
22. Dahlöf B, Sever PS, Poulter NR *et al.*; ASCOT Investigators. Prevention of cardiovascular events with an antihypertensive regimen of amlodipine adding perindopril as required versus atenolol, adding bendroflumethiazide as required, in the Anglo-Scandinavian Cardiac Outcomes Trial - Blood Pressure Lowering Arm (ASCOT-BPLA): a multicentre randomised controlled trial. *Lancet* 2005; 366:895–906.
23. LIPID Study Group. Long-term effectiveness and safety of pravastatin in 9014 patients with coronary heart disease and average cholesterol levels: the LIPID trial follow-up. *Lancet* 2002; 359:1379–1387.
24. Munro E, Patel M, Chan P *et al.* Inhibition of human vascular smooth muscle cell proliferation by lovastatin: the role of isoprenoid intermediates of colesterol síntesis. *Eur J Clin Invest* 1994; 24:766–772.
25. Bright R. Guy's Hospital Reports, 1836.
26. Riva-Rossi S. Un Nuova Sfigmomanometro. *Gazz Med di Torino* 1896; 981–1001.
27. Anitschkow NN. Experimental arteriosclerosis in animals. In: *Arteriosclerosis: A survey of the problem.* Cowdry, EV. (ed.). MacMillan, New York , 1933, pp 271–322.
28. Keys A, Taylor HL, Blackburn H, Brozek J, Anderson JT, Simonson E. Coronary heart disease among Minnesota business and professional men followed 15 years. *Circulation* 1963; 28:381.
29. Keys A (ed.). Coronary heart disease in seven countries. *Circulation* 1970; 41(4 suppl).
30. Kannel WB *et al.* (eds). The Framingham Study. An Epidemiologic Investigation of Cardiovascular Disease. Section 30: some characteristics related to the incidence of cardiovascular disease and death: >18-year follow-up. DHEW publications No, (NIH) 74-599, Government Printing Office, Washington DC, 1974.
31. Kagan A, McGee DL, Yano K, Rhoads GG, Nomura A. Serum cholesterol and mortality in a Japanese-American population: The Honolulu Heart Program. *Am J Epidemiology* 1981; 114:11–20.
32. Pooling Project Research Group. Relationship of blood pressure, serum cholesterol, smoking habit, relative weight and ECG abnormalities to incidence of major coronary events. Final Report of the Pooling Project. *J Chronic Dis* 1978; 31:201–306.
33. Novello FC, Sprague JM. Benzothiadiazine dioxides as novel diuretics. *J Am Chem Soc* 1957; 79:2028.
34. Hypertension Detection and Follow-up Program Cooperative Group. Five-year findings of the hypertension detection and follow-up program. Reduction in mortality of persons with high blood pressure, including mild hypertension. *JAMA* 1979; 242:2562–2571.
35. Australian National Blood Pressure Study (ANBP); the Australian Therapeutic trial in mild hypertension. *Lancet* 1980; 1:1261.
36. Schoenfeld MR, Goldberger E. Hypercholesterolemia induced by thiazides: a pilot study. *Curr Ther Res Clin Exp* 1964; 6:180–184.
37. Multiple Risk Factor Intervention Trial Research Group. Multiple Risk Factor Intervention Trial – risk factor changes and mortality results. *JAMA* 1982; 248:1465–1477.

38. Smith WF. The effects of thiazide diuretics on plasma lipids. Multiple Risk Factor Intervention Trial Research Group. In: Annual Conference Council on Cardiovascular Disease Epidemiology. Orlando, FL, 1978.

39. Goldman AI, Steele BW, Schnaper HW, Fitz AE, Frohlich ED, Perry HM Jr. Serum lipoprotein levels during chlorthalidone therapy. Veterans Administration, National Heart, Lung, and Blood Institute Cooperative Study on Antihypertensive Therapy: Mild Hypertension. *JAMA* 1980; 244:1691–1695.

40. Ames RP, Hill P. Elevation of serum lipids during diuretic therapy of hypertension. *Am J Med* 1976; 61:748–757.

41. Ames RP, Hill P. Raised serum-lipids during treatment of hypertension with chlorthalidone. *Lancet* 1976; 1:721–723.

42. Ames RP, Hill P. Raised serum lipid concentrations during diuretic treatment of hypertension: a study of predictive indeces. *Clin Sci Mol Med* 1978; 4:311S–314S.

43. Schnaper H, Fitz A, Frohlich E, Goldman A, Perry HM Jr, Steele B. Chlorthalidone and serum cholesterol. *Lancet* 1977; 2:295.

44. Grimm RH *et al.* Results of a randomized dosage reduction of diuretics in hypertensive men: The Multiple Risk Factor Intervention Trial (MRFIT). *Circulation* 1981; 64.

45. Grimm RH. The effects of diuretics on blood lipids and lipoproteins in mildly hypertensive men: implications for cardiovascular risk, a PhD thesis. Doctor of Philosophy. In: Laboratory of Physiological Hygiene. University of Minnesota: Minneapolis, 1984.

46. Cohen JD, Grimm RH Jr, Smith WM. Multiple Risk Factor Intervention Trial (MRFIT), VI, Intervention on Blood Pressure. *Prev Med* 1981; 10:501–518.

47. Leren TP. Doxazosin increases low-density lipoprotein receptor activity. *Acta Medica Toxicol* 1985; 56:269–272.

48. Harvard CW, Kokhar AM, Flax JS. Open assessment of the effect of prazosin on plasma lipids. *J Cardiovasc Pharmacol* 1982; 4(suppl 2):S238–S241.

49. Beinart IW, Cramp DG, Pearson RM, Harvard CW. The effect of metoprolol on plasma lipids. *Postgrad Med J* 1979; 55:709–711.

50. Lehtonen A, Hietanen E, Marniemi J, Peltonen P, Niskanen J. Effect of prindolol on serum lipids and lipid metabolizing enzymes. *Brit J Clin Pharmacol* 1982; 13(suppl 2):445S–447S.

51. Streja D, Mymin D. Effect of propranolol on HDL-cholesterol concentrations. *Br Med J* 1978; 2:1495.

52. Lithell H, Vessby B. Effect of prazosin on lipoprotein metabolism in premenopausal hypertensive women. *J Cardiovasc Pharmacol* 1981; 3(suppl 3):223.

53. Grimm RH Jr, Leon AS, Hunninghake DB, Lenz K, Hannan P, Blackburn H. Effects of thiazide diuretics on plasma lipids and lipoproteins in mildly hypertensive patients. *Ann Intern Med* 1981; 94:7–11.

54. Grimm RH Jr, Flack JM, Grandits GA *et al.* Long-term effects on plasma lipids of diet and drugs to treat hypertension. *JAMA* 1996; 275:1549–1556.

55. Kjeldsen SE, Eide I, Leren P, Foss OP, Holme I, Eriksen IL. The effect on HDL cholesterol of oxprenolol and atenolol. *Scand J Clin Lab Invest* 1982; 42:449–453.

56. Cutler R. Effect of antihypertensive agents on lipid metabolism. *Am J Cardiol* 1983; 51:628–631.

57. Krone W, Nägele H. Effects of antihypertensives on plasma lipids and lipoprotein metabolism. *Am Heart J* 1988; 116:1729–1734.

58. Caggiula AW, Christakis G, Farrand M *et al.* The Multiple Risk Factor Intervention Trial. IV. Intervention on blood lipids. *Prev Med* 1981; 10:443–475.

59. SHEP Cooperative Research Group. Prevention of stroke by antihypertensive drug treatment in older persons with isolated systolic hypertension. Final results of the Systolic Hypertension in the Elderly Program (SHEP). *JAMA* 1991; 265:3255–3264.

60. MRC Working Party. Medical Research Council trial of treatment of hypertension in older adults: principal results. *Br Med J* 1992; 304:405–412.

61. Dahlöf B, Devereux RB, Kjeldsen SE *et al.*; LIFE Study Group. Cardiovascular morbidity and mortality in the Losartan Intervention for Endpoint reduction in hypertension study (LIFE): a randomized trial against artenolol. *Lancet* 2002; 359:995–1003.

9

Treatment of familial hypercholesterolaemia

R. Huijgen, H. J. Avis, B. A. Hutten, M. N. Vissers, J. J. P. Kastelein

INTRODUCTION

Familial hypercholesterolaemia (FH) is the most common monogenetic disorder of lipid metabolism. In 1939, the Norwegian Carl Müller was one of the first to describe FH as a clinical entity that is characterised by the familial expression of xanthomatosis, hypercholesterolaemia and heart disease. Later studies revealed the autosomal dominant inheritance of FH and, more than 30 years later, Michael Brown and Joseph Goldstein elucidated the underlying molecular defect. In 1985, they won the Nobel Prize for their discovery of a single gene responsible for the expression of a specific low-density lipoprotein cholesterol (LDL-C) receptor (LDLR) [1].

The average prevalence of the heterozygous form of FH is 1 in 500 individuals [2], resulting in nearly 10 million patients worldwide. In some populations, this frequency is strikingly higher due to founder effects [3]. Homozygous FH is rare, affecting one in a million individuals.

The clinical characteristics of FH are most profound in homozygous patients, but they are often also evidently present in heterozygous patients. LDL-C is elevated about 10-fold in homozygous-and 3-fold in heterozygous patients. The high LDL-C levels lead to deposition of cholesterol in various tissues, presenting as tendon xanthomas, xanthelasmata and arcus cornealis. Accumulation of cholesterol in the arterial walls finally leads to premature atherosclerotic cardiovascular disease (CVD) [2]. In untreated heterozygous patients, about 50% of males and 30% of females develop CVD before the age of 60 years [4], whereas homozygous patients are already suffering from CVD events in the second decade of life [2]. Although FH is a monogenetic disorder, the phenotypic expression in terms of dyslipidaemia and CVD burden varies considerably [5].

The LDLR is abundantly present on the surface of liver cells where it specifically clears LDL-C from the circulation. Nowadays, more than a 1000 mutations in the LDLR gene or its promoter region are known to result in an absence or dysfunction of the LDLR, leading to FH in the majority of cases [6]. Aside from the LDLR, the core protein of LDL-C, apolipoprotein B100 (apoB100), also plays a role in the receptor-mediated uptake of LDL-C [7]. Five mutations

Roeland Huijgen, MD, MSc, Department of Vascular Medicine, Academic Medical Center, Amsterdam, The Netherlands

Hans J. Avis, MD, Department of Vascular Medicine, Academic Medical Center, Amsterdam, The Netherlands

Barbara A. Hutten, PhD, Clinical Epidemiologist, Department of Clinical Epidemiology, Biostatistics and Bioinformatics, Academic Medical Center, Amsterdam, The Netherlands

Maud N. Vissers, PhD, Scientific Researcher / Nutritionist, Department of Vascular Medicine, Academic Medical Center, Amsterdam, The Netherlands

John J. P. Kastelein, MD, PhD, Professor of Medicine; Chairman, Department of Vascular Medicine, Academic Medical Center, Amsterdam, The Netherlands

in *APOB* cause FH, in this form also known as 'familial defective apolipoprotein B' [7, 8]. In general, *LDLR* mutations lead to a more severe phenotype than mutations in the *APOB* gene [9, 10]. A third putative cause for FH is a gain-of-function mutation in the proprotein convertase subtilisin/kexin type 9 (PCSK9) gene [11]. Increased levels, or an increased activity of PCSK9 are hypothesised to result in hypercholesterolaemia due to decreased recycling of the LDLR after LDL-C uptake to the cell surface of the hepatocytes and increased redistribution of LDLR to lysosomes where they are subsequently destroyed. Overall, specific mutations in the genes for LDLR, apoB or PCSK9 result in an impaired clearance of LDL particles by hepatocytes and subsequently cause elevations in LDL-C plasma levels that are characteristic of FH [2].

FH is usually diagnosed by means of clinical features. Several diagnostic tools have been developed based on cholesterol levels, medical history, presence of xanthomas, and family history [12]. However, when diagnosis based on clinical criteria is compared with the genetic diagnosis, it becomes apparent that these tools do not necessarily provide consistent sensitivity and specificity [13]. The only way to unequivocally diagnose FH is to demonstrate a causative functional mutation by DNA analysis.

Patients with FH are at a high risk of premature atherosclerosis and CVD and they should be treated with lipid-lowering medication, preferably from childhood onwards [14]. Although no controlled clinical trials have evaluated the effect of lipid-lowering treatment on cardiovascular endpoints in FH specifically, the relationship between hypercholesterolaemia and the risk of CVD is indisputable. Furthermore, treatment with most LDL-C lowering agents has been proven to reduce the risk [15]. In this chapter, current and possible future treatment modalities for FH patients are discussed. The treatment options for special groups of FH patients will also be considered.

TREATMENT OF FH

TREATMENT GOALS

High levels of LDL-C have consistently been shown to be associated with coronary heart disease (CHD) risk [16]. Furthermore, the link between LDL-C lowering and the reduction of CVD risk has been clearly established, and *'the lower, the better'* has become a paradigm in the management of hypercholesterolaemia.

Although no clear goals have been defined for treatment of the FH population, LDL-C targets can be deduced from the recently adapted National Cholesterol Education Program (NCEP) and European guidelines. Those guidelines recommend a stringent LDL-C target of below 1.8 mmol/l for very high-risk patients (those with multiple CHD risk factors who have an absolute 10-year risk for major coronary events of >20%) [17, 18]. These targets can also apply to FH patients with manifest CVD or to those with a severe family history of premature CVD. For most FH patients, the LDL-C goal for 'normal' high-risk patients (<2.6 mmol/l) is acceptable as a minimum treatment target. In the United Kingdom, a target of >50% LDL-C reduction is recommended [19].

As the first step, FH patients are advised to adhere to a healthy lifestyle including diet, frequent physical activity and no smoking. However, often these lifestyle modifications alone do not result in targeted LDL-C levels and therefore the vast majority of patients with FH depend on pharmacological interventions to lower LDL-C levels. In untreated FH subjects, LDL-C levels are typically in the range of 5–10 mmol/l. Consequently, reductions of 50–75% are required to reach an LDL-C target level of ≤2.6 mmol/l [20].

CURRENT TREATMENT OPTIONS

Since the second half of the 20th century, efficacious pharmacological interventions for FH patients have only gradually become available. Without effective treatment, patients with a severe FH phenotype at first relied on radical measures such as portocaval shunting, ileal bypass and liver transplantation. Because of major advancements in pharmacological treatment of FH, these surgical modalities are only occasionally used in treatment-resistant FH patients today.

In this section, the commonly used registered pharmacological interventions are discussed, with a focus on the treatment of heterozygous FH patients. Alternative treatment options in paediatric, pregnant or homozygous FH patients are also outlined.

Statins

Statins – or 3-hydroxy 3-methylglutaryl coenzyme A (HMG CoA) reductase inhibitors – play a central role in the primary and secondary prevention of CVD and are currently considered the most effective drugs for lowering plasma LDL-C levels. By inhibiting the rate-limiting step of cholesterol synthesis, where HMG CoA is converted to mevalonate (Figure 9.1), statins decrease the hepatic cholesterol pool, which in turn stimulates the production of mRNA for the LDLR gene [21].

Enhanced LDL-C liver uptake via the LDLR results in increased LDL-C clearance and lower plasma LDL-C levels [2]. Results of a meta-analysis, which included the data from 164 randomised, placebo-controlled trials on LDL-C reduction, demonstrated that the six commonly used statins in their most potent doses yielded LDL-C reductions between 33 and 58% [22]. In a series of primary as well as secondary prevention trials using various statins it was consistently shown that reductions in LDL-C were associated with a clear decrease in the cardiovascular event rate. In fact, the relationship between LDL-C reduction and event rate was strikingly predictable, every 1 mmol/l (39 mg/dl) reduction in LDL-C being associated with a 23% reduction in CHD risk [23]. As a consequence, statin-induced LDL-C reduction has become the cornerstone of current treatment guidelines for cardiovascular prevention [17, 20].

Although there were no randomised, placebo-controlled clinical trials specifically investigating patients with FH, the clinical efficacy of statins in reducing CHD events was highlighted in the large Simon Broome cohort with clinically diagnosed FH subjects. The timeframe of this study, which overlaps the introduction of statins, allowed observations and comparison between treated and non-treated FH patients in 1999. Treatment was found to effectively lower the risk of CHD in patients with clinical FH as shown by the declined relative risk for coronary mortality from 1992 onwards [24, 25]. In line with these findings is the robust reduction in CHD risk induced by statin treatment, which was observed in a large FH cohort in the Netherlands [26].

One of the trials with statins that showed beneficial effects in FH subjects is the ASAP trial [27], in which the intima-media thickness of the carotid artery (cIMT) was used as an endpoint. cIMT as measured by ultrasonography is a surrogate marker for atherosclerosis and a validated predictor for cardiovascular events [28]. Two-year treatment with atorvastatin 80 mg/day reduced LDL-C by 51%, accompanied by a decrease in cIMT of 0.031 mm. Treatment with simvastatin 40 mg/day reduced LDL-C by 41%, but in contrast to the findings in the atorvastatin arm, cIMT increased by 0.036 mm (Figure 9.2). These results suggest the benefit of more aggressive lipid lowering in FH patients.

Ezetimibe

Ezetimibe is the first of a new class of drugs that selectively inhibits cholesterol absorption. This agent inhibits cholesterol uptake and transport through the enterocyte most likely by blocking the Niemann–Pick C1-like 1 (NPC1L1) transporter in enterocytes [29] (Figure 9.3). This reduces the fractional cholesterol absorption by 54% [30] and results in reduced cholesterol transport from the intestine to the liver via chylomicrons. By way of compensation, LDLR expression is upregulated and clearance of LDL-C from plasma increased [30]. In patients with primary hypercholesterolaemia, ezetimibe monotherapy reduced LDL-C levels by 17–20% [30, 31].

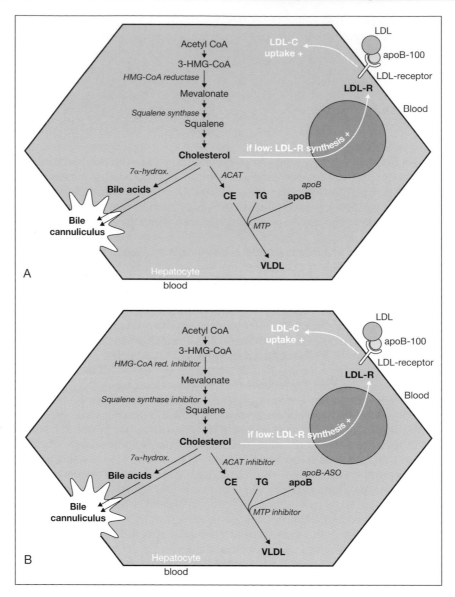

Figure 9.1 Cholesterol and VLDL-C synthesis and inhibitory agents in these pathways. (A) Shows the cholesterol, bile acid, and VLDL cholesterol synthesis with the enzymes catalysing these processes. (B) Demonstrates the site of action of agents which can impair the cholesterol or VLDL synthesis. Under conditions of low hepatic cholesterol, LDLR synthesis is increased, which results in LDL-C clearance from plasma via the LDLR pathway. Cholesterol can be esterified and stored as cholesteryl esters in the hepatocytes, packaged into VLDL particles and secreted into the plasma, secreted directly into the bile, or converted to bile acids by cholesterol 7α-hydroxylase and subsequently secreted into the bile. 7α-hydrox = cholesterol 7α-hydroxylase (CYP7A1); ACAT = acyl-coenzyme A:cholesterol acyltransferase; apoB100 = apolipoprotein B100; ASO = antisense oligonucleotides; CE = cholesteryl esters; HMG-CoA = hydroxy 3-methylglutaryl coenzyme A; LDL-C = low-density lipoprotein cholesterol; LDLR = LDL-C receptor; MTP = microsomal triglyceride transfer protein; TG = triglycerides; VLDL = very low-density lipoprotein.

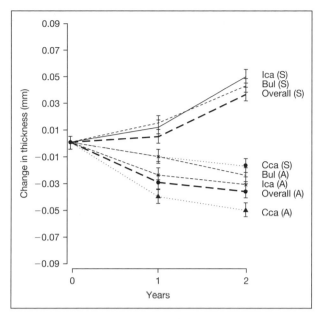

Figure 9.2 Change in intima-media thickness (IMT) (mm) in the different segments of the carotid artery after 1 and 2 years of treatment with simvastatin (40 mg/day) or atorvastatin (80 mg/day) in patients with heterozygous familial hypercholesterolaemia. (A) = atorvastatin; (S) = simvastatin; Bul = carotid bifurcation; Cca = common carotid artery; Ica = internal carotid artery; Vertical bars = standard deviation. The lines represent the combined measurements of intima-media thickness measurements of the right and left carotid arteries (with permission from [27]).

Combination therapy of ezetimibe with several statins resulted in 12–23% incremental decrease in LDL-C when compared to statin treatment alone [32, 33]. The safety profile does not differ between combination and statin monotherapy, but combination therapy allows significantly more patients to achieve their LDL-C goals as statin monotherapy (71.5% vs. 18.9%) [34]. Moreover, the combination of ezetimibe with a low-dose statin has a similar effect on LDL-C as high-dose statins, which is of considerable benefit in patients who do not tolerate high doses of statins [32]. However, the long-term effects of the addition of ezetimibe to statin treatment remain to be elucidated. A randomised, controlled trial in 720 FH patients, the ENHANCE (Ezetimibe and Simvastatin in Hypercholesterolemia Enhances Atherosclerosis Regression) trial, compared the 2-year efficacy of daily therapy with 80 mg/day simvastatin in all subjects in combination with 10 mg/day of ezetimibe or with placebo. The addition of ezetimibe to 80 mg/day simvastatin did not reduce cIMT, the primary outcome measure in this cohort of FH patients, despite a 16% incremental reduction in LDL-C (Table 9.1). The reason why this incremental LDL-C reduction did not beneficially affect cIMT remains unclear [35]. Thus, the outcomes of the ongoing clinical endpoint trial, IMPROVE IT, which evaluates the effect of addition of ezetimibe, are eagerly awaited.

Bile acid sequestrants
Bile acid sequestrants lower cholesterol levels by binding bile acids in the intestine and thereby interrupting the enterohepatic cycle (Figure 9.3). As a consequence of the diminished return of bile acids to the liver, hepatic bile acid synthesis from cholesterol by cholesterol 7 alpha hydroxylase (cytochrome P450, family 7, subfamily A, polypeptide 1) (CYP7A1) is increased in order to maintain constant bile acid levels [36]. The decrease in hepatic

Table 9.1 Ongoing, recently completed or discontinued randomised controlled phase III or IV trials in FH patients

Clinical trial	Phase	Inclusion criteria	Treatment	Duration (wks)	Primary endpoint	Start date	Results
PLUTO [92]	III	HeFH 10–17 y	n = 177, randomised (1:1:1:1) between: **rosuvastatin** dose 5, 10, 20 mg or placebo 3 mo double-blind, 9 mo open-label dose titration	52	ΔLDL-C	June 2006	Results expected in 2009
WEL–410 [86]	IV	HeFH 10–17 y	n = 97, treatment-naïve or statin monotherapy + **colesevelam** n = 97, treatment-naïve or statin monotherapy + placebo	26	ΔLDL-C	November 2005	Results expected in 2009
PO2579 [85]	III	HeFH 10–17 y	n = 248, randomised between: simvastatin dose 10, 20, 40 mg + **ezetimibe** 10 mg or placebo 6 wks 10/10 or 20/10 or 40/10 double-blind, 40/10 mg 26 wks double-blind, 10/10 or 20/10 mg 20 wks open-label	52	ΔLDL-C	August 2005	~ 15% additional LDL-C reduction with ezetimibe; no adverse safety outcomes
RADIANCE 1 [56]	III	HeFH 18–70 y	n = 450, atorvastatin + **torcetrapib** n = 454, atorvastatin + placebo	104	ΔcIMT	December 2003	No benefit of torcetrapib on IMT; see text [56]
TRIPLE [43]	IV	HeFH 18–75 y	n = 40, current therapy (including ezetimibe) + **colesevelam** n = 40 current therapy (including ezetimibe) + placebo 3 mo double blind, 9 mo open-label	56	ΔLDL-C	August 2007	Results expected in 2009
ACHIEVE [53]	III	HeFH 18–70 y LDL-C ≥2.6 mmol/l	n = 450, intensive lipid-lowering treatment + **MK0524A** n = 450, intensive lipid-lowering treatment + placebo	96*	ΔcIMT	October 2006	Prematurely discontinued in 2008

	Phase	Population	Treatment		Endpoint	Date	Comments
ENHANCE [35]	III	HeFH 30–75 y	n = 357, simvastatin 80 mg + **ezetimibe** n = 363, simvastatin 80 mg+ placebo	104	ΔcIMT	June 2002	No benefit of ezetimibe addition to simvastatin 80 mg on cIMT; see text [35]
CAPTIVATE [93]	III	HeFH 40–75 y LDL-C ≥2.5 mmol/L	n = 443, current therapy + CS-505 (**pactimibe**) n = 438, current therapy + placebo	65*	ΔcIMT	February 2004	More cIMT progression in treatment group. *Premature discontinuation after 15 mo; see text [67]
TAK-475-016 [61]	III	HoFH >8 y	n = 20, current therapy + **lapaquistat** 100 mg (50 mg) n = 20, current therapy + placebo	24 + ext*	ΔLDL-C	November 2005	Prematurely discontinued due to liver toxicity in 2008; see text [63]

Δ = from baseline; * = premature discontinuation; cIMT = carotid intima-media thickness; ext = extension period; HeFH = heterozygous FH; HoFH = homozygous FH; LDL-C = low-density lipoprotein cholesterol; mg = milligram; mo = months; wks = weeks; y = year. Only trials which intended to only include patients with FH are described in this table. These trials were found in the online databases www.clinicaltrials.gov, www.controlled-trials.com and EudraCD, using the search terms "Familial hypercholesterolemia" and "Primary hypercholesterolemia" and limits "Phase III and/or Phase IV-trials".

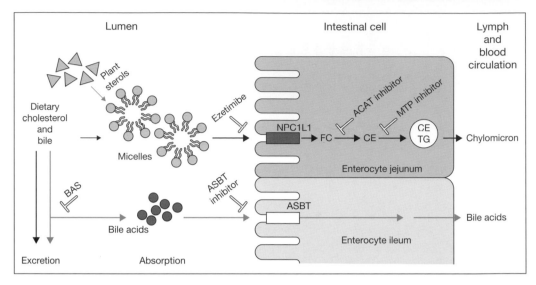

Figure 9.3 Intestinal cholesterol and bile acid uptake and inhibitory agents in these pathways. Dietary cholesterol and bile acids can be absorbed in the small intestine. NPC1L1 is critical for intestinal cholesterol absorption and ASBT for bile acids. Cholesterol and bile acid (re-uptake as well as the formation of chylomicrons can be inhibited by several (future) treatment modalities as shown in this figure. ACAT = acyl-coenzyme A:cholesterol acyltransferase; ASBT = ileal apical sodium-dependent bile acid transporter; BAS = bile acid sequestrants; CE = cholesteryl esters; FC = free cholesterol; MTP = microsomal triglyceride transfer protein; NPC1L1 = Niemann–Pick C-1-like1 protein; TG = triglycerides.

intracellular cholesterol levels due to the conversion to bile acids leads to lower hepatic cholesterol concentrations and increased hepatic LDLR expression, which subsequently decreases plasma LDL-C levels [37] (Figure 9.1).

Colestyramine, colestipol and colesevelam are the most widely used agents in this class of cholesterol-lowering drugs and they reduce LDL-C on average by 15% [36]. Colestyramine was the first lipid-lowering drug to show a survival benefit in hypercholesterolaemic patients in a large placebo-controlled trial [39]. However, colestyramine and colestipol are associated with gastrointestinal side-effects, in particular constipation and flatulence, making long-term compliance poor. Colesevelam, a newly engineered bile acid sequestrant, has a greater potency to bind bile acids per gram of product, thereby providing a much better tolerability profile than the other sequestrants. Colesevelam in doses of 3.75 g/day has been shown to reduce LDL-C by 13–19% when taken as monotherapy [38, 40] and up to an additional 16% when taken in combination with atorvastatin [41]. If combined with ezetimibe, it reduced LDL-C by an additional 11% [42].

Colesevelam is currently being tested in FH patients in a phase IV trial – the TRIPLE study. In this trial, colesevelam is combined with a statin and ezetimibe to provide additional LDL-C lowering in FH patients who have not reached the LDL-C target despite maximal tolerated dose of statin and ezetimibe [41] (Table 9.1).

LDL apheresis

Although the use of LDL apheresis is primarily reserved for homozygous FH patients, it is sometimes employed for heterozygous FH patients (e.g. in patients with a severe phenotype who do not respond to conventional drug treatment, or in pregnant women with heterozygous FH and CVD, in whom the use of conventional drugs is contraindicated [42]). LDL apheresis is a safe procedure that can transiently reduce LDL-C levels. A small number of trials have demonstrated that apheresis could lower LDL-C by about 55%, but none of these trials has demonstrated a significant effect on surrogate cardiovascular endpoints [45, 46]. Furthermore, LDL apheresis is expensive and must be performed every 1–2 weeks [12].

Plant sterols and stanols

Foods enriched with plant sterols or stanols can also inhibit the uptake of dietary and biliary cholesterol from the small intestine. Plant sterols and stanols presumably displace choles-terol from mixed micelles and thereby reduce intestinal absorption, but the exact mechanism is unknown (Figure 9.3). Abundant evidence shows that consuming 2 g/day of plant sterols and stanols reduces LDL-C by about 10% [47]. Consumption of foods rich in plant sterols or stanols is generally recognised as safe [47]. However, any adverse effects of the absorption of plant sterols into the circulation are currently unknown, and no trials have directly tested the effects of sterols and stanols on cardiovascular risk. Nevertheless, based on current evi-dence, the NCEP-ATPIII reports recommend a diet designed for maximal LDL-C lowering including foods enriched with plant sterols/stanols (2 g/day) [17].

TREATMENT IN DEVELOPMENT

Nicotinic acid

Recent meta-analyses have shown that even the most aggressive treatment with statins reduces the cardiovascular risk by only 30%, which leaves a considerable residual CVD risk [23]. High-density lipoprotein cholesterol (HDL-C) levels were inversely associated with subsequent recurrent CVD in patients who had reached LDL-C levels <1.8 mmol/l with intensive statin treatment [48]. Also in FH patients, a low HDL-C was strongly associated with the progression of atherosclerosis as measured by intima-media thickness (IMT) [49] and with the risk for clinically documented coronary artery disease [50]. Those data sug-gested that HDL-C raising strategies could have an important therapeutic role in FH patients, especially in those with low HDL-C levels.

Among currently-registered drugs with the capacity to increase HDL-C, nicotinic acid derivative compounds are the most accepted, and the HDL-C increase is accompanied by a decrease in LDL-C and very low-density lipoprotein cholesterol (VLDL-C). Niacin is such a nicotinic acid derivate and treatment with niacin has been demonstrated to result in a rise in HDL-C of about 21% as well as a decrease in the IMT [51]. Despite these favourable out-comes, niacin has several side-effects, of which the most important is flushing. These flushes limit the wider clinical use of niacin. Flushes can be suppressed by MK0524 (also known as laropiprant) which antagonises the prostaglandin D_2 receptor 1 [52]. In 2006, a phase III clinical trial was launched to evaluate the efficacy and tolerability of niacin in combination with laropiprant in FH subjects who had not reached the target LDL-C level (<2.6 mmol/l) using other medicinal options (the Assessment of Coronary Health Using an Intima-Media Thickness Endpoint for Vascular Effects (ACHIEVE) trial [53]) (Table 9.1). However, this trial was discontinued in 2008 based on the disappointing results of the ENHANCE trial that had also been designed with cIMT in treated heterozygous FH patients [35, 54].

CETP inhibitors

Cholesteryl ester transfer protein (CETP) plays an important role in cholesterol metabolism because it is responsible for the transfer of cholesteryl esters from high-density lipoprotein (HDL) to very low-density lipoproteins (VLDL) and low-density lipoproteins (LDL). As a consequence, CETP inhibition is expected for raising HDL-C and lower LDL-C, thereby providing a therapeutic option for reducing the risk of CVD. FH patients with high CETP levels were demonstrated not only to have a more atherogenic lipid profile that was less receptive to statin treatment, but also to show an increased progression of IMT [55]. The CETP-inhibiting agent torcetrapib has been tested in a phase III study (RADIANCE 1). In this 2-year parallel study, 850 FH subjects were randomised to receive either atorvastatin plus torcetrapib or atorvastatin alone. Despite a significant and robust increase of 52% in HDL-C and a significant decrease of 21% in LDL-C, the addition of torcetrapib to atorvastatin did not inhibit the progression of atherosclerosis. In fact, the secondary endpoint (i.e. the annual change in mean IMT for the common carotid) showed an increase of 0.0038 mm/year in the torcetrapib–atorvastatin group compared to a decrease of 0.0014 mm/year in the atorvastatin monotherapy group [56]. Furthermore, the addition of torcetrapib increased the average systolic blood pressure by 2.8 mmHg. In a simultaneously initiated study on 15 000 (non-FH) patients, the addition of torcetrapib to atorvastatin treatment was demonstrated to lead to excess mortality at interim analysis [57]. This led to early termination of the study and the withdrawal of torcetrapib at the end of 2006.

At this moment, the key question is whether the adverse effect on cardiovascular outcome caused by the addition of torcetrapib was due to CETP inhibition itself or to agent-specific toxicity. Currently, other CETP inhibitors (e.g. dalcetrapib and anacetrapib) are in the final stages of development. Results of phase III studies with these novel CETP inhibitors are eagerly awaited to answer this crucial question.

Squalene synthase inhibitors

A step further than the conversion of HMG-CoA to mevalonate in the cholesterol biosynthetic pathway is the conversion of farnesyl pyrophosphate into squalene by squalene synthase (Figure 9.1). Squalene synthase inhibitors impede this conversion. Unlike HMG-CoA reductase inhibitors, squalene synthase inhibitors do not lower the levels of mevalonate, which is not only the precursor of cholesterol, but also of, e.g., coenzyme Q10, a key component of the mitochondrial respiratory chain. It was therefore postulated that selective inhibition of squalene synthase might result in better tolerability when compared to statins because of fewer liver abnormalities and myopathy related to depletion of non-squalene-metabolites of mevalonate [58]. Animal studies have shown promising results [59, 60] and the squalene synthase inhibitor lapaquistat (TAK-475) is now in phase III development (Table 9.1). Several studies with lapaquistat in combination with statins and ezetimibe are currently ongoing in both homozygous FH patients as well as in patients with primary hypercholesterolaemia [61, 62]. As a result of liver toxicity issues, clinical development of the squalene synthase inhibitors was discontinued in 2008 [63].

ACAT inhibitors

Acyl-coenzyme A:cholesterol acyltransferase (ACAT) is responsible for cholesterol esterification (Figure 9.1; Figure 9.3). There are two isoforms of this enzyme, ACAT1 and ACAT2. ACAT1 is expressed ubiquitously and regulates cholesterol homeostasis in the brain, macrophages and adrenal glands. ACAT2 is expressed in the liver and small intestine, where it esterifies cholesterol, thereby regulating hepatic lipoprotein and cholesterol absorption. ACAT inhibitors have been shown to decrease plasma cholesterol levels and to have beneficial effects on the arterial wall in experimental animal models [64]. Avasimibe and pactimibe are non-selective ACAT inhibitors that have both reached phase III clinical trials. However, both pactimibe and avasimibe failed to show beneficial effects, and treatment with these compounds even resulted in increased coronary plaque volume as assessed by intravascular ultrasound (IVUS) [65, 66]. Furthermore, pactimibe increased IMT progression in FH subjects [67]. The conclusion of these negative findings was that non-selective ACAT inhibition is unable to inhibit the progression of atherosclerosis and may even promote atherogenesis. As a consequence, further development with avasimibe and pactimibe for cardiovascular prevention in humans was discontinued in 2003 and 2005, respectively.

Selective inhibition of isoform hepatic ACAT2 by antisense oligonucleotides (ASOs) remains under development. ACAT2 specific inhibition has been shown to effectively reduce atherosclerosis in animal models [68], but the consequences in humans are still unknown.

MTP inhibitors

In the absence of functional microsomal triglyceride transfer protein (MTP), as in the rare recessive genetic disorder abetalipoproteinaemia, the liver cannot synthesise VLDL, leading to an absence of all lipoproteins containing apoB in the plasma [69]. Due to the decreased levels of the atherogenic apoB particles such as VLDL and LDL, inhibition of MTP was hypothesised to slow the progression of atherosclerosis. Phase I trials with MTP inhibitors such as BMS-201038 have shown promise, since the highest doses reduced plasma LDL-C by more than 50% [70]. However, further development of BMS-201038 was discontinued due to significant hepatic fat accumulation at even moderately effective doses [70]. Accumulation of liver fat is likely to be intrinsically linked to the mechanism of action of MTP inhibitors (Figure 9.1), which is in accordance with the increased incidence of steatosis demonstrated in subjects with familial hypobetalipoproteinaemia [69]. Such accumulation could present a serious barrier to the clinical use of this class of agents. However, a new MTP inhibitor, JTT-130, is currently being tested in phase II trials. In animal models, this compound did not result in significant lipid accumulation [71].

ApoB antisense

Selective inhibition of messenger ribonucleic acid (mRNA) by ASOs is an entirely new approach to modifying cholesterol levels (Figure 9.1). Administration of ASOs to human apoB that interferes with the synthesis of apoB100 mRNA is in advanced development and has shown striking results in phase II studies both as monotherapy and in combination with statins. ISIS 301012 is the apoB antisense drug that is in the most advanced stage of development. Data generated over the last year with the ISIS 301012 phase II trials in all types of patients with elevated LDL-C have shown dramatic efficacy across all patient types. The antisense inhibitor ISIS 301012 is a 20-mer oligonucleotide, complementary to part of the coding region of human apoB100 mRNA. The drug is administered subcutaneously once a week or less and appears to have a substantial LDL-C lowering efficacy of ~50% in FH patients, and also when added to existing maximal lipid-lowering therapy. Thus far, the use of apoB antisense has proven safe [72]. The most common adverse events were mild injection site reactions that did not affect adherence to the protocol and a modest alanine aminotransferase increase. Currently, the effect of ISIS 301012 on the accumulation of hepatic triglyceride is evaluated using magnetic resonance spectroscopy [72, 73].

PRE-CLINICAL PHASE

Apical sodium-dependent bile acid transporter (ASBT) inhibition

A new strategy to impair ileal bile acid reclamation is to inhibit the intestinal bile acid transporter (Figure 9.3). Several inhibitors have been tested in animal models, resulting in a reduction of plasma LDL-C [36], but no data from human trials are available thus far.

PCSK9 inhibition

Statins upregulate both *LDLR* and *PCSK9* expression [74]. The increased expression of PCSK9 may attenuate the LDL-C lowering effect of statins. Inhibition of *PCSK9* activity could therefore enhance the effects of statins [75]. Indeed, animal models showing the effect of ASOs targeting *PCSK9* make PCSK9 an attractive target for LDL-C lowering therapy [76], but human studies have not been performed to date.

Gene therapy

Liver-directed gene transfer of the LDL-C receptor is theoretically attractive but awaits the development of better and safer vectors. Furthermore, the use of gene therapy is currently hindered by the lack of a physiological control mechanism that protects the hepatocytes from pathological accumulation of lipids and cholesterol [77].

TREATMENT OF SPECIFIC GROUPS

Children with FH

In the last decade, a plethora of studies have focussed on the clinical characteristics and treatment of children with FH. Clinical cardiovascular events are very rare in children with heterozygous FH but do occur in homozygous patients. However, morphological and func-tional changes of the vessel wall are already present in children with heterozygous FH [78, 79] underlining the early initiation of the process of atherosclerosis. Morphological changes in children with FH are illustrated by an increased cIMT when compared with non-affected siblings. The impaired endothelial function in children with FH is reflected by a decreased flow-mediated dilatation (FMD) [78]. In addition, as in adults with CVD, inflammatory markers are increased [80].

The early vascular changes in children with FH suggest that treatment should be started at young age. Recent guidelines advocate pharmacological therapy from 8 years of age onwards. LDL-C levels at which treatment should be initiated and LDL-C treatment goals depend on the presence of other risk factors for CVD [81]. As in adults, statins are the cor-nerstone of treatment for children with FH. Several studies have been performed in children and a meta-analysis on the efficacy and safety of statin therapy in children with FH showed that the efficacy of statins was similar to that observed in adults. Moreover, it did not show any clinically-relevant differences between statin-and placebo-treated children with respect to the occurrence of adverse events, growth and sexual maturation (Figure 9.4), and liver-and muscle toxicity [82].

One study in children with heterozygous FH showed that 2 years of treatment with pravastatin led to a decreased cIMT progression when compared to placebo [83]. After this study, children who were on placebo changed to statin treatment and the children in the pravastatin group remained on statin therapy. The cIMT was assessed again after an aver-age treatment period of 4.5 years. Those data revealed that the age of statin initiation was an independent predictor of cIMT after follow-up, indicating that earlier initiation of sta-tin treatment delays the progression of cIMT in adolescents and young adults [14]. Treatment with simvastatin was demonstrated to restore endothelial function, as mea-sured by FMD, in children with FH, which suggests that early treatment can also norma-lise endothelial dysfunction [78]. However, there are no data available on the effect of (statin) therapy initiated in childhood on the occurrence of cardiovascular events later in life.

Besides statins, there are several other options for the treatment of children with FH. Coadministration of ezetimibe with simvastatin 10, 20 or 40 mg led to approximately 15% additional lowering of LDL-C in comparison to simvastatin alone without untoward safety outcomes in children and adolescents (10–17 years of age) with FH [84, 85]. Another study is currently investigating the effect of colesevelam in paediatric FH patients, either as mono-therapy or added to a statin [86] (Table 9.1). Food products enriched with plant sterols have been shown to reduce LDL-C by a moderate 9–18% in children with FH, and this may also be an effective and safe additional therapy for this patient group [87]. Other agents, such as the traditional bile acid binding resins and nicotinic acid derivates are not considered a treatment option for children [84].

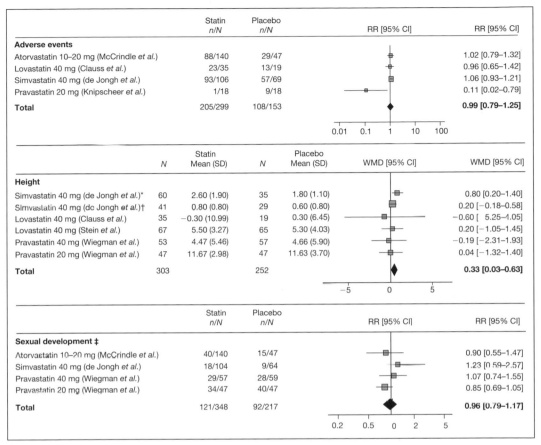

	Statin n/N	Placebo n/N	RR [95% CI]	RR [95% CI]
Adverse events				
Atorvastatin 10–20 mg (McCrindle *et al.*)	88/140	29/47		1.02 [0.79–1.32]
Lovastatin 40 mg (Clauss *et al.*)	23/35	13/19		0.96 [0.65–1.42]
Simvastatin 40 mg (de Jongh *et al.*)	93/106	57/69		1.06 [0.93–1.21]
Pravastatin 20 mg (Knipscheer *et al.*)	1/18	9/18		0.11 [0.02–0.79]
Total	205/299	108/153		**0.99 [0.79–1.25]**

	N	Statin Mean (SD)	N	Placebo Mean (SD)	WMD [95% CI]	WMD [95% CI]
Height						
Simvastatin 40 mg (de Jongh *et al.*)*	60	2.60 (1.90)	35	1.80 (1.10)		0.80 [0.20–1.40]
Simvastatin 40 mg (de Jongh *et al.*)†	41	0.80 (0.80)	29	0.60 (0.80)		0.20 [−0.18–0.58]
Lovastatin 40 mg (Clauss *et al.*)	35	−0.30 (10.99)	19	0.30 (6.45)		−0.60 [5.25–1.05]
Lovastatin 40 mg (Stein *et al.*)	67	5.50 (3.27)	65	5.30 (4.03)		0.20 [−1.05–1.45]
Pravastatin 40 mg (Wiegman *et al.*)	53	4.47 (5.46)	57	4.66 (5.90)		−0.19 [−2.31–1.93]
Pravastatin 20 mg (Wiegman *et al.*)	47	11.67 (2.98)	47	11.63 (3.70)		0.04 [−1.32–1.40]
Total	303		252			**0.33 [0.03–0.63]**

	Statin n/N	Placebo n/N	RR [95% CI]	RR [95% CI]
Sexual development ‡				
Atorvastatin 10–20 mg (McCrindle *et al.*)	40/140	15/47		0.90 [0.55–1.47]
Simvastatin 40 mg (de Jongh *et al.*)	18/104	9/64		1.23 [0.59–2.57]
Pravastatin 40 mg (Wiegman *et al.*)	29/57	28/59		1.07 [0.74–1.55]
Pravastatin 20 mg (Wiegman *et al.*)	34/47	40/47		0.85 [0.69–1.05]
Total	121/348	92/217		**0.96 [0.79–1.17]**

Figure 9.4 Forest plots of the occurrence of adverse events, height change, and sexual development in statin-and placebo-treated children with familial hypercholesterolaemia. * = Male participants; † = female participants; ‡ = sexual development was measured as the number of participants that proceeded one or more Tanner stages during the study; CI = confidence interval; *n* = the number of patients with an 'event'; *N* = the total number of participants per group; RR = relative risk; WMD = weighted mean difference (with permission from [82]).

Pregnancy

As a result of screening programmes [85], more individuals are diagnosed with FH during or even before adolescence. One of the consequences of this is that an increased number of women of childbearing age is being identified. The question arises as to whether (and how) to treat women who wish to become pregnant, who are currently pregnant, or who are breastfeeding their newborns. Currently, it is recommended to stop lipid-lowering drugs because of possible teratogenic effects. As a consequence, cholesterol levels will rise during this period, which may have adverse effects for both mother and child. For instance, both animal and human studies have suggested that a high cholesterol environment *in utero* is associated with an increased progression of atherosclerotic lesions later in life [89, 90]. Furthermore, the influence of intermittent treatment cessation before and during pregnancy on CVD risk in humans is unknown. Future studies should further investigate the risk for mother and child in relation to maternal hypercholesterolaemia as well as the teratogenicity of various lipid-lowering drugs.

LDL apheresis has been suggested as a non-pharmacological alternative for the treatment of patients at evident cardiovascular risk and severely elevated LDL-C levels during pregnancy [44].

Homozygous FH

Homozygous FH is caused by a loss-of-function mutation in both alleles of the *LDLR* gene, and consequently, patients with homozygous FH have plasma cholesterol levels >13 mmol/l. This condition is associated with early, widespread and severe atherosclerosis. If untreated, patients have CVD before 20 years of age and generally do not survive past 30 years of age.

Since patients with homozygous FH do not have any functional LDLRs, they usually respond poorly to statin-and other conventional drug therapies that require upregulation of LDLRs to exert their effect. Treatment with the most potent registered statin doses reduced LDL-C by only 21% and did not reach desirable cholesterol levels [91]. Recently, the use of LDL apheresis has become the standard treatment for homozygous FH that is not responding to conventional drug treatment.

CONCLUSIONS

FH is a prevalent inherited disorder that gives rise to premature CVD. Early diagnosis gives the opportunity to initiate preventive measures and pharmacological interventions early in life.

Lowering LDL-C is the mainstay of treatment for FH. First choice agents are HMG-CoA-reductase inhibitors (statins), most often atorvastatin, rosuvastatin or simvastatin at maximally tolerated doses in order to reach the LDL-C target of <2.6 mmol/l.

In several FH carriers, statins or the higher doses of statins cannot be used due to side-effects, reduced efficacy or contraindications such as pregnancy. Monotherapy or combination therapy with agents targeting cholesterol absorption or interrupting the enterohepatic cycle of bile acids can further lower LDL-C.

In order to raise HDL-C, CETP inhibitors, such as dalcetrapib and anacetrapib, and extended release nicotinic acid in combination with laropiprant are in advanced stages of clinical development for FH patients.

Novel cholesterol synthesis inhibitors that target squalene synthase and inhibitors of VLDL-C synthesis such as ACAT and MTP inhibition have recently been tested in late phase II or III trials in FH patients. The clinical development of these compounds has currently been discontinued.

The combination of statin therapy with ezetimibe and apoB mRNA inhibition has the potential to finally enable the vast majority of FH patients to reach their target LDL-C goals.

Disclosures

JJP Kastelein has received consulting fees from ISIS, Pfizer, AstraZeneca, Merck, Schering-Plough and Roche; lecture fees from Pfizer, AstraZeneca, Merck/Schering-Plough and Roche; and research grants from Pfizer, AstraZeneca, Merck, Schering-Plough, Roche and Sanofi.

REFERENCES

1. Steinberg D. Thematic review series: the pathogenesis of atherosclerosis. An interpretive history of the cholesterol controversy: part I. *J Lipid Res* 2004; 45:1583–1593.
2. Goldstein JL, Hobbs HH, Brown MS. The metabolic and molecular bases of inherited disease. McGraw-Hill, New York, 2001.
3. Leitersdorf E, Tobin EJ, Davignon J, Hobbs HH. Common low-density lipoprotein receptor mutations in the French Canadian population. *J Clin Invest* 1990; 85:1014–1023.

4. Stone NJ, Levy RI, Fredrickson DS, Verter J. Coronary artery disease in 116 kindred with familial type II hyperlipoproteinemia. *Circulation* 1974; 49:476–488.

5. Koeijvoets KC, Wiegman A, Rodenburg J, Defesche JC, Kastelein JJ, Sijbrands EJ. Effect of low-density lipoprotein receptor mutation on lipoproteins and cardiovascular disease risk: a parent–offspring study. *Atherosclerosis* 2005; 180:93–99.

6. Leigh SE, Foster AH, Whitall RA, Hubbert CS, Humphries SE. Update and analysis of the University College London low-density lipoprotein receptor familial hypercholesterolaemia database. *Ann Hum Genet* 2008; 72:485–498.

7. Pullinger CR, Hennessy LK, Chatterton JE *et al*. Familial ligand-defective apolipoprotein B. Identification of a new mutation that decreases LDL receptor binding affinity. *J Clin Invest* 1995; 95:1225–1234.

8. Fouchier SW, Kastelein JJ, Defesche JC. Update of the molecular basis of familial hypercholesterolemia in The Netherlands. *Hum Mutat* 2005; 26:550–556.

9. Miserez AR, Keller U. Differences in the phenotypic characteristics of subjects with familial defective apolipoprotein B-100 and familial hypercholesterolemia. *Arterioscler Thromb Vasc Biol* 1995; 15:1719–1729.

10. Souverein OW, Defesche JC, Zwinderman AH, Kastelein JJ, Tanck MW. Influence of LDL-receptor mutation type on age at first cardiovascular event in patients with familial hypercholesterolaemia. *Eur Heart J* 2007; 28:299–304.

11. Abifadel M, Varret M, Rabès JP *et al*. Mutations in PCSK9 cause autosomal dominant hypercholesterolemia. *Nat Genet* 2003; 34:154–156.

12. Marks D, Thorogood M, Neil HA, Humphries SE. A review on the diagnosis, natural history, and treatment of familial hypercholesterolaemia. *Atherosclerosis* 2003; 168:1–14.

13. Damgaard D, Larsen ML, Nissen PH *et al*. The relationship of molecular genetic to clinical diagnosis of familial hypercholesterolemia in a Danish population. *Atherosclerosis* 2005; 180:155–160.

14. Rodenburg J, Vissers MN, Wiegman A *et al*. Statin treatment in children with familial hypercholesterolemia: the younger, the better. *Circulation* 2007; 116:664–668.

15. Prospective Studies Collaborators. Blood cholesterol and vascular mortality by age, sex, and blood pressure: a meta-analysis of individual data from 61 prospective studies with 55 000 vascular deaths. *Lancet* 2007; 370:1829–1839.

16. Castelli WP, Garrison RJ, Wilson PW, Abbott RD, Kalousdian S, Kannel WB. Incidence of coronary heart disease and lipoprotein cholesterol levels. The Framingham Study. *JAMA* 1986; 256:2835–2838.

17. Third Report of the National Cholesterol Education Program (NCEP) Expert Panel on Detection, Evaluation, and Treatment of High Blood Cholesterol in Adults (Adult Treatment Panel III) final report. *Circulation* 2002; 106:3143–3421.

18. Grundy SM, Cleeman JI, Merz CN *et al*. Implications of recent clinical trials for the National Cholesterol Education Program Adult Treatment Panel III guidelines. *Circulation* 2004; 110:227–239.

19. Wierzbicki, AS, Humphries SL, Minhas R. Familial hypercholesterolaemia: summary of NICE guidelines. *Br Med J* 2008; 337:a1095.

20. Civeira F. Guidelines for the diagnosis and management of heterozygous familial hypercholesterolemia. *Atherosclerosis* 2004; 173:55–68.

21. Ma PT, Gil G, Sudhof TC, Bilheimer DW, Goldstein JL, Brown MS. Mevinolin, an inhibitor of cholesterol synthesis, induces mRNA for low density lipoprotein receptor in livers of hamsters and rabbits. *Proc Natl Acad Sci USA* 1986; 83:8370–8374.

22. Law MR, Wald NJ, Rudnicka AR. Quantifying effect of statins on low density lipoprotein cholesterol, ischaemic heart disease, and stroke: systematic review and meta-analysis. *Br Med J* 2003; 326:1423.

23. Baigent C, Keech A, Kearney PM *et al*. Efficacy and safety of cholesterol-lowering treatment: prospective meta-analysis of data from 90 056 participants in 14 randomised trials of statins. *Lancet* 2005; 366:1267–1278.

24. Risk of fatal coronary heart disease in familial hypercholesterolaemia. Scientific Steering Committee on behalf of the Simon Broome Register Group. *Br Med J* 1991; 303:893–896.

25. Mortality in treated heterozygous familial hypercholesterolaemia: implications for clinical management. Scientific Steering Committee on behalf of the Simon Broome Register Group. *Atherosclerosis* 1999; 142:105–112.

26. Versmissen J, Oosterveer DM, Yazdanapanah M *et al*. Efficacy of statins in familial hypercholesterolaemia: a long term cohort study. *Br Med J* 2008; 337:a2423.

27. Smilde TJ, Van Wissen S, Wollersheim H, Trip MD, Kastelein JJ, Stalenhoef AF. Effect of aggressive versus conventional lipid lowering on atherosclerosis progression in familial hypercholesterolaemia (ASAP): a prospective, randomised, double-blind trial. *Lancet* 2001; 357:577–581.

28. Duivenvoorden R, Nederveen AJ, de Groot E, Kastelein JJ. Atherosclerosis imaging as a benchmark in the development of novel cardiovascular drugs. *Curr Opin Lipidol* 2007; 18:613–621.

29. Altmann SW, Davis HR Jr, Zhu LJ et al. Niemann-Pick C1 Like 1 protein is critical for intestinal cholesterol absorption. *Science* 2004; 303:1201–1204.

30. Sudhop T, Lutjohann D, Kodal A et al. Inhibition of intestinal cholesterol absorption by ezetimibe in humans. *Circulation* 2002; 106:1943–1948.

31. Dujovne CA, Ettinger MP, McNeer JF et al. Efficacy and safety of a potent new selective cholesterol absorption inhibitor, ezetimibe, in patients with primary hypercholesterolemia. *Am J Cardiol* 2002; 90:1092–1097.

32. Ballantyne CM, Houri J, Notarbartolo A et al. Effect of ezetimibe coadministered with atorvastatin in 628 patients with primary hypercholesterolemia: a prospective, randomized, double-blind trial. *Circulation* 2003; 107:2409–2415.

33. Pearson TA, Denke MA, McBride PE et al. Effectiveness of ezetimibe added to ongoing statin therapy in modifying lipid profiles and low-density lipoprotein cholesterol goal attainment in patients of different races and ethnicities: a substudy of the Ezetimibe add-on to statin for effectiveness trial. *Mayo Clin Proc* 2006; 81:1177–1185.

34. Pearson TA, Denke MA, McBride PE, Battisti WP, Brady WE, Palmisano J. A community-based, randomized trial of ezetimibe added to statin therapy to attain NCEP ATP III goals for LDL cholesterol in hypercholesterolemic patients: the ezetimibe add-on to statin for effectiveness (EASE) trial. *Mayo Clin Proc* 2005; 80:587–595.

35. Kastelein JJ, Akdim F, Stroes ES et al. Simvastatin with or without ezetimibe in familial hypercholesterolemia. *N Engl J Med* 2008; 358:1431–1443.

36. Li H, Xu G, Shang Q et al. Inhibition of ileal bile acid transport lowers plasma cholesterol levels by inactivating hepatic farnesoid X receptor and stimulating cholesterol 7 alpha-hydroxylase. *Metabolism* 2004; 53:927–932.

37. Huff MW, Telford DE, Edwards JY et al. Inhibition of the apical sodium-dependent bile acid transporter reduces LDL cholesterol and apoB by enhanced plasma clearance of LDL apoB. *Arterioscler Thromb Vasc Biol* 2002; 22:1884–1891.

38. Davidson MH, Dillon MA, Gordon B et al. Colesevelam hydrochloride (cholestagel): a new, potent bile acid sequestrant associated with a low incidence of gastrointestinal side effects. *Arch Intern Med* 1999; 159:1893–1900.

39. The Lipid Research Clinics Coronary Primary Prevention Trial results. I. Reduction in incidence of coronary heart disease. *JAMA* 1984; 251:351–364.

40. Insull W Jr, Toth P, Mullican W et al. Effectiveness of colesevelam hydrochloride in decreasing LDL cholesterol in patients with primary hypercholesterolemia: a 24-week randomized controlled trial. *Mayo Clin Proc* 2001; 76:971–982.

41. Hunninghake D, Insull W Jr, Toth P, Davidson D, Donovan JM, Burke SK. Coadministration of colesevelam hydrochloride with atorvastatin lowers LDL cholesterol additively. *Atherosclerosis* 2001; 158:407–416.

42. Bays H, Rhyne J, Abby S, Lai YL, Jones M. Lipid-lowering effects of colesevelam HCl in combination with ezetimibe. *Curr Med Res Opin* 2006; 22:2191–2200.

43. A Phase 4 Randomised, Double-Blind, Placebo-Controlled, Parallel-Group, Multi-Centre Study of Colesevelam as Add-on Therapy in Patients with Familial Hypercholesterolaemia. EUDRACT Number: 2007-000582-37.

44. Cashin-Hemphill L, Noone M, Abbott JF, Waksmonski CA, Lees RS. Low-density lipoprotein apheresis therapy during pregnancy. *Am J Cardiol* 2000; 86:1160, A10.

45. Thompson GR, Maher VM, Matthews S et al. Familial Hypercholesterolaemia Regression Study: a randomised trial of low-density-lipoprotein apheresis. *Lancet* 1995; 345:811–816.

46. Park JW, Merz M, Braun P. Effect of HELP-LDL-apheresis on outcomes in patients with advanced coronary atherosclerosis and severe hypercholesterolemia. *Atherosclerosis* 1998; 139:401–409.

47. Katan MB, Grundy SM, Jones P, Law M, Miettinen T, Paoletti R. Efficacy and safety of plant stanols and sterols in the management of blood cholesterol levels. *Mayo Clin Proc* 2003; 78:965–978.

48. Barter P, Gotto AM, LaRosa JC et al. HDL cholesterol, very low levels of LDL cholesterol, and cardiovascular events. *N Engl J Med* 2007; 357:1301–1310.

49. Junyent M, Cofan M, Nunez I, Gilabert R, Zambon D, Ros E. Influence of HDL cholesterol on preclinical carotid atherosclerosis in familial hypercholesterolemia. *Arterioscler Thromb Vasc Biol* 2006; 26:1107–1113.

50. Neil HA, Seagroatt V, Betteridge DJ *et al*. Established and emerging coronary risk factors in patients with heterozygous familial hypercholesterolaemia. *Heart* 2004; 90:1431–1437.

51. Taylor AJ, Lee HJ, Sullenberger LE. The effect of 24 months of combination statin and extended-release niacin on carotid intima-media thickness: ARBITER 3. *Curr Med Res Opin* 2006; 22:2243–2250.

52. Cheng K, Wu TJ, Wu KK *et al*. Antagonism of the prostaglandin D2 receptor 1 suppresses nicotinic acid-induced vasodilation in mice and humans. *Proc Natl Acad Sci USA* 2006; 103:6682–6687.

53. Carotid IMT (intima-media thickening) study with MK0524A in subjects with familial hypercholesterolemia: Identifier NCT00384293. Available at www.clinicaltrials.gov (accessed 2 January, 2008).

54. Vergeer M, Zhou R, Duivervoorden R *et al*. Carotid intima media thickness progression is modest in statin-treated familial hypercholesterolaemia patients—results from a patient level meta-analysis of 1257 patients. Abstract AHA 2008 # 2223. *Circulation* 2008; 118:S687b.

55. de Grooth GJ, Smilde TJ, van Wissen S *et al*. The relationship between cholesteryl ester transfer protein levels and risk factor profile in patients with familial hypercholesterolemia. *Atherosclerosis* 2004; 173:261–267.

56. Kastelein JJ, van Leuven SI, Burgess L *et al*. Effect of torcetrapib on carotid atherosclerosis in familial hypercholesterolemia. *N Engl J Med* 2007; 356:1620–1630.

57. Barter PJ, Caulfield M, Eriksson M *et al*. Effects of torcetrapib in patients at high risk for coronary events. *N Engl J Med* 2007; 357:2109–2122.

58. Bliznakov EG. Lipid-lowering drugs (statins), cholesterol, and coenzyme Q10. The Baycol case – a modern Pandora's box. *Biomed Pharmacother* 2002; 56:56–59.

59. Hiyoshi H, Yanagimachi M, Ito M *et al*. Effect of ER-27856, a novel squalene synthase inhibitor, on plasma cholesterol in rhesus monkeys: comparison with 3-hydroxy-3-methylglutaryl-coa reductase inhibitors. *J Lipid Res* 2000; 41:1136–1144.

60. Ugawa T, Kakuta H, Moritani H *et al*. YM-53601, a novel squalene synthase inhibitor, reduces plasma cholesterol and triglyceride levels in several animal species. *Br J Pharmacol* 2000; 131:63–70.

61. The Effect of TAK-475 or Placebo co-Administration With Current Lipid-Lowering Treatment on Blood Cholesterol Levels in Subjects With Homozygous Familial Hypercholesterolemia, identifier NCT00263081. Available at www.clinicaltrials.gov (accessed 2 January, 2008).

62. Effect of TAK-475 or Placebo on Blood Cholesterol Levels in Subjects co-Administered High-Dose Statin. Available at www.clinicaltrials.gov (accessed 2 January, 2008).

63. TAKEDA provides update on development status of TAK-475, an investigational compound for treatment of hypercholesterolemia. www.takeda.com (accessed 29 October, 2007).

64. Nicolosi RJ, Wilson TA, Krause BR. The ACAT inhibitor, CI-1011 is effective in the prevention and regression of aortic fatty streak area in hamsters. *Atherosclerosis* 1998; 137:77–85.

65. Tardif JC, Grégoire J, L'Allier PL *et al*. Effects of the acyl coenzyme A:cholesterol acyltransferase inhibitor avasimibe on human atherosclerotic lesions. *Circulation* 2004; 110:3372–3377.

66. Nissen SE, Tuzcu EM, Brewer HB *et al*. Effect of ACAT inhibition on the progression of coronary atherosclerosis. *N Engl J Med* 2006; 354:1253–1263.

67. Meuwese MC, Duivenvoorden R, Zwinderman AH *et al*. Effect of ACAT inhibition on carotid atherosclerosis in familial hypercholesterolemia. *J Clin Lipidol* XVI DALM Symposium NY 2007; 1:382.

68. Bell TA III, Brown JM, Graham MJ, Lemonidis KM, Crooke RM, Rudel LL. Liver-specific inhibition of acyl-coenzyme a:cholesterol acyltransferase 2 with antisense oligonucleotides limits atherosclerosis development in apolipoprotein B100-only low-density lipoprotein receptor-/-mice. *Arterioscler Thromb Vasc Biol* 2006; 26:1814–1820.

69. Whitfield AJ, Barrett PH, Robertson K, Havlat MF, van Bockxmeer FM, Burnett JR. Liver dysfunction and steatosis in familial hypobetalipoproteinemia. *Clin Chem* 2005; 51:266–269.

70. Cuchel M, Bloedon LT, Szapary PO *et al*. Inhibition of microsomal triglyceride transfer protein in familial hypercholesterolemia. *N Engl J Med* 2007; 356:148–156.

71. Aggarwal D, West KL, Zern TL, Shrestha S, Vergara-Jimenez M, Fernandez ML. JTT-130, a microsomal triglyceride transfer protein (MTP) inhibitor lowers plasma triglycerides and LDL cholesterol concentrations without increasing hepatic triglycerides in guinea pigs. *BMC Cardiovasc Disord* 2005; 5:30.

72. Kastelein JJ, Wedel MK, Baker BF *et al*. Potent reduction of apolipoprotein B and low-density lipoprotein cholesterol by short-term administration of an antisense inhibitor of apolipoprotein B. *Circulation* 2006; 114:1729–1735.

73. Akdim F, Stroes ES, Kastelein JJ. Antisense apolipoprotein B therapy: where do we stand? *Curr Opin Lipidol* 2007; 18:397–400.

74. Dubuc G, Chamberland A, Wassef H *et al*. Statins upregulate PCSK9, the gene encoding the proprotein convertase neural apoptosis-regulated convertase-1 implicated in familial hypercholesterolemia. *Arterioscler Thromb Vasc Biol* 2004; 24:1454–1459.

75. Rashid S, Curtis DE, Garuti R *et al*. Decreased plasma cholesterol and hypersensitivity to statins in mice lacking Pcsk9. *Proc Natl Acad Sci USA* 2005;102:5374–5379.

76. Frank-Kamentsky M, Grefhorst A, Anderson NN *et al*. Therapeutic RNA: targeting PCSK9 acutely lowers plasma cholesterol in rodents and LDL cholesterol in non-human primates. *Proc Natl Acad Sci USA* 2008; 105:11915–11920.

77. Rader DJ. Gene therapy for familial hypercholesterolemia. *Nutr Metab Cardiovasc Dis* 2001; 11(suppl 5):40–44.

78. de Jongh S, Lilien MR, op't Roodt J, Stroes ES, Bakker HD, Kastelein JJ. Early statin therapy restores endothelial function in children with familial hypercholesterolemia. *J Am Coll Cardiol* 2002; 40:2117–2121.

79. Wiegman A, de Groot E, Hutten BA *et al*. Arterial intima-media thickness in children heterozygous for familial hypercholesterolaemia. *Lancet* 2004; 363:369–370.

80. Ueland T, Vissers MN, Wiegman A *et al*. Increased inflammatory markers in children with familial hypercholesterolaemia. *Eur J Clin Invest* 2006; 36:147–152.

81. Daniels SR, Greer FR. Lipid screening and cardiovascular health in childhood. *Pediatrics* 2008;122:198–208.

82. Avis HJ, Vissers MN, Stein EA *et al*. A systematic review and meta-analysis of statin therapy in children with familial hypercholesterolemia. *Arterioscler Thromb Vasc Biol* 2007; 27:1803–1810.

83. Wiegman A, Hutten BA, de Groot E *et al*. Efficacy and safety of statin therapy in children with familial hypercholesterolemia: a randomized controlled trial. *JAMA* 2004; 292:331–337.

84. McCrindle BW, Urbina EM, Dennison BA *et al*. Drug therapy of high-risk lipid abnormalities in children and adolescents: a scientific statement from the American Heart Association Atherosclerosis, Hypertension, and Obesity in Youth Committee, Council of Cardiovascular Disease in the Young, with the Council on Cardiovascular Nursing. *Circulation* 2007; 115:1948–1967.

85. Van der Graaf A, Cuffie-Jackson C, Vissers MN *et al*. Efficacy and safety of coadministration of ezetimibe and simvastatin in adolescents with heterozygous familial hypercholesterolemia. *J Am Coll Cardiol* 2008; 52:1421–1429.

86. Efficacy and Safety of Colesevelam in Pediatric Patients with Genetic High Cholesterol, Identifier NCT00145574. Available at www.clinicaltrials.gov (accessed 2 January, 2008).

87. Jakulj L, Vissers MN, Rodenburg J, Wiegman A, Trip MD, Kastelein JJ. Plant stanols do not restore endothelial function in pre-pubertal children with familial hypercholesterolemia despite reduction of low-density lipoprotein cholesterol levels. *J Pediatr* 2006; 148:495–500.

88. Umans-Eckenhausen MA, Defesche JC, Sijbrands EJ, Scheerder RL, Kastelein JJ. Review of first 5 years of screening for familial hypercholesterolaemia in the Netherlands. *Lancet* 2001; 357:165–168.

89. Napoli C, Glass CK, Witztum JL, Deutsch R, D'Armiento FP, Palinski W. Influence of maternal hypercholesterolaemia during pregnancy on progression of early atherosclerotic lesions in childhood: Fate of Early Lesions in Children (FELIC) study. *Lancet* 1999; 354:1234–1241.

90. Alkemade FE, Gittenberger-de Groot AC, Schiel AE *et al*. Intrauterine exposure to maternal atherosclerotic risk factors increases the susceptibility to atherosclerosis in adult life. *Arterioscler Thromb Vasc Biol* 2007; 27:2228–2235.

91. Marais AD, Raal FJ, Stein EA *et al*. A dose-titration and comparative study of rosuvastatin and atorvastatin in patients with homozygous familial hypercholesterolaemia. *Atherosclerosis* 2008; 197:400–406.

92. PLUTO: Pediatric Lipid-redUction Trial of rOsuvastatin, identifier NCT00355615. Available at www.clinicaltrials.gov (accessed 2 January, 2008).

93. Efficacy and Safety of the ACAT Inhibitor CS-505 (Pactimibe) for Reducing the Progression of Carotid Artery Disease. (CAPTIVATE): identifier: NCT00151788. Available at www.clinicaltrials.gov (accessed 2 January, 2008).

10

Lipid lowering in chronic kidney disease

V. Perkovic, M. J. Jardine, M. Gallagher, A. Cass

INTRODUCTION

Chronic kidney disease (CKD) most often manifests as the presence of proteinuria or a reduced glomerular filtration rate (GFR), and is highly prevalent in the community. Population based studies have suggested that CKD affects 10–15% of the adult population [1–3]. Sufferers are at substantially higher risk of cardiovascular disease than people with normal kidney function, and their level of risk increases with reducing kidney function [4, 5]. In the most severe form of CKD – end-stage kidney disease (ESKD) – regular dialysis or kidney transplantation are required to maintain life. ESKD affects approximately 0.1% of the population and is associated with annual mortality rates at least 20-fold greater than age- and sex-matched controls, mostly resulting from premature cardiovascular disease [6, 7]. Restoration of kidney function by renal transplantation results in better survival compared with people on dialysis, but cardiovascular disease remains a major problem [8]. Because of the high prevalence of CKD in the community and the associated excess burden of cardio-vascular mortality and morbidity, there is great interest in exploring the mechanisms by which this cardiovascular risk might be reduced.

Dyslipidaemia is common in patients with CKD, but the nature of the lipid disturbance in CKD is quite different to that commonly seen in the general population. The characteristic lipid abnormality in CKD is an increase in triglyceride levels – a consequence of the reduced clearance of triglyceride-rich particles from the blood [9]. In addition, HDL cholesterol (HDL-C) levels are suppressed due to reduced production of the apolipoproteins AI and AII. Overall total cholesterol and LDL cholesterol (LDL-C) values are typically similar to those in the general population but the pattern of the lipid subfractions is changed into one that is more atherogenic, with greater concentrations of small, dense LDL particles [10]. The divergence from the general population increases with the severity of renal dysfunction.

In people with ESKD, the total cholesterol levels appear to be influenced by the form of dialysis employed: patients treated with haemodialysis tend to have similar total cholesterol

Vlado Perkovic, MBBS, PhD, FRACP, Co-director, Renal Division, The George Institute for International Health, University of Sydney, Sydney, Australia

Meg J. Jardine, MBBS, PhD, FRACP, Nephrologist and Senior Research Fellow, The George Institute for International Health, University of Sydney, Sydney, Australia

Martin Gallagher, MBBS, FRACP, MPH, Nephrologist and Senior Research Fellow, The George Institute for International Health, University of Sydney, Sydney, Australia

Alan Cass, MBBS, PhD, FRACP, Co-director, Renal Division, The George Institute for International Health, University of Sydney, Sydney, Australia

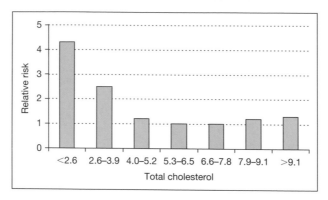

Figure 10.1 The relative risk of cardiovascular death according to serum total cholesterol levels among 12 000 patients receiving haemodialysis in the United States of America (with permission from [12]).

levels to those observed in the general population, while patients receiving peritoneal dialysis often have a particularly atherogenic lipid profile, characterised by even greater elevations in triglycerides and LDL-C and greater reductions in HDL-C, which may be related to the greater glucose exposure from the treatment [11].

LIPIDS AND CARDIOVASCULAR DISEASE IN CKD – OBSERVATIONAL STUDIES

Much of the uncertainty concerning the efficacy of lipid-lowering therapies in CKD has arisen from the results of observational studies examining the relationship between total cholesterol levels and the risk of cardiovascular death amongst dialysis patients. The first such analysis, from the United States Renal Data System (USRDS), which included 12 000 patients on dialysis [12], found an inverse relationship between lipid levels and the risk of cardiovascular mortality (Figure 10.1); patients with the lowest cholesterol levels had the highest risk of death [12]. This generated concern about the safety and efficacy of lipid lowering in dialysis patients. Many argued, however, that the findings resulted from reverse causality, whereby dialysis patients who were unwell from other causes had both a low cholesterol level and a high risk of cardiovascular death, rather than the low cholesterol being a causal factor. Similar relationships have subsequently been noted in other dialysis registries.

In addition to concerns that lowering of cholesterol levels might not reduce cardiovascular risk in CKD, there has been significant uncertainty regarding the safety of statin therapy in this population. In particular, concerns have been expressed that higher rates of myopathy, rhabdomyolysis and liver toxicity might occur. As a result, studies assessing the efficacy and safety of lipid lowering in CKD patients have become a research priority.

LIPID LOWERING IN ESKD PATIENTS RECEIVING DIALYSIS: DIE DEUTSCHE DIABETES DIALYSE (4D) STUDY

The 4D study is the largest completed trial conducted among ESKD patients requiring dialysis [13]. It involved 178 centres in Germany, enrolling 1522 people with diabetes who had commenced dialysis within the preceding 2 years and who had LDL-C levels between 2.1 and 4.9 mmol/l. Of these, 1255 were eventually randomised in a double-blind fashion to receive either atorvastatin 20 mg/day or a matching placebo. They were followed for a mean duration of approximately 4 years. The participants were at very high risk for cardiovascular events at baseline, as evidenced by nearly one-third having established coro-

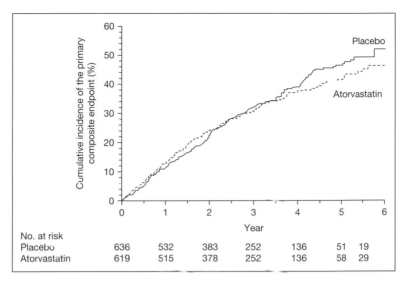

Figure 10.2 Cumulative incidence of the primary endpoint according to randomised group in the 4D trial (with permission from [13]).

nary heart disease, more than one-sixth having pre-existing cerebrovascular disease and more than 40% having documented peripheral vascular disease. The mean LDL-C level was 3.13 mmol/l at study initiation. This was reduced by 1.86 mmol/l (42%) in the active therapy arm within 4 weeks of randomisation but remained essentially unchanged in the placebo arm. Over the entire duration of the trial, the mean difference in LDL-C levels between the active and placebo study groups was approximately 1 mmol/l.

The primary endpoint chosen in the 4D study was a composite of non-fatal myocardial infarction and death due to cardiac causes or stroke. This occurred in 469 patients during the follow-up period. In the atorvastatin-treated group, 226 patients reached the primary endpoint compared with 243 in the placebo group (Figure 10.2). The relative risk (RR) for the primary endpoint (0.92) did not reach statistical significance (95% confidence interval [CI] 0.77–1.10; $P = 0.37$). Among the prespecified secondary endpoints, a significant 18% reduction in all cardiac events was observed (95% CI 1–32%), but no effect was demonstrated upon either total or cause-specific mortality. No effect was demonstrated for stroke overall (RR 1.12; CI 0.81–1.55), but an increase in the frequency of fatal stroke was observed (RR 2.03; CI 1.05–3.93) in the active treatment arm.

The effect of atorvastatin on cardiac events in this trial was consistent with that seen in studies in the general population; however, the effect on stroke events was not, and remains unexplained. The excess strokes were classified as ischaemic rather than haemorrhagic, results which were at odds with those seen in the SPARCL (Stroke Prevention by Aggressive Reduction in Cholesterol Levels) study [14] and the broader data in the general population [15]. Importantly, the 4D study did not demonstrate any increase in muscle-or liver-related adverse effects in ESKD patients receiving dialysis.

Since significant uncertainty persists about the efficacy of statin therapy in ESKD, the results of ongoing trials are awaited with interest [16, 17].

LIPID LOWERING IN RECIPIENTS OF KIDNEY TRANSPLANTS

Only one large-scale study of lipid lowering in transplant recipients has been completed – the ALERT (Assessment of Lescol in Renal Transplantation) study, undertaken in Europe

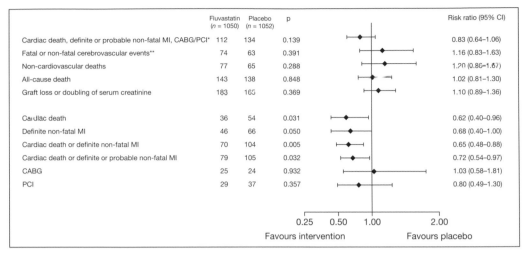

	Fluvastatin (n = 1050)	Placebo (n = 1052)	p	Risk ratio (95% CI)
Cardiac death, definite or probable non-fatal MI, CABG/PCI*	112	134	0.139	0.83 (0.64–1.06)
Fatal or non-fatal cerebrovascular events**	74	63	0.391	1.16 (0.83–1.63)
Non-cardiovascular deaths	77	65	0.288	1.20 (0.86–1.67)
All-cause death	143	138	0.848	1.02 (0.81–1.30)
Graft loss or doubling of serum creatinine	183	165	0.369	1.10 (0.89–1.36)
Cardiac death	36	54	0.031	0.62 (0.40–0.96)
Definite non-fatal MI	46	66	0.050	0.68 (0.40–1.00)
Cardiac death or definite non-fatal MI	70	104	0.005	0.65 (0.48–0.88)
Cardiac death or definite or probable non-fatal MI	79	105	0.032	0.72 (0.54–0.97)
CABG	25	24	0.932	1.03 (0.58–1.81)
PCI	29	37	0.357	0.80 (0.49–1.30)

0.25   0.50   1.00   2.00

Favours intervention   Favours placebo

Figure 10.3 ALERT study endpoints associated with fluvastatin use vs. placebo (with permission from [18]). * = study primary endpoint; ** = fatal or non-fatal stroke, transient ischaemic attack, reversible ischaemic neurological deficit, subarachnoid haemorrhage; CABG = coronary artery bypass graft; PCI = percutaneous coronary intervention.

and Canada [18]. ALERT enrolled 2102 adult recipients of stable renal or renal–pancreas transplants of at least 6 months' standing, who had a total cholesterol between 4.0 and 9.0 mmol/l. In this double-blind trial, participants were assigned initially to 40 mg fluvastatin or to a matching placebo. In an effort to increase the separation in LDL-C levels between the groups, dosage was increased to 80 mg fluvastatin or placebo at a mean of 2.8 years of follow-up. All participants received cyclosporine-based immunosuppressive therapy.

The study population was at relatively low overall cardiovascular risk. At baseline, the mean age of the participants was 50 years; the mean blood pressure was 144/86 and mean body mass index (BMI) was 25.8 kg/m². Diabetes was present in 19% of participants and 3% had a history of myocardial infarction. The mean baseline creatinine was 145 μmol/l and mean LDL-C was 4.1 mmol/l. Participants were excluded if they had had a recent episode of transplant rejection (within the previous 3 months) or a recent myocardial infarction (within 6 months). Participants were followed up for a mean of 5.1 years, during which an average difference between the groups of 1.0 mmol/l LDL-C was noted.

ALERT did not show a significant reduction in the primary endpoint of major cardiac events (cardiac death, non-fatal myocardial infarction or coronary revascularisation procedure) with active therapy (risk ratio 0.83; CI 0.64–1.06; P = 0.139). Statistically significant beneficial effects for some secondary endpoints were demonstrated (Figure 10.3). The event rate during the study was substantially lower than had been anticipated (12.7% achieved compared to 25% anticipated), so that the trial had less power to identify a significant effect; this is likely to have contributed to the non-significant result. Safety data showed similar rates of adverse events, infection and malignant disease in the treatment and placebo groups.

A number of *post hoc* analyses have been performed on this large study of renal transplant recipients. Further analyses of graft function parameters confirmed the lack of a benefit of the intervention on graft outcomes.

LIPID LOWERING IN EARLIER STAGE CKD

To date, large-scale trials specifically designed to investigate the effects of lipid lowering on the risk of cardiovascular events in people with earlier stage CKD have not been completed.

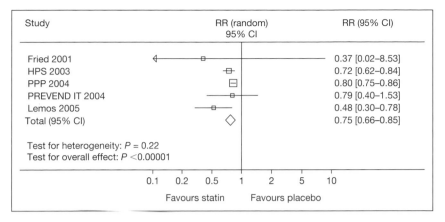

Figure 10.4 A meta-analysis of the effects of lipid lowering on major cardiovascular events among individuals with early CKD (adapted with permission from [19]).

Most trials in the broader non-CKD population, however, have included substantial numbers of participants with early stage CKD (stages 1–3a); several analyses of these subgroups have now been reported.

A recently reported Cochrane group systematic review analysed data from the trials in the general population which have included patients with early CKD [19]. The largest amount of data came from the Prospective Pravastatin Pooling (PPP) project, which pooled data from three placebo-controlled trials of pravastatin: the West of Scotland Coronary Prevention Study (WOSCOPS), Cholesterol and Recurrent Events (CARE) and Long-Term Intervention with Pravastatin in Ischaemic Disease (LIPID) studies. Additional data were obtained from the Heart Protection Study (HPS) and several smaller trials. The summary results showed a highly significant 25% reduction in the risk of major cardiovascular events among individuals with CKD who were receiving statins (CI 15–34%; P <0.001) (Figure 10.4). A significant 20% reduction in the risk of cardiovascular mortality (CI 10–30%; P <0.001) and a 19% reduction in the risk of total mortality (CI 11–26%; P <0.001) were also noted. These study results provide no evidence of heterogeneity for any of these endpoints.

These findings provide strong support for the use of statins in people with early kidney disease. However, few of the individuals with CKD in each of these studies had advanced stage CKD. For example, only 27 of the 19 700 participants in the PPP study had an estimated GFR <30 ml/min, and these people were excluded from the analyses according to kidney function. Since most of the individuals with CKD in these analyses are likely to have had a GFR >45 ml/min, the generalisability of these results to individuals with more advanced CKD remains uncertain.

The question of statin dose in CKD has had relatively little attention, but an important paper describing *post hoc* analyses from the Treat to New Targets (TNT) trial has shed some light on this issue [20]. This trial, conducted among 10 001 participants with established coronary heart disease, randomised participants to therapy with either 10 mg or 80 mg of atorvastatin. A total of 3107 participants had CKD at baseline, namely an estimated GFR <60 ml/min. The additional LDL-C reductions seen with atorvastatin 80 mg compared with 10 mg were similar in the CKD subgroup. Among the participants with CKD, the primary endpoint of major cardiovascular events occurred in 149 participants randomised to atorvastatin 80 mg, compared to 202 patients randomised to atorvastatin 10 mg. This highly significant 32% relative risk reduction (CI 16–45%; P = 0.0003) translated into an

9.   Attman PO, Samuelsson O, Johansson AC, Moberly JB, Alaupovic P. Dialysis modalities and dyslipidemia. *Kidney Int* 2003; 84:S110–S112.

10. Baigent C, Burbury K, Wheeler D. Premature cardiovascular disease in chronic renal failure. *Lancet* 2000; 356:147–152.

11. Weiner DE, Sarnak MJ. Managing dyslipidemia in chronic kidney disease. *J Gen Intern Med* 2004; 19:1045–1052.

12. Lowrie EG, Lew NL. Death risk in hemodialysis patients: the predictive value of commonly measured variables and an evaluation of death rate differences between facilities. *Am J Kidney Dis* 1990; 15:458–482.

13. Wanner C, Krane V, Marz W *et al.* Atorvastatin in patients with type 2 diabetes mellitus undergoing hemodialysis. *N Engl J Med* 2005; 353:238–248.

14. Amarenco P, Bogousslavsky J, Callahan A 3rd *et al.* High-dose atorvastatin after stroke or transient ischemic attack. *N Engl J Med* 2006; 355:549–559.

15. Baigent C, Keech A, Kearney PM *et al.* Efficacy and safety of cholesterol-lowering treatment: prospective meta-analysis of data from 90 056 participants in 14 randomised trials of statins. *Lancet* 2005; 366:1267–1278.

16. Baigent C, Landry M. Study of Heart and Renal Protection (SHARP). *Kidney Int* 2003; 84:S207–S210.

17. Fellstrom BC, Holdaas H, Jardine AG. Why do we need a statin trial in hemodialysis patients? *Kidney Int* 2003; 84:S204–S206.

18. Holdaas H, Fellstrom B, Jardine AG *et al.* Effect of fluvastatin on cardiac outcomes in renal transplant recipients: a multicentre, randomised, placebo-controlled trial. *Lancet* 2003; 361:2024–2031.

19. Strippoli GF, Navaneethan SD, Johnson DW *et al.* Effects of statins in patients with chronic kidney disease: meta-analysis and meta-regression of randomised controlled trials. *Br Med J* 2008; 336:645–651.

20. Shepherd J, Kastelein JJP, Bittner V *et al.* Intensive lipid lowering with atorvastatin in patients with coronary heart disease and chronic kidney disease: the TNT (Treating to New Targets) study. *J Am Coll Cardiol* 2008; 51:1448–1454.

21. Sandhu S, Wiebe N, Fried LF, Tonelli M. Statins for improving renal outcomes: a meta-analysis. *J Am Soc Nephrol* 2006; 17:2006–2016.

11

Statins and heart failure

J. Kjekshus

INTRODUCTION

The Scandinavian Simvastatin Survival Study (4S) [1] was the first clinical trial to convincingly document that the 3-hydroxy 3-methylglutaryl coenzyme A (HMG-CoA) reductase inhibitor simvastatin reduced cardiovascular events, including fatal and non-fatal myocardial infarction, sudden death, the need for coronary revascularisation and stroke in high-risk patients with arteriosclerotic disease. A number of statins have now been tested in a multitude of clinical trials involving more than 90 000 low- and high-risk patients, confirming and expanding the positive role of statins in preventing atherosclerotic diseases in different populations [2]. Despite this evidence, there has been marked uncertainty over the role of lipid-lowering regimens in heart failure patients due to epidemiological observations showing an inverse relationship between cholesterol concentrations and prognosis, and because of undefined pleiotropic effects. Patients with more severe manifestations of heart failure were typically excluded from the earlier landmark trials, and until recently there was virtually no clinical evidence for the use of statins in heart failure patients.

However, prospective randomised clinical studies have shown that statin treatment reduces incident heart failure in patients with coronary artery disease, probably as a result of delaying progression or possibly even causing the regression of coronary artery stenoses. In the 4S trial, 4444 patients without coronary heart disease and with no evidence of heart failure were randomised to simvastatin 20–40 mg/day or matching placebo. Among the patients who received simvastatin, 8.3% had incident *de novo* heart failure compared with 10.3% of patients who were treated with placebo ($P = 0.015$). More patients who developed heart failure had a myocardial infarction during the last 3 months before heart failure was diagnosed [3]. Prevention of current myocardial damage with recurrent myocardial infarction may therefore have decreased incident heart failure. More recently, the PROVE IT-TIMI 22 study investigated among its endpoints whether intensive statin therapy reduced hospitalisation for heart failure after an acute coronary syndrome. The study showed that more aggressive lowering of low-density lipoprotein cholesterol (LDL-C) with atorvastatin 80 mg as compared to pravastatin 40 mg was associated with a significant reduction in the rate of hospitalisation for heart failure (1.6% vs. 3.1%; $P = 0.016$). This was independent of the occurrence of recurrent myocardial infarction or previous episodes of heart failure [4]. These studies suggested a favourable and 'dose-dependent' role for statins in the prevention of heart failure in patients with coronary artery disease and with no previous history of heart failure. Although the 4S trial also demonstrated that patients in the placebo group

John Kjekshus, MD, PhD, Professor, Department of Cardiology, University of Oslo, Rikshospitalet University Clinic, Oslo, Norway

who developed heart failure had higher mortality compared with those in the simvastatin group, the two groups were no longer balanced, and this result cannot therefore be translated to patients with established heart failure.

POTENTIAL CLINICAL EFFECTS OF STATINS IN HEART FAILURE PATIENTS

When coronary heart disease is complicated by heart failure, the overall cardiovascular event rate increases 3–4-fold, despite effective blockade of neurohormonal activation with other heart failure therapies [3].

The concept that progressive coronary atherosclerosis is the driving mechanism in heart failure is controversial. Although coronary artery disease is the most important cause of new onset of heart failure, non-fatal and fatal myocardial infarction has been reported infrequently relative to the overall event rate in previous clinical trials. However, the actual incidence of patients dying from acute myocardial infarction remains constant.

Heart failure patients mostly die from progressive heart failure and sudden arrhythmic death initiated by ventricular tachycardia originating at the borderzone of scar tissue. The pathogenesis of these events in heart failure is different from that in patients without heart failure. This is because acute coronary occlusion is less important than mechanisms related to the loading conditions of the dysfunctional ventricle, remodelling processes, ventricular extrasystolic depolarisation and autonomic imbalance.

On the other hand, autopsy studies have suggested that unrecognised coronary syndromes may often underlie sudden death and even death related to pump failure. This suggests a potentially important role for statins in patients with heart failure. Evidence of myocardial ischaemia or infarction has been observed in 42% of autopsies in heart failure patients who died suddenly [5].

Similarly, an acute myocardial infarction was reported in 55% of sudden arrhythmic deaths and in 81% death classified as due to progressive heart failure [6]. Accordingly, there is a potential role for statins to prevent ischaemic events and progression of heart failure and sudden death.

Unfortunately, conclusions cannot safely be drawn from autopsy studies because they are highly selective and represent less than 20% of all deaths. Furthermore, evidence of myocardial ischaemia in heart failure patients dying suddenly may be secondary to rapid ventricular tachycardia before it deteriorates into ventricular fibrillation.

EPIDEMIOLOGICAL DATA

Heart failure patients have lower cholesterol concentrations than patients without heart failure. In contrast to patients without heart failure, a low cholesterol level also portends a poor prognosis in heart failure [7–10].

This inverse epidemiology, observed in ischaemic as well as non-ischaemic heart failure, may reflect the fact that low cholesterol in heart failure and more generally in old, frail, high-risk patients is a marker of incipient risk associated with low cardiac output, low albumin, renal failure, cancer and other factors [10, 11].

Since clinical evidence for the benefit of statins in coronary heart disease is largely related to a marked reduction of LDL-C and regression of vascular atherosclerosis [12], the prevention of myocardial infarction and the overall effect on cardiovascular outcome in heart failure might therefore be confounded by the inverse effect of low cholesterol in overall outcome.

PLEIOTROPIC EFFECTS OF STATINS WHICH MIGHT BE BENEFICIAL

The favourable effects of statins in reducing adverse cardiovascular outcomes in non-heart failure patients has largely been attributed to retarding the progression of coronary stenoses and stabilisation of unstable coronary plaques. This effect is clearly dose-dependent, as demonstrated in the ASTEROID (A Study to Evaluate the Effect of Rosuvastatin on Intravascular Ultrasound-Derived Coronary Atheroma Burden) trial by the monitoring of coronary atherosclerotic progression using intravascular ultrasound. Rosuvastatin 40 mg/day reduced LDL-C concentrations by 53% and increased high-density lipoprotein cholesterol (HDL-C) by 15%, resulting in a significant average regression of the coronary atheroma volume by 6.8%. This study strongly suggested that aggressive lipid-modulating treatment could actually reverse the atherosclerotic disease process [12].

However, heart failure is a syndrome that involves broad activation of the inflammatory system, including pro- and anti-inflammatory cytokines, cell adhesion molecules, the complement system and cardiac auto-antibodies. C-reactive protein (CRP) and tumour necrosis factor-alpha (TNF-α) are predictors of cardiovascular morbidity and mortality and are also assumed to be directly involved in the pathogenic process.

In addition to plaque stabilisation and regression of lipid-rich stenoses, statins possess unique effects that improve endothelial function, increase vascular nitric oxide (NO) and reduce oxidative stress, not observed with other cholesterol-lowering agents [13]. These pleiotropic effects of statins are attributed mostly to inhibition of intermediate products in alternative pathways to those leading to cholesterol synthesis. Some intermediate products activate intracellular signalling molecules, which release inflammatory mediators. Many of these inflammatory markers (e.g. CRP, TNF-α, interleukin [IL]-6) are markedly increased in heart failure patients and predict cardiovascular morbidity and mortality [14]. Reducing cholesterol synthesis with HMG-CoA reductase inhibitors lowers inflammatory markers [15], although this has not been observed in all studies [16]. Statins have also been postulated to exert a dual effect as a modulator of the immune system and they may activate as well as inhibit pro-inflammatory cytokines [17].

It has been suggested that intermolecular differences between statins contribute to differences in pleiotropic effects such as NO bio-availability, anti-inflammatory activity and inhibition of oxidative stress [18].

In experimental and clinical studies, statins may inhibit neurohormonal activation, restore autonomic balance [19], prevent arrhythmias [20] and reverse left ventricular remodelling [15]. However, it has not been established clearly that a reduction of inflammatory markers by statins alone may reverse the pathogenic remodelling that occurs in post-ischaemic heart failure or prevent new coronary events such that patient prognosis is improved. Epidemiological studies of the association between LDL-C concentrations and cardiovascular disease in non-heart failure populations demonstrated a 30% lower mortality from ischaemic heart disease for each 1 mmol/l lower cholesterol [21]. This is greater than the 21% reduction observed in a meta-analysis of statin trials with a similar reduction in cholesterol [2]. Thus, at least in non-heart failure patients, it is unlikely that the pleiotropic anti-inflammatory effects of statins are of major importance. Specific anti-inflammatory interventions have been tested in large prospective heart failure trials, which could not demonstrate any favourable effects on cardiovascular events [22, 23]. This does not exclude the possible role of a more universal suppression of the inflammatory system.

Functional improvements have been observed in ischaemic and non-ischaemic cardiomyopathies. Indeed, initial preliminary studies of statin treatment in non-ischaemic cardiomyopathies have demonstrated improvements of ejection fraction by 4–7% [15, 24].

POSSIBLE HARMFUL EFFECTS OF STATIN TREATMENT

LDL-C and HDL-C have been hypothesised to play an important role in advanced heart failure by binding to and detoxifying endotoxins entering the circulation through the oedematous and leaky intestinal wall. A reduction of lipoproteins might therefore worsen the prognosis [25]. Statins also inhibit the mevalonate pathway, which depresses the synthesis of coenzyme Q10, which is in turn important for the mitochondrial generation of adenosine triphosphate (ATP). This could also worsen myocardial function. Low levels of coenzyme Q10 have been linked to a progressive cardiomyopathy and also to myalgias observed in some heart failure patients treated with statins [26]. Supplementation of coenzyme Q10 has been described to have a beneficial effect on myalgias, but no consistent effect has been observed on ejection fraction, peak oxygen consumption or exercise duration in patients with congestive heart failure [27]. In the LIPID (Long-Term Intervention with Pravastatin in Ischaemic Disease) study [28], pravastatin reduced coenzyme Q10 concentrations, but this reduction did not influence the risk of recurrent cardiovascular events.

The inhibition of the mevalonate pathway will also inhibit downstream the activation of selenocystein-tRNA. This reduction in selenoprotein production has been postulated to cause skeletal and cardiac muscle myopathy [29], but the clinical importance of this is yet to be determined.

CLINICAL OUTCOME TRIALS OF STATINS IN HEART FAILURE

There has been great uncertainty about the clinical role of statins in patients with heart failure and this has been reflected in treatment guidelines in which recommendations regarding the use of statins for heart failure are at best inconsistent.

Observational data from clinical heart failure trials have suggested that concurrent treatment with statins has favourable effects on left ventricular function and clinical endpoints such as NYHA (New York Heart Association) functional class and mortality [24, 30–36] (Figure 11.1). Furthermore, these studies have suggested that there is a favourable interaction between statins and β-adrenergic blocking agents [37, 38]. The effect observed with simvastatin in observational studies is characterised by an effect on mortality that is similar in patients with dilated cardiomyopathy and with heart failure with preserved ejection fraction [39]. The alleged effect is also independent of whether heart failure has an ischaemic or non-ischaemic aetiology and of the mode of death.

However, the selection of patients for statin treatment in non-randomised trials introduces the possibility of significant bias in such studies which cannot easily be adjusted for. This is reflected in sometimes dramatic reductions in mortality ranging from 13–57%. In a recent meta-analysis, Ramasubbu and colleagues [40] analysed 12 non-randomised and one randomised study and estimated an overall relative reduction in mortality of 26% (Figure 11.1). Stratified analysis of trials with non-ischaemic and ischaemic aetiology of heart failure suggested similar protective effects among both patient groups. In summary, although the results from these observational studies have consistently favoured statin treatment, the results have limited value as proof of concept because of the selection bias in treatment with statins and other optional drugs.

The place of statin treatment can only be settled by large, prospective, randomised, controlled outcome trials. Two such studies have now been completed; CORONA [41] and GISSI-HF [42, 43]. The results from these trials did not confirm the favourable effects suggested in retrospective observational studies.

THE CORONA STUDY

The CORONA study was undertaken specifically to examine the long-term efficacy and tolerability of rosuvastatin in patients with documented stable heart failure due to coronary heart disease. Rosuvastatin is a novel statin which very effectively reduces LDL-C and is also associated with a modest increase in HDL-C. It also suppresses markers of inflammatory activity, such as CRP, TNF-α and IL-6 [15]. The study was multinational and had a randomised, double-blind, parallel group design which assessed the efficacy and safety of rosuvastatin 10 mg against matching placebo in patients with symptomatic heart failure in

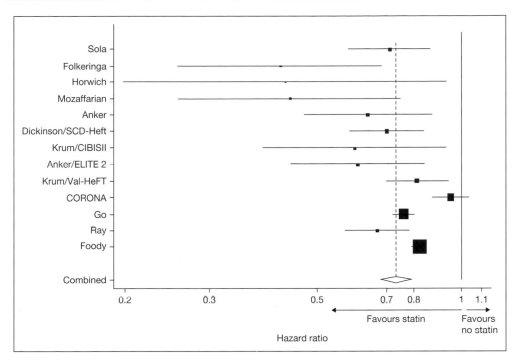

Figure 11.1 Mortality among patients with heart failure according to statin treatment in twelve non-randomised and one randomised prospective trial (adapted with permission from [40]).

NYHA Class II–IV. Patients were eligible if they were older than 60 years of age, were not being treated with, or in need of treatment with, a statin and had an ejection fraction <40% (or <35% if in NYHA class II) . The study included 5011 patients and follow-up was driven by the estimated need for 1422 patients to have sufficient endpoints and power to address reliably the effect on the primary endpoint. This primary endpoint was the time to first event of cardiovascular death, non-fatal myocardial infarction or non-fatal stroke. The median follow-up time was 32.8 months.

Rosuvastatin resulted in a marked net reduction of LDL-C (34%) and of CRP (37%) at the closing visit. The primary endpoint occurred in 11.4 per 100 patient-years in those in the rosuvastatin arm compared to 12.3 per 100 patient-years in those assigned placebo. This reduction in the primary endpoint was not significant (Figure 11.2). The trend to benefit was consistent across all patient subgroups and was accounted for by a decrease in non-fatal myocardial infarction (172 compared with 207) and non-fatal non-haemorrhagic strokes (88 compared with 106). A total of 728 patients in the rosuvastatin group and 759 in the placebo group died. A numeric difference favouring rosuvastatin was observed for sudden death (316 vs. 327), coronary events (554 vs. 588), fatal infections (54 vs. 68), pulmonary embolism (2 vs. 8) and aortic aneurysm (2 vs. 8). Rosuvastatin significantly reduced hospitalisations for all causes compared to placebo (3694 vs. 4074; $P = 0.007$) and for a cardiovascular cause (2193 vs. 2564; $P < 0.001$).

Post hoc analyses must be interpreted with caution. However, in a retrospective analysis of 'atherothrombotic' events (fatal and non-fatal myocardial infarction and fatal and non-fatal non-ischaemic strokes) there was a significant difference favouring rosuvastatin (227 vs. 284; hazard ratio [HR] 0.84; confidence interval [CI] 0.70–1.00; $P = 0.05$). Recent subgroup analysis demonstrated that NT-proBNP but not CRP added substantial independent predictive

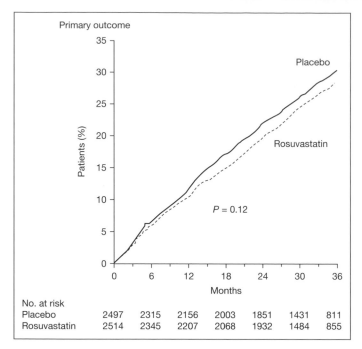

Figure 11.2 Kaplan-Meier estimates for the primary composite endpoint of death from cardiovascular causes, non-fatal myocardial infarction and non-fatal stroke in the CORONA trial (adapted with permission from [41]).

information, both short- and long-term, for all cardiovascular endpoints. Analysis of treatment effects according to NT-proBNP clearly showed a favourable effect for the primary composite (HR 0.65; 95% CI 0.47–0.88) and coronary endpoints (HR 0.74; 95% CI 0.55–1.00) in patients with NT-proBNP lower than 102 pmol/l (850 pg/ml) (Cleland J *et al*. Abstract; ESC 2008). It is general knowledge that elevated CRP concentrations are associated with worse outcomes in heart failure. Retrospective analysis of the CORONA database demonstrated that CRP >2.0 mg/l (median 5.6 mg/l) has been associated with 50% higher cardiovascular event rates compared to patients with CRP <2.0 mg/l (median 1.1 mg/l). Furthermore, rosuvastatin treatment has been associated with significantly better cardiovascular outcomes in patients with CRP >2.0 mg/l, (McMurray J *et al*. Abstract; AHA 2008).

It is important that the observed adverse events including permanent discontinuation of study drug were significantly less among rosuvastatin patients compared to placebo, despite this being an old and fragile patient population (490 vs. 546; $P = 0.03$). No case of rhabdomyolysis was observed.

The overall consistency of a numeric effect in favour of rosuvastatin in all subgroups, the statistically significant effect on fatal and non-fatal myocardial infarction and non-haemorrhagic stroke, the beneficial effect on hospitalisation and the effect in subgroups characterised by low brain natriuretic peptide (BNP) concentrations support the concept that rosuvastatin reduces events related to atherothrombosis. However, these events were overwhelmed by other events in this patient population (sudden and progressive heart failure deaths) which are not sensitive to statins. Assuming rosuvastatin did reduce the risk of acute atherothrombotic events, the results of CORONA imply that the major aetiology of cardiovascular deaths in this vulnerable population of otherwise well-treated patients with advanced systolic heart failure may be a primary electrical event, related to ventricular dilatation and scarring, rather than an atherothrombotic event. Sudden death in heart failure is probably not due to an acute coronary occlusion and in this respect differs from sudden death in non-heart failure populations in which statins confer marked benefit on sudden death [1].

The finding of a significant beneficial effect on cardiovascular outcomes among patients with CRP >2.0 mg/l may support the hypothesis of a pleiotropic effect of rosuvastatin. Conversely, an elevated CRP may be indicative of a phenotype in which the arteries are particularly sensitive to LDL, or that LDL is modified to become more toxic. Consequently, lowering of LDL may be particular important, even in patients with low LDL levels, as long as CRP is elevated.

GISSI-HF

The GISSI-HF trial had a factorial design and compared rosuvastatin 10 mg/day to placebo and n-3 PUFAs 1 g/day to placebo in 6975 patients (4574 only randomised to the rosuvastatin/placebo arm). The study included patients with heart failure of non-ischaemic as well as ischaemic aetiology and some patients with preserved left ventricular ejection fraction. Only 37% were in NYHA Class III/IV compared to 63% of the cohort in CORONA and only 1250 of the GISSI-HF patients fulfilled the inclusion criteria for CORONA.

Patients in GISSI-HF were followed for a median of 3.9 years. The primary endpoints for both arms of the trial were time to death, and time to death or admission to hospital for cardiovascular reasons. The results are summarised in Figure 11.3. Concerning the rosuvastatin arm, there was no effect on clinical outcome in patients for any prespecified subgroups by age, aetiology of heart failure or according to ejection fraction. As in CORONA, safety data were reassuring, with no signal that treatment could be harmful.

The rationale for testing n3-PUFA is patients with heart failure derived from experimental studies which had shown favourable effects on inflammatory processes, platelet aggregation, blood pressure and heart rate, ventricular function, autonomic effects and arrhythmias [44, 45], and from epidemiological studies, which had shown that fish consumption might decrease coronary heart disease death. In addition, n3-PUFA had been shown to decrease cardiovascular events, particularly sudden death in 11 323 survivors of myocardial infarction in the GISSI-Prevenzione study [46]. In GISSI-Prevenzione, the absolute benefits of n3-PUFA were also greater in those with lower ejection fraction [47]. Benefits of n3-PUFA had also been shown in other earlier studies.

Although the benefits of n3-PUFA in GISSI HF were modest, they were observed on a background of recommended therapies for heart failure were consistent across all prespecified subgroups. n3-PUFA were also safe, and such treatment is relatively cheap.

CONCLUSIONS

Basic science data suggest mechanisms by which statins may exert both beneficial and deleterious effects in patients with heart failure. Epidemiological data that show an inverse relationship between serum cholesterol level and outcome could reflect the poor general health of patients with advanced heart failure.

Observational data have shown improved outcomes with statin use in those with heart failure, but such data may be confounded. This emphasizes the need for randomised, controlled clinical trials in this important group who were excluded from the initial studies of statins in patients with coronary heart disease. The CORONA and GISSI-HF trials did not show a significant reduction in the primary endpoint, but treatment was safe. In CORONA, some secondary endpoints were reduced.

One reason for not reaching the anticipated effect, despite the marked reduction in LDL-C and CRP, may be that the heart failure populations, particularly in CORONA, were too sick to respond to the lipid-lowering and pleiotropic effects of statins.

	Rosuvastatin/Placebo	N3-PUFA/Placebo
n	4574	6975
Mean age (years)	68	67
Previous AMI	33%	42%
NYHA (Class II)	63%	63%
All deaths (adjusted HR) P value	1.00 (95.5% CI 0.90–1.12) 0.94	0.91 (95.5% CI 0.83–1.00) 0.04
Death or CVD hospitalisation (adjusted HR) P value	1.01 (99% CI 0.91–1.11) 0.90	0.92 (99% CI 0.85–1.00) 0.009

Figure 11.3 Key baseline characteristics and primary endpoints in the two arms of the GISSI-HF trial (with permission from [42, 43]). AMI = acute myocardial infarction; CVD = cardiovascular disease; HR = hazard ratio; NYHA = New York Health Association; PUFA = polyunsaturated fatty acids

In the 4S trial, which included patients with coronary artery disease but excluded all patients with heart failure, 4444 patients were randomised to placebo or simvastatin 20–40 mg [1]. LDL-C was reduced by 35% in the treatment group. All major coronary events (coronary death, myocardial infarction and resuscitated cardiac arrest) were reduced by 34% and total mortality by 30%. Furthermore, sudden death was reduced by 41%. However, the proportion of patients suffering a fatal myocardial infarction was 26.6% compared to the smaller proportion of 1.2% in CORONA, for example. Worsening heart failure and sudden death were more frequent in CORONA than in 4S. Rates of stroke and non-cardiovascular death were comparable in the two trials (Figure 11.4). Patients in CORONA were older and more frail, although representative of heart failure patients. Although the correct cause of death is difficult to ascertain, the discrepancies in effect between non-heart failure and heart failure patients suggest that the substrate for statin treatment is different among the two populations. The improvement of prognosis in severe heart failure by implantable defibrillator and resynchronisation devices also strongly suggest that the mechanisms for sudden death and progressive heart failure in this population are different from those in non-heart failure patients [48]. Indeed, in CORONA, there was a trend for greater effect on cardiovascular endpoints among patients with lesser degree of cardiac dysfunction (younger patients with better preserved ejection fraction, body mass index and blood pressure). Importantly, retrospective analysis demonstrated that rosuvastatin consistently improved primary and secondary endpoints in a subset of patients with mild heart failure as defined by NT-proBNP <102 pmol/l and also that elevated CRP may be a marker of patients who are particularly sensitive to the beneficial effects of statin treatment.

WHERE DO THE FINDINGS IN CORONA AND GISSI-HF LEAVE US?

Statin treatment should not be stopped when heart failure develops in patients with ischaemic heart disease because of potential benefit, although this may be limited to a reduction of atherosclerotic events (fatal and non-fatal myocardial infarction or non-haemorrhagic stroke) and hospitalisation. For prevention of other cardiovascular events, which accounted for much of the morbidity and mortality in heart failure patients in CORONA and GISSI-HF, and which were not influenced by rosuvastatin, the focus for treatment should be on causes and mechanisms for arrhythmic death and progression of heart failure. However, there is suggestive evidence of an indication to commence statins in patients with mild systolic heart

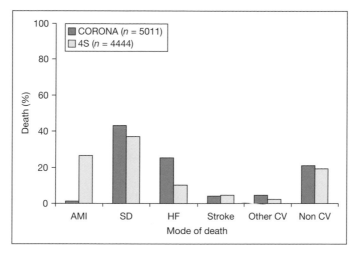

Figure 11.4 Mode of deaths in the CORONA (heart failure) [41] and 4S (non-heart failure) [1] trials.

failure of ischaemic aetiology when NT-proBNP is <150 pmol/l and with CRP >2.0 mg/l. The hypotheses raised by these apparent therapeutic effects in such patients with heart failure need to be confirmed in prospective randomised trials.

In GISSI-HF, n3-PUFA was associated with a modest but significant reduction in death, and death or hospitalisation for cardiovascular reasons. In the light of these findings, guidelines for heart failure treatment probably need to be reviewed with respect to this therapeutic approach and further research should address the dose and mode of intake of n3-PUFA.

SUMMARY

Statins are effective in the prevention of coronary heart disease and accordingly have been shown to reduce incident heart failure. However, in patients with established heart failure, the pathogenic mechanisms are more complex and in addition to coronary ischaemia, involve neurohormonal activation, ventricular remodelling, electrical instability and marked inflammatory activation. Myocardial infarction is relatively infrequent compared to progressive heart failure and arrhythmic death, which may not be amenable to statin treatment. Patients with more severe heart failure were also usually excluded from the early landmark clinical trials. Experimental and clinical studies are not consistent, but have suggested that statins may improve myocardial function, partly accounted for by their pleiotropic effects. Retrospective non-randomised studies have demonstrated benefit for statin users compared to non-statin users. Nevertheless, the clinical effect among heart failure patients has not been properly evaluated in randomised prospective outcome trials until recently. The CORONA (Controlled Rosuvastatin Multinational Study in Heart Failure) trial did not confirm a general benefit of rosuvastatin on cardiovascular outcome in heart failure patients with ischaemic heart disease. Rosuvastatin reduced the number of hospitalisations and an effect was also observed on non-fatal and fatal myocardial infarction and stroke. *Post hoc* analyses demonstrated an effect on the cardiovascular outcomes, which was limited to the patients with mild heart failure as evidenced by N-terminal prohormone brain natriuretic peptide (NT-proBNP) <102 pmol/l. No effect was observed on sudden death and death from progressive heart failure. More recently, the GISSI-HF (Gruppo Italiano per lo Studio della Sopravvivenza nell'Infarto Miocardico Heart Failure) trial showed benefit of n3-polyunsaturated fatty acids (n3-PUFA) but not rosuvastatin in a broader cohort of patients with heart failure with either ischaemic or non-ischaemic aetiology. These results have clinical implications with respect to the role of such agents in heart failure treatment.

REFERENCES

1. Scandinavian Simvastatin Survival Study Group. Randomised trial of cholesterol lowering in 4444 patients with coronary heart disease: the Scandinavian Simvastatin Survival Study (4S). *Lancet* 1994; 344:1383–1389.
2. Cholesterol Treatment Trialist Collaborators. Efficacy and safety of cholesterol-lowering treatment: prospective meta-analysis of data from 90 056 participants in 14 randomised trials of statins. *Lancet* 2005; 366:1267–1278.
3. Kjekshus J, Pedersen TR, Olsson AG, Faergeman O, Pyörälä K. The effects of simvastatin on the incidence of heart failure in patients with coronary heart disease. *J Card Fail* 1997; 3:249–254.
4. Scirica BM, Morrow DA, Cannon CP *et al.*; for the PROVE IT-TIMI 22 investigators. Intensive statin therapy and the risk of hospitalization for heart failure after an acute coronary syndrome in the PROVE IT-TIMI 22 study. *J Am Coll Cardiol* 2006; 47:2326–2331.
5. Uretsky BF, Thygesen K, Armstrong PW *et al*. Acute coronary findings at autopsy in heart failure patients with sudden death: results from the assessment of treatment with lisinopril and survival (ATLAS) trial. *Circulation* 2000; 102:611–616.
6. Ørn A, Cleland JGF, Romo M, Kjekshus J, Dickstein K. Recurrent infarction is the most common cause of death in patients with left ventricular dysfunction following myocardial infarction. *Am J Med* 2005; 118:752–775.
7. Horwich TB, Hamilton MA, Maclellan, Fonarow GC. Low serum total cholesterol is associated with marked increase in mortality in advanced heart failure. *J Card Fail* 2002; 8:216–224.
8. Kronmal RA, Cain KC, Ye Z, Omen GS. Total serum cholesterol levels and mortality risk as a function of age. A report based on the Framingham data. *Arc Intern Med* 2003; 152:1065–1073.
9. Rauchhaus M, Clark AL, Doehner W *et al*. The relationship between cholesterol and survival in patients with chronic heart failure. *J Am Coll Cardiol* 2003; 43:1933–1940.
10. Kalantar-Zadeh K, Block G, Horwich T, Fonarow GC. Reverse epidemiology of conventional cardiovascular risk factors in patients with chronic heart failure. *J Am Coll Cardiol* 2004; 43:1439–1444.
11. Corti M-C, Guralnik JM, Salive ME *et al*. Clarifying the direct relation between total cholesterol levels and death from coronary heart disease in older persons. *Ann Intern Med* 1997; 126:753–760.
12. Nissen SE, Nicholls SJ, Sipahi I *et al* ; for the ASTEROID investigators. Effect of very high-intensity statin therapy on regression of coronary atherosclerosis: the ASTEROID trial. *JAMA* 2006; 295:1556–1565.
13. Landmesser U, Bahlmann F, Mueller M *et al*. Simvastatin versus ezetemibe. Pleiotropic and lipid-lowering effects on endothelial function in humans. *Circulation* 2005; 111:2356–2363.
14. Yndestad A, Damås K, Øie E *et al*. Role of inflammation in the progression of heart failure. *Curr Cardiol Rep* 2007; 9:236–241.
15. Sola S, Mir MQ, Lerakis S *et al*. Atorvastatin improves left ventricular systolic function and serum markers of inflammation in nonischemic heart failure. *J Am Coll Cardiol* 2006; 47:332–337.
16. Bleske BE, Nicklas JM, Bard RL *et al*. Neutral effect on markers of heart failure, inflammation, endothelial activation and function, and vagal tone after high-dose HMG-CoA reductase inhibition in non-diabetic patients with non-ischemic cardiomyopathy and average low-density lipoprotein level. *J Am Coll Cardiol* 2006; 47:338–341.
17. Kiener PA, Davis PM, Murray JL *et al*. Stimulation of inflammatory responses in vitro and in vivo by lipophilic HMG-CoA reductase inhibitors. *Int Immunopharmacol* 2001; 1:105–118.
18. Mason RP, Walter MF, Day CA, Jacob RF. Intermolecular differences of 3-hydroxy-3-methylglutaryl coenzyme A reductase inhibitors contribute to distinct pharmacologic and pleiotropic actions. *Am J Cardiol* 2005; 96(suppl):11F–23F.
19. Pliquett RU, Cornish KG, Peuler JD, Zucker IH. Simvastatin normalizes autonomic neural control in experimental heart failure. *Circulation* 2003; 107:2493–2498.
20. Goldberger JJ, Subacius H, Schaechter A *et al*.; for the DEFINITE investigators. Effects of statin therapy on arrhythmic events and survival in patients with nonischemic dilated dardiomyopathy. *J Am Coll Cardiol* 2006; 48:1228–1233.

21. Prospective Studies Collaboration. Blood cholesterol and vascular mortality by age, sex, and blood pressure: a meta-analysis of individual data from 61 prospective studies with 55 000 vascular deaths. *Lancet* 2007; 370:1829–1839.

22. Chung ES, Packer M, Lo KH, Fasanmade AA, Willerson JT; Anti TNF Therapy Against Congestive Heart Failure Investigators. Randomized, double-blind, placebo-controlled, pilot trial of infliximab, a chimeric monoclonal antibody to tumor necrosis factor α, in patients with moderate-to-severe heart failure (ATTACH) trial. *Circulation* 2003; 107:3133–3140.

23. Mann DL, McMurray JJV, Packer M *et al*. Targeted anticytokine therapy in patients with chronic heart failure: results of the randomized etanercept worldwide evaluation (RENEWAL). *Circulation* 2004; 109:1594–1602.

24. Node K, Fujita M, Kitakaze M Hori M, Liao JK. Short-term statin therapy improves cardiac function and symptoms in patients with idiopathic dilated cardiomyopathy. *Circulation* 2003; 108:839–843.

25. Rauchhaus M, Coats AJ, Anker SD. The endotoxin-lipoprotein hypothesis. *Lancet* 2000; 356:930–933.

26. Marcoff L, Thompson PD. The role of coenzyme Q10 in statin-associated myopathy: a systematic review. *J Am Coll Cardiol* 2007; 49:2231–2237.

27. Khatta M, Alexander BS, Krichten CM *et al*. The effect of coenzyme Q10 in patients with congestive heart failure. *Ann Int Med* 2000; 132:636–640.

28. Stocker R, Pollicino C, Gay CA *et al*. Neither plasma coenxyme Q10 concentration, nor its decline during pravastatin therapy, is linked to recurrent cardiovascular disease events:A prospective case-control study from the LIPID study. *Atherosclerosis* 2006; 187:198–204.

29. Moosmann B, Behl C. Selenoprotein synthesis and side-effects of statins. *Lancet* 2004; 363:892–894.

30. Horwich TB, MacLellan R, Fonarow GC. Statin therapy is associated with improved survival in ischemic and non-ischemic heart failure. *J Am Coll Cardiol* 2004; 43:642–648.

31. Ray GR, Gong Y, Sykora K, Tu JV. Statin use and survival outcomes in elderly patients with heart failure. *Arch Intern Med* 2005; 165:62–67.

32. Krum H, Latini R, Maggioni AP *et al*. Statins and symptomatic chronic systolic heart failure: a post-hoc analysis of 5010 patients enrolled in Val-HeFT. *Int J Cardiol* 2007; 119:48–53.

33. Go AS, Lee WY, Yang J, Lo JC, Gurwitz JH. Statin therapy and risks for death and hospitalization in chronic heart failure. *JAMA* 2006; 296:2105–2111.

34. van der Harst P, Voors AA, van Gilst WH, Böhm M, van Veldhuisen DJ. Statins in the treatment of chronic heart failure: a systematic review. *PLoS Med* 2006; 3:e333.

35. Martin JH, Krum H. Statins and clinical outcomes in heart failure. *Clin Sci (Lond)* 2007; 113:119–127.

36. Krum H, Ashton E, Reid C *et al*. Double-blind, randomized, placebo-controlled study of high-dose HMG CoA reductase inhibitor therapy on ventricular remodeling, pro-inflammatory cytokines and neurohormonal parameters in patients with chronic systolic heart failure. *J Card Fail* 2007; 13:1–7.

37. Hognestad A, Dickstein K, Myhre E, Snapinn S, Kjekshus J; for the OPTIMAAL investigators. Effect of combined statin and beta-blocker treatment on one-year morbidity and mortality after acute myocardial infarction associated with heart failure. *Am J Cardiol* 2004; 93:603–606.

38. Krum H, Bailey M, Meyer W *et al*. Impact of statin therapy on clinical outcomes in chronic heart failure patients according to beta-blocker use: Results of CIBIS II. *Cardiology* 2007; 108:28–34.

39. Shah R, Wang Y, Foody JM. Effects of statins, angiotensin-converting enzyme inhibitors, and beta blockers on survival in patients ≥65 years of age with heart failure and preserved left ventricular systolic function. *Am J Cardiol* 2008; 101:217–222.

40. Ramasubbu K, Estep J, White D *et al*. Experimental and clinical basis for the use of statins in patients with ischemic and nonischemic cardiomyopathy. *J Am Coll Cardiol* 2008; 51:415–426.

41. Kjekshus J, Apetrei E, Barrios V *et al*. A randomized placebo-controlled trial of the efficacy and safety of rosuvastatin on cardiovascular outcomes in 5011 older patients with low ejection fraction, ischemic, moderate and severe heart failure. *N Eng J Med* 2007; 357:2248–2261.

42. GISSI-HF Investigators. Effect of rosuvastatin in patients with chronic heart failure (the GISSI-HF trial): a randomised, double-blind, placebo-controlled trial. *Lancet* 2008; published online DOI: 10.1016/S0140-6736(08)61240-4.

43. GISSI-HF Investigators. Effect of n-3 polyunsaturated fatty acids in patients with chronic heart failure (the GISSI-HF trial): a randomised, double-blind, placebo-controlled trial. *Lancet* 2008; published online DOI: 10.1016/S0140-6736(08)61239-8.

44. Simopoulos AP. Omega-3 fatty acids in health and disease and growth and development. *Am J Clin Nutr* 1991; 54:438–463.

45. He K, Song Y, Daviglus M *et al.* Accumulated evidence on fish consumption and coronary heart disease mortality: a meta-analysis of cohort studies. *Circulation* 2004; 109:2705–2711.

46. GISSI-Prevenzione Investigators. Dietary supplementation with n-3 polyunsaturated fatty acids and vitamin E after myocardial infarction: results of the GISSI-Prevenzione trial. *Lancet* 1999; 354:447–455.

47. Macchia A, Levantesi G, Franzosi MG *et al.* Left ventricular systolic dysfunction, total mortality and sudden death in patients with myocardial infarction treated with n-3 polyunsaturated fatty acids. *Eur J Heart Fail* 2005; 7:904–909.

48. Lindenfeld JA, Feldman AM, Saxon L *et al.* Effects of cardiac resynchronization therapy with or without a defibrillator on survival and hospitalizations in patients with New York Heart Association class IV heart failure. *Circulation* 2007; 115:204–212.

12

Absolute risk assessment in the general population

L. Chen, A. M. Tonkin

INTRODUCTION

Cardiovascular disease (CVD) represents the major health problem for the world. CVD, particularly coronary heart disease (CHD) and stroke, is the leading cause of death, accounting for 30% of all deaths worldwide [1]. This number approximates the proportion of deaths from communicable diseases, maternal and perinatal conditions and nutritional deficiencies added together [1].

Furthermore, CHD and stroke are among the ten leading causes of disease burden in the world. According to the World Health Report 2004 [2], covering 192 member states of the World Health Organization, CVD was responsible for the loss of 148 million disability-adjusted life years (DALYs), equivalent to 9.9% of all DALYs lost. CVD also imposes a great economic health burden. The annual direct and indirect health system costs of CVD were estimated to equal about 1.7% of Australia's gross domestic product in 2004 [3] and to cost $448.5 billion in the United States in 2008 [4]. In European countries, the estimated total costs of CVD were €169 billion in 2003 [5].

The first presentation of CHD in more than 25% of patients is with fatal myocardial infarction (MI) or sudden death [6]. Of those who present with a first stroke, the case-fatality rate within 1 month is around 23% [7]. Moreover, it has been recognised that atherosclerosis, the major underlying cause of CVD, develops silently over decades before clinical presentation [8].

A framework for cardiovascular health strategies is shown in Figure 12.1 [9]. Although those with clinical manifestations associated with atherosclerosis or with diabetes are at highest risk for future CVD events, up to one-half of all events occur in the general population without such previous events. This underpins the need to develop tools to predict the risk of future events. Such an approach will inform the most effective and cost-effective use of preventive therapies.

Lei Chen, MD, MMed, Endocrinologist, Department of Epidemiology and Preventive Medicine, School of Public Health and Preventive Medicine, Monash University, Melbourne, Australia

Andrew M. Tonkin, MBBS, MD, FRACP, FCSANZ, Professor of Medicine; Consultant Cardiologist; Head, Cardiovascular Research Unit, Department of Epidemiology and Preventive Medicine, School of Public Health and Preventive Medicine, Monash University, Melbourne, Australia

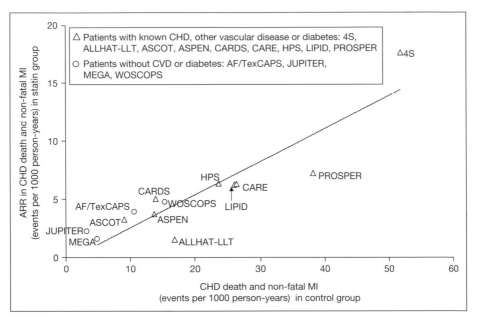

Figure 12.2 Relationship between absolute risk reduction (ARR) and event rates in the control group in thirteen statin trials. Some outcomes were substituted for 4S: major coronary events including coronary death, non-fatal definite or probable MI, silent MI, or resuscitated cardiac arrest; AFCAPS, acute major coronary events including fatal or non-fatal MI, unstable angina, sudden cardiac death; ASPEN, fatal or non-fatal MI; CARDS, acute coronary heart disease event including MI, unstable angina, acute CHD death, or resuscitated cardiac arrest; JUPITER, any MI; MEGA: CHD including fatal or non-fatal MI, cardiac sudden death, angina, or coronary revascularisation. Abbreviations: 4S = Scandinavian Simvastatin Survival Study; AF/TexCAPS = Air Force / Texas Coronary Atherosclerosis Prevention Study; ALLHAT-LLT = Antihypertensive and Lipid-Lowering Treatment to Prevent Heart Attack Trial; ASCOT-LLA = Anglo-Scandinavian Cardiac Outcomes Trial – Lipid Lowering Arm; ASPEN = Atorvastatin Study for Prevention of Coronary Heart Disease Endpoints in Non-Insulin-Dependent Diabetes Mellitus; CARDS = Collaborative Atorvastatin Diabetes Study; CARE = Cholesterol And Recurrent Events; HPS = Heart Protection Study; LIPID = Long-term Intervention with Pravastatin in Ischaemic Disease; JUPITER = Justification for the Use of statins in Prevention: an Intervention Trial Evaluating Rosuvastatin; MEGA = Management of Elevated Cholesterol in the Primary Prevention Group of Adult Japanese Study; PROSPER = PROspective Study of Pravastatin in the Elderly at Risk; WOSCOPS = West of Scotland Coronary Prevention Study.

Absolute and relative risk reduction: number needed to treat

Relative risk reduction measures the reduction in event rates with an intervention in relative terms, while absolute risk reduction measures an arithmetic reduction in event rates [23]. They can be used to evaluate the benefit of an intervention, such as the reduction in the number of CVD events associated with lipid-lowering therapy compared with standard therapy or placebo. Meta-analysis of trials of statins in primary prevention of CVD showed that the reduction in the risk of major CHD events was related to CHD risk at baseline [16]. However, this relationship is found in all patient groups. Figure 12.2 shows the relationship between rates of the composite of CHD death and non-fatal MI per 1000 person-years in the control group and the absolute risk reduction in this endpoint in those assigned a statin in the thirteen published large-scale, controlled clinical trials [24–36]. A linear relationship between risk in the control groups and absolute risk reduction is observed across the trials. Therefore, absolute risk reduction is greatest in those with the highest baseline risk [37]. The number needed to treat is simply the inverse of the absolute risk reduction and describes the number of patients that need to be treated to prevent one adverse event during a given time interval.

APPROACHES TO ABSOLUTE RISK ASSESSMENT

CARDIOVASCULAR RISK PREDICTION TOOLS DERIVED FROM THE FRAMINGHAM HEART STUDY

The Framingham Heart Study was initiated in 1948 in Framingham, Massachusetts. It has been a seminal study in the identification of CVD risk factors, and also in the development of tools predicting the risk of future CVD events. The first risk prediction function was introduced in the 1960s and a series of risk equations or scoring systems have subsequently followed. These risk assessment tools allow an estimation of the risk of general and separate manifestations of CVD, including CHD, stroke, intermittent claudication and heart failure [38–53].

Most of these algorithms are used for the prediction of risk in people without previous history of CVD. Only one equation specifically considers estimation of the risk of subsequent CHD in patients with a history of CHD or ischaemic stroke [49].

For flexibility of use, risk prediction tools have been presented not only as exact equations using continuous variables, but also in the form of a point scoring system or score sheet using categorical variables. Furthermore, a simplified CHD prediction model [47] was formulated based on blood pressure, TC and LDL-C categories proposed by the United States Joint National Committee and National Cholesterol Education Program (NCEP). The accuracy of this categorical approach was comparable to that using continuous variables. This point scoring system – the Framingham risk score – was later modified and incorporated in the National Cholesterol Education Program Adult Treatment Panel III (NCEP-ATPIII) guidelines [54].

The risk prediction equations for CVD and CHD developed by Anderson and colleagues in 1991 [42, 43] are the other functions that have been incorporated into clinical practice [55–59]. In general, these tools allow an estimation of absolute risk of CHD or CVD over 5 or 10 years in people aged from 30–74 years, although the risk factors and related categories on which these tools are based are not identical. For example, the New Zealand charts, also often used in Australia, incorporate the ratio of TC and HDL-C instead of their separate levels [56]. Other tools based on the 1991 Anderson equations are the risk prediction charts incorporated in the 2nd Joint British Societies (JBS) Guidelines [57], the Sheffield table [58] and the Canadian nomogram [59].

Of particular note, the Framingham researchers have updated their general CVD risk algorithms and have recently published two risk prediction scores on the basis of a large number of CVD events in a more contemporary time period [52]. The general CVD risk functions were found to have good discrimination and calibration both for predicting global CVD risk and for predicting the risk of individual manifestations of CVD.

THE EXTERNAL VALIDITY OF FRAMINGHAM RISK EQUATIONS IN OTHER DIFFERENT POPULATIONS

The Framingham risk prediction equations were developed from a study that mainly comprised a white, middle-class population from a single location in the United States, and was initiated around the peak of CHD incidence. This raises concerns about whether they can be generalised to other populations.

Testing of the Framingham functions in six prospective cohort studies in the United States showed that they performed reasonably well for the prediction of CHD events over a 5-year period for both white and black men and women [50]. However, for Japanese-American and Hispanic men and Native American women, CHD risk was systematically overestimated. After recalibration for differing prevalence of risk factors and underlying rates of CHD events, the Framingham functions also worked well in these populations [50]. Thus, the Framingham authors argued that it would be necessary to obtain cross-sectional data on risk factor prevalence as well as population data on CHD events over time before applying the Framingham prediction equations in other populations. Interestingly, the Framingham risk function is well calibrated to predict the risk of first coronary events in Australia and New Zealand cohorts [60–62].

Two recently published meta-analyses [63, 64] have compared the predicted risk of CHD or CVD based on the commonly used Framingham risk equations [42, 43, 47] with observed risk. Although the studies included in these two meta-analyses are not identical, both found that the ratio of predicted and observed risk varied across the studies. For prediction of the risk of CHD, the predicted to observed ratio ranged from under-prediction of 0.43 (95% confidence interval [CI] 0.27–0.67) to over-prediction of 2.87 (95% CI 1.91–4.31) [63]. In general, the Framingham risk equations tend to over-predict risk in populations with a low risk or which have experienced a decline in CVD, and under-predict risk in a high-risk population (e.g. people in lower socioeconomic classes) [65, 66], or with a history of diabetes, reduced renal function, a family history of premature CVD, or in populations where the incidence of CVD has increased.

ABSOLUTE RISK ASSESSMENT TOOLS FROM POPULATIONS OTHER THAN THE FRAMINGHAM HEART STUDY PARTICIPANTS

Improving CVD and CHD risk prediction has become a hot topic in the field of cardiovascular epidemiology over the last decade. Of particular note, the study populations from which CVD risk prediction equations are developed have been greatly extended. One example is the risk calculator for CHD developed from American-Indians, a population with a high risk for diabetes and albuminuria [67]. Additionally, the study populations are not only based on predefined cohorts, but also come from data routinely collected from general practice, such as the QRISK score [68–69].

The SCORE risk charts were generated from a pool of 12 datasets from European cohort studies with over 2.7 million years of follow-up and allow an estimation of 10-year risk of cardiovascular death [70]. This important project provided separate risk charts for prediction of fatal CVD over 10 years for high-risk and low-risk European populations, taking into account the difference in the prevalence of risk factors and incidence of CVD events. The high-risk model was based on the baseline survival function for cohorts from Denmark, Finland and Norway, and the low-risk model was based on data from Belgium, Italy and Spain. The SCORE authors and the 4th European Joint Task Force Guidelines recommend that a middle-aged adult with a 10-year risk of fatal CVD over 5% be considered at high risk [22].

However, a recent population study in Norway showed that, for men, the SCORE high-risk function overestimated and the low-risk model underestimated the CVD mortality as compared to the observed 10-year risks; both functions underestimated mortality in young women and over-predicted it in older women [71]. The high-risk model was also found to overestimate the risk of fatal CVD in Germany [72], and the low-risk model over-predicted the risk of fatal CVD in Austrian men and women [73]. Therefore, before implementation of the SCORE charts in clinical practice, proper recalibration to allow for time trends in both mortality and risk factor distribution is required. To date, updated and recalibrated charts are now available for Belgium, Germany, Greece, The Netherlands, Poland, Spain and Sweden [22].

In addition, the SCORE risk charts are based on total atherosclerotic CVD mortality and do not include non-fatal and, therefore, total CVD or CHD events, and so might not truly reflect the burden of atherosclerotic risk. With respect to this issue, the 4th European Joint Task Force Guidelines state that a 5% risk of CVD death approximates a 10% risk of the combination of fatal and non-fatal CVD events. This was based on examination of the FINRISK MONICA data and Markov modelling of Dutch data [22]. Of note, a recent study from Iceland showed that the 10-year risk threshold of 5% for fatal CVD corresponds to a 12% risk for CHD morbidity [74].

Since there is no universal risk prediction tool that is suitable for application in different populations, a series of population-specific prediction functions have been generated, particularly in those populations considered at low risk for CVD, such as the Italian [75–76], Chinese [77, 78] and Japanese [79]. The most common or recently published tools are summarised in Table 12.1.

Specifically, there are two recently published tools from Asian countries. One describes the 10-year risk of ischaemic CVD, including ischaemic stroke and coronary events from 17 years of follow-up from the USA-PRC Collaborative Study of Cardiovascular Epidemiology cohort in China [78]. Another risk chart for the prediction of fatal CVD, CHD or stroke over a 10-year period was generated in a Japanese population aged over 30 years from the NIPPON DATA80 study [79]. However, the performance and applicability of these equations from individual countries in cohorts other than the derived dataset are still unclear. Furthermore, resources for risk factor screening are limited in many Asian countries in which the incidence of CVD has been dramatically increasing. Interestingly, an analysis by the Asia Pacific Cohort Studies Collaboration showed that a low-information Framingham CVD risk prediction equation, based on age, sex, smoking status, systolic blood pressure and TC – after recalibration using contemporary data from Asia – is likely to estimate future risk of CVD with similar accuracy in Asian populations as tools derived from Asian local cohorts [80]. This provides another insight into the use of assessment tools in low- or middle-income countries in which costly cohort studies are not easily funded.

SOME IMPORTANT TRENDS IN THE DEVELOPMENT OF RISK PREDICTION FUNCTIONS

Prediction of risk in younger adults

Traditional risk prediction functions such as the Framingham equations are usually generated from populations aged at least 30 years and they tend to underestimate risk in young adults. Age is the major determinant of risk of CVD events. However, the emphasis on age may overlook the important contributions that modifiable risk factors make in young adults. One study from the United States showed that the Framingham risk score remained <10% for all participants aged 18–29 years and only reached 12% in people aged 30–39 years in the highest decile of predicted risk [81]. In dealing with the under-prediction of risk in younger adults, a new risk scoring system has been derived from the Pathobiological Determinants of Atherosclerosis in Youth study [82]. It allows an estimation of the probability of atherosclerotic lesions in the coronary artery or abdominal aorta at autopsy in individuals aged 15 34 years [67]. This risk function was based on traditional risk factors, including age, sex, HDL-C and non-HDL-C, smoking, blood pressure, obesity and hyperglycaemia. The approach is useful in identifying young individuals with a high probability of already having atherosclerosis.

Additionally, estimation of relative risk [22] or lifetime risk [83] in conjunction with absolute risk assessment are two further approaches that might help identify a subset of younger individuals with low absolute risk but high relative risk or significant lifetime risk for CVD due to the cumulative effects of multiple risk factors or changes in risk factors over time. Briefly, lifetime risk relates to the risk of developing a specific disease before death.

Improvement in risk prediction for women

Women are usually estimated to be at lower risk than men of the same age, and inspection of the SCORE risk charts shows that their risk is merely deferred by 10 years [22]. However, women at older ages will carry a greater CVD risk burden as life expectancy increases and it does so particularly in women. Ultimately, more women than men die from CVD. The new Reynolds risk score for women developed from the Women's Health Study of 24 558 women followed up for a median of 10.2 years might help improve CVD risk prediction in women [84]. Three new variables were significant and incorporated into this new score compared

Table 12.1 Representative and recently published prediction tools for CVD or CHD

Study	Features of derivation cohorts	Predicted outcomes	Risk factors	Statistical methods	Available electronic format
ASSIGN score [104]	30–74 yrs, 6540 men and 6757 women free of CVD	CVD; 10 yrs	Age, sex, smoking, SBP, TC, HDL-C, diabetes, family history, index of social status	Cox proportional hazards model	An electronic calculator is available at: http://www.assign-score.com/
Copenhagen Risk Score [98]	22–93 yrs, 11 765 men and women	MI; 10 yrs	Age, sex, smoking, SBP, TC, HDL-C, BMI, diabetes, previous history of MI, family history of CVD	Cox proportional hazards model	PRECARD@ program allows an estimation of risk of MI in 5, 10 and 20 years (not online)
CUORE equation [76]	35–69 yrs, 6865 men free of CHD	CHD; 10 yrs	Age, smoking, SBP, anti-hypertensive medication, TC, HDL-C, diabetes, family history of CHD	Cox proportional hazards model	
DECODE risk scores [96]	30–74 yrs, 16 506 men and 8907 women	Fatal CVD; 5 or 10 yrs	Age, state of glucose tolerance, fasting glucose, (for prediction of 5-yr risk only: smoking, SBP, TC, HDL-C)	Cox proportional hazards model	
Dubbo equation [61]	≥45 yrs, 2102 men and women free of CHD, stroke	CVD; 5 and 10 yrs	Age, sex, smoking, SBP, anti-hypertensive medication, TC, HDL-C, diabetes	Logistic regression model	
FINRISK equation [97]	30–59 yrs, men and women	'Hard' CHD; 10 yrs	Age, sex, smoking, SBP, total and HDL cholesterol, diabetes	Logistic regression model	
Framingham equations –Anderson et al. 1991 [42, 43]	30–74 yrs, 2590 men and 2983 women free of CVD	CHD, MI, fatal CHD, stroke, CVD, fatal CVD; 4–12 yrs	Age, sex, smoking, SBP or DBP, TC, HDL-C, diabetes, ECG-LVH	Weibull accelerated failure time model	It has been built into New Zealand CVD risk prediction charts, Sheffield table, Risk Prediction Charts incorporated in the 2nd JBS guidelines

Model	Population	Outcome; time	Risk factors	Statistical model	Notes
Framingham equations – Wilson et al. 1998 [47]	30–74 yrs, 2849 men and 2856 women free of CHD	CHD; 10 yrs	Age, sex, smoking, SBP and DBP, TC or LDL-C, HDL-C, diabetes	Cox proportional hazards model	An electronic calculator is available at: http://hp2010.nhlbihin.net/atpiii/calculator.asp
Framingham equations – D'Agostino et al. 2000 [49]	35–74 yrs, 4823 men and 5333 women free of CVD	CHD; 1–4 yrs	Age, sex, smoking, SBP, anti-hypertensive medication, TC, HDL-C, diabetes, (women only: menopause, alcohol, with and without triglyceride)	Weibull accelerated failure time model	
Framingham equations – D'Agostino et al. 2000 [49]	35–74 yrs, 718 men and 458 women with history of CHD or ischaemic stroke	CHD; 1–4 yrs	Age, sex, smoking (women only), SBP (women only), TC, HDL-C, diabetes	Weibull accelerated failure time model	
Framingham equations – D'Agostino et al. 2008 [52]	30–74 yrs, 3969 men and 4522 women free of CVD	CVD; 10 yrs	Based on traditional risk factors: age, sex, smoking, SBP, anti-hypertensive medication, TC, HDL-C, diabetes	Cox proportional hazards model	
			Based on non-laboratory predictors: age, sex, smoking, anti-hypertensive medication, BMI, diabetes		
NIPPON DATA80 risk chart [79]	≥30 yrs, 4098 men and 5255 women free of CVD	Fatal CHD, fatal stroke, and fatal CVD; 10 yrs	Age, sex, smoking, SBP, total cholesterol, glucose	Cox proportional hazards model	
PROCAM risk score [99]	20–78 yrs, 18460 men and 8515 women free of CVD	'Hard' CHD; 10 yrs	Age, sex, smoking, SBP, HDL and HDL cholesterol, triglycerides, diabetes, fasting glucose, family history of CVD	Weibull proportional hazards model	

Table 12.1 Continued

Study	Features of derivation cohorts	Predicted outcomes	Risk factors	Statistical methods	Available electronic format
QRISK2 score [69]	35–74 yrs, 636 753 men and 646 421 women free of CVD and diabetes	CVD; 10 yrs	Age, sex, ethnicity, smoking, SBP, antihypertensive medication, TC/HDL-C, BMI, family history of CHD, index of social status	Cox proportional hazards model	An electronic calculator is available at: http://qr2.dyndns.org/
Reynolds risk score for women [84]	≥45 yrs, 16 400 women free of CVD and cancer	CVD; 10 yrs	Age, smoking, SBP, TC, HDL-C, hs CRP, HbA$_{1c}$ (in people with diabetes), parental history of MI	Cox proportional hazards model	An electronic calculator is available at: http://www.Reynoldsriskscore.org
Reynolds risk score for men [114]	≥50 yrs, 10 724 men free of CVD, diabetes and cancer	CVD; 10 yrs	Age, smoking, SBP, TC, HDL-C, hsCRP, parental history of MI	Cox proportional hazards model	An electronic calculator is available at: http://www.Reynoldsriskscore.org
Riskard risk chart [75]	45–74 yrs, 8517 men and 3 473 women free of CVD	CVD; 10 yrs	Age, sex, smoking, SBP, TC, diabetes	Weibull accelerated failure time model	
Riskard risk software [75]	45–74 yrs, 11 039 men and 4777 women free of CVD	CVD, CHD and stroke; 5, 10 and 15 yrs	Age, sex, smoking, mean BP, HDL-C, non-HDL-C, diabetes, BMI, heart rate	Weibull accelerated failure time model	
SCORE risk charts [70]	19–80 yrs, 11 709 men and 88 080 women free of CHD	Fatal CVD, fatal CHD, fatal non-CHD; 10 yrs	Age, sex, smoking, SBP, TC or TC/HDL-C	Weibull proportional hazards model	Separate sex-specific charts for populations at high and low risk of CVD An electronic version (HeartScore) is available at: http://www.heartscore.org/Pages/welcome.aspx

UKPDS risk engine [89]	25–65 yrs, 2643 men and 1897 women with newly diagnosed type 2 diabetes and free of CHD	'Hard' CHD; 4–20 yrs	Age at diagnosis of diabetes, smoking, SBP, TC/HDL-C, HbA$_{1c}$, ethnicity	Maximum likelihood estimation	An electronic calculator is available at: http://www.dtu.ox.ac.uk/
Wu et al. [78]	35–59 yrs, 4890 men and 5013 women free of MI and stroke	CVD: 10 yrs	Age, sex, smoking, SBP, TC, diabetes, BMI	Cox proportional hazards model	An electronic program is available at: http://www.healthyheart-china.com
Zhang et al. [77]	18–74 yrs, 3000 male steelworkers	CHD, ischaemic and hemorrhagic stroke; 10 yrs	CHD: age, smoking, SBP, TC, BMI

Ischaemic stroke: age, smoking, SBP, TC

Haemorrhagic stroke: age, SBP, DBP, TC | Cox proportional hazards model | |

Note: 'Hard' CHD includes myocardial infarction or coronary death.
Abbreviations: BMI = body mass index; BP = blood pressure; CHD = coronary heart disease; CVD = cardiovascular disease; DBP = diastolic blood pressure; ECG-LVH = electrocardiographically determined left ventricular hypertrophy; HbA$_{1c}$ = haemoglobin A$_{1c}$; HDL-C = high-density lipoprotein cholesterol; hs CRP = high-sensitivity C-reactive protein; LDL-C = low-density lipoprotein cholesterol; MI = myocardial infarction; SBP = systolic blood pressure; TC = total cholesterol.

with the Framingham risk score. These were the parental history of premature CHD, high-sensitivity C-reactive protein (hs CRP) and glycosylated haemoglobin A_{1c} (HbA$_{1c}$) in people with diabetes. Using this new score, 40–50% of women who were estimated to be at intermediate risk (5–20%) according to the Framingham risk score were reclassified into higher or lower risk categories. These findings are consistent with another publication from this study about 1 year ago [85].

Risk assessment in people with diabetes

People with diabetes are at increased risk of cardiovascular events not only because of the risk inherently associated with diabetes but also because other CVD risk factors such as dyslipidaemia and high blood pressure are more common. The NCEP-ATPIII, 2nd JBS and 4th European Joint Task Force guidelines recommend that people with type 2 or type 1 diabetes should be regarded as at high risk [22, 54, 57, 86, 87]. Moreover, the 4th European Joint Task Force guidelines state that CVD risk may be 5-fold higher in women with diabetes and 3-fold higher in men with diabetes compared to those without diabetes [22].

However, absolute CVD risk varies within individuals with diabetes, and further risk stratification might help decide the intensity of risk reduction therapies. The UKPDS (United Kingdom Prospective Diabetes Study) risk engine is the best known model for predicting risk of CHD or stroke in people with type 2 diabetes [88, 89]. It incorporates the duration of diabetes and the plasma level of HbA$_{1c}$ in the prediction models compared to the Framingham equations. Subsequently, another two models have been developed from population cohort studies in the United Kingdom and the United States [90, 91]. Furthermore, a scoring system for future macrovascular risk was developed from 2136 patients with type 1 diabetes using the Royal College of Physicians of Edinburgh Diabetes Register [94].

Some have argued against the above approaches to estimating risk in people with diabetes. Results from a meta-analysis of 33 cohort studies in the Asia Pacific region suggested that CHD risk prediction tools should account for diabetes simply by including a variable for diabetes in the equations [95]. In addition, the authors stated that there is no justification for generating separate risk prediction models for people with diabetes, nor for assuming that everyone with diabetes should be regarded as high risk. This concept is reflected in a series of prediction models from different populations [61, 75, 76, 79, 84, 96–99], which include either a variable indicating the status of diabetes, or the measures of glucose level, such as fasting or casual glucose level, or HbA$_{1c}$. However, it is noteworthy that all of the risk prediction tools described are based on analysis of subsequent first CVD events. In people with diabetes, a first CVD event is more likely to be fatal, however, and the subsequent prognosis is worse in those who survive.

Inclusion of new risk markers in the risk prediction tools

A series of novel biomarkers have been suggested to be independently associated with the risk of CHD or stroke, e.g. C-reactive protein (CRP), fibrinogen, microalbuminuria, B-type natriuretic peptide and homocysteine. Some new risk factors have also been incorporated into the recently published tools, e.g. BMI, CRP, albuminuria and area measures of social deprivation. However, their additive prognostic value beyond traditional risk factors on CVD is still questioned.

As one example, a number of observational studies and meta-analyses have found that CRP is independently associated with increased risk for CVD after adjustment for potential confounding factors [100]. However, its incremental value in the prediction of CHD beyond traditional risk factors, as assessed by the measures of area under the receiver-operating characteristic curve or Harrell's c-statistic has been small and most results were not statistically significant [101]. Conversely, researchers in the Women's Health Study found that although the addition of CRP had a minimal effect on the c-statistic after accounting for age, smoking and blood pressure, the effect was nonetheless greater than that of TC, LDL-C or HDL-C, which suggested that the measures of discrimination may not be sufficiently sensitive in evaluating risk prediction models [85].

Many have argued that the major focus of research on the area under the receiver-operating characteristic curve or c-statistic in determining whether or not a factor is important ignores the role of other analyses such as testing calibration, the relationship between predicted and observed event notes [102]. Indeed, because the commonly used methods may lack the power to identify the incremental value of new markers in the prediction model at an individual level, even if these markers have been shown to be significantly associated with CVD events, researchers have commenced investigation of new methods to quantify the improved prognostic value of new markers. Pencina and colleagues [103] described two new approaches to evaluating the usefulness of a new marker, one termed the net reclassification improvement, and the other the integrated discrimination improvement which might assess the new model's ability to improve integrated (average) sensitivity without sacrificing integrated (average) specificity.

Another important refinement of multivariate risk prediction models is the inclusion of measures of socioeconomic status. Numerous studies have found that CVD mortality and related risk factors are associated with socioeconomic status. However, such a measure was not included in earlier prediction tools such as the Framingham risk scores. Furthermore, studies have found that the Framingham risk scores underestimated risk in socioeconomically deprived groups in the United Kingdom and also in the Australian Aboriginal people [65, 66].

ASSIGN and QRISK scores from Scotland and the United Kingdom, respectively, are two of the most recently published CVD prediction tools, both of which include a measure of social deprivation [68, 69, 104]. The QRISK score is derived from a large database from general practices in the United Kingdom and adds BMI, family history of premature CHD and area measure of social deprivation to a set of standard risk factors. An external validation of the QRISK score showed a larger proportion of patients at high risk in the most deprived when compared with the most affluent subgroup using the QRISK score, but a much smaller deprivation gradient for the Framingham equation [105]. More recently, the QRISK score has been updated with additional risk factors: ethnicity, type 2 diabetes, renal disease, atrial fibrillation and rheumatoid arthritis [69].

GUIDELINES RELATED TO LIPID THERAPY USING ABSOLUTE RISK ASSESSMENT

Cholesterol is a major determinant of the development of atherosclerosis. It has been estimated that at least 4.4 million people in the world die each year as a result of raised TC levels [1]. Total cholesterol above an 'ideal' of 3.8 mmol/l is estimated to account for 56% of global ischaemic heart disease and 18% of global stroke burden [106].

There has been a paradigm shift in cardiovascular risk management. Increasing data indicate that treatment decisions should be based primarily on absolute estimates of cardiovascular risk rather than a single risk factor such as cholesterol. Recent modelling of a large Canadian national survey suggested that a 'high baseline risk strategy', using the recommendations of the New Zealand CVD prevention guidelines would prevent more than twice the number of CHD deaths than a treatment strategy based on high TC concentration (>6.2 mmol/l), despite the fact that only slightly more people would be treated under the 'high baseline risk strategy' compared to the number with elevated TC level (12.9% vs. 11.1%) [107]. Moreover, the absolute risk approach to the management of cholesterol level is more cost-effective than treatment based on the measured cholesterol level, as calculated by the ratio of total costs and the total health effects in terms of DALYs averted [108]. Importantly, studies have also shown that the cost-effectiveness of statin treatment is strongly related to the absolute risk of CHD and that statin therapy is cost-effective for people with an estimated annual CHD risk >4% [109].

Table 12.2 Representative guidelines for HMG-CoA reductase inhibitor (statin) treatment for prevention of CHD or CVD events

	4th European Joint Task Force, 2007 [22]	2nd Joint British Societies, 2005 [57]	US NCEP ATP III, updated in 2004 [110]	Canadian Cardiovascular Society position statement, 2006 [111]	NHFA/CSANZ position statement on lipid management, 2005 [86]	New Zealand guidelines on the assessment and management of cardiovascular risk, 2003 [112]
Absolute risk assessment tool incorporated in the guideline	The SCORE risk charts [70]	The CVD risk prediction charts based on the 1991 Framingham equations – Anderson et al. 1991 [42]	Framingham Risk Score based on the Framingham equations – Wilson et al. 1998 [47]	Framingham Risk Score based on the Framingham equations – Wilson et al. 1998 [47]	The New Zealand risk prediction charts based on the 1991 Framingham equations – Anderson et al. [42]	The New Zealand risk prediction charts based on the 1991 Framingham equations – Anderson et al. [42]
Predicted outcome	Fatal CVD, 10 yrs	CVD, 10 yrs	'Hard' CHD, 10 yrs	'Hard' CHD, 10 yrs	CVD, 5 yrs	CVD, 5 yrs
Risk factors required for absolute risk assessment	Age, sex, smoking, SBP, TC or TC/HDL-C	Age, sex, smoking, SBP, TC/HDL-C	Age, sex, smoking, SBP, anti-hypertensive medication, TC, HDL-C	Age, sex, smoking, SBP, anti-hypertensive medication, TC, HDL-C	Age, sex, smoking, SBP, TC/HDL-C, diabetes	Age, sex, smoking, SBP, TC/HDL-C, diabetes
High-risk population determined by clinical manifestations	Known CVD; Type 2 and type 1 diabetes with microalbuminuria; Markedly increased single risk factors especially if associated with end-organ damage; Close relatives of patients with premature CVD or of those at particularly high risk	Known CVD; Type 1 or type 2 diabetes; TC/HDL-C ratio ≥6; BP ≥160/100 mmHg or lesser elevated BP with target organ damage; Familial hypercholesterolaemia or other inherited dyslipidaemias	Known CHD or other forms of clinical atherosclerotic disease; Diabetes	Known CVD; Type 1 or type 2 diabetes; Chronic kidney disease with GFR <30 ml/min/1.73m².	Known CVD; Diabetes; Chronic kidney disease; Familial hypercholesterol-aemia; Aboriginal and Torres Strait Islander peoples	Known CVD; Familial lipid disorders; Diabetes with overt nephropathy or other renal disease

	10-year risk of fatal CVD ≥5%	10-year risk of CVD ≥20%	Multiple (2+) CHD risk factors with 10-year risk of 'hard' CHD ≥20%	10-year risk of 'hard' CHD ≥20%	5-year risk of CVD ≥15%, or 5-year risk of CVD 10–15% with concomitant metabolic syndrome or family history of premature CHD	5-year risk of CVD ≥15%
High-risk population determined by the absolute risk assessment						
Lipid targets	TC <4.5 mmol/l (or <4.0 mmol/l if feasible) LDL-C <2.5 mmol/l (or <2.0 mmol/l if feasible)	TC <4.0 mmol/l or a ≥5% reduction LDL-C <2.0 mmol/l or a 30% reduction	LDL-C <2.5 mmol/l (or <1.8 mmol/l if feasible)	LDL-C <2.0 mmol/l TC/HDL-C <4.0	LDL-C <2.5 mmol/l (or <2.0 mmol/l if feasible) HDL-C >1.0 mmol/l Triglycerides <1.5 mmol/l	There is no normal or ideal lipid level. The goal is to reduce 5-year CVD risk to less than 15%

Notes: 'Hard' CHD includes MI or coronary death. The major risk factors identified in risk factor counting in the NCEP-ATPIII guidelines include: cigarette smoking, hypertension (BP ≥140/90 mmHg or on anti-hypertensive medication), low HDL-C (<40 mg/dl), family history of premature CHD (CHD in male first-degree relative <55 years of age; CHD in female first-degree relative <65 years of age), and age (men ≥45 years; women ≥55 years).

Abbreviations: BP = blood pressure; CHD = coronary heart disease; CVD = cardiovascular disease; GFR = glomerular filtration rate; HDL-C = high-density lipoprotein cholesterol; LDL-C = low- density lipoprotein cholesterol; NCEP ATPIII = National Cholesterol Education Program Adult Treatment Panel III; NHFA/CSANZ = National Heart Foundation of Australia and Cardiac Society of Australia and New Zealand; SBP = systolic blood pressure.

The principle of absolute risk assessment was first used in 1993 by New Zealand groups in guidelines for the management of raised blood pressure [55]. The approach has been quickly adopted by other influential groups. To date, many clinical practice guidelines have incorporated absolute risk assessment approaches for predicting risk in people without known CVD and diabetes [22, 54, 57, 86, 110–112]. These new guidelines recommend that people at highest CVD risk should be given the highest priority as they derive the greatest absolute risk reduction and net benefit with an effective intervention. Table 12.2 lists the most recently published guidelines related to lipid therapy for CVD prevention.

All of these guidelines use the Framingham risk prediction functions [42, 47], except the 4th European Joint Task Force guidelines which are based on the SCORE risk charts. The outcome of interest and timeframe over which risk for these events is estimated also vary. Most use 10-year risk assessment, although the Australian and New Zealand guidelines propose predicting CVD risk over 5 years. Furthermore, the current United States and Canadian guidelines recommend the use of the Framingham risk scores and suggest those with a 10-year risk of MI or coronary death over 20% are at high risk, while other guidelines emphasise total cardiovascular risk assessment, not CHD only. CHD, stroke and peripheral vascular disease share many common risk factors, particularly related to atherosclerosis. Drug interventions as well as lifestyle modification, such as smoking cessation, also reduce the risk in different vascular territories. It therefore appears reasonable to target general CVD rather than one specific manifestation of CVD. The choice of a general risk function for predicting the first manifestations of CVD is also strengthened in the most recently published paper from the Framingham Heart Study [52].

Ideally, risk prediction models incorporated in guidelines should allow more accurate targeting of statin prescribing to those individuals who are accurately identified to be at high risk. Manuel and colleagues [113] compared the potential effectiveness and efficiency of six national or international guidelines for statin treatment to reduce deaths from CHD in a Canadian population. The effectiveness and efficiency of guidelines were assessed by whether they recommended treatment to fewer people while at the same time preventing more deaths from CHD or CVD. The investigators found that the Australian and British guidelines were the most effective, potentially avoiding the most deaths, while the New Zealand guideline was the most efficient, potentially avoiding almost as many deaths while recommending treatment of fewer individuals. However, it should be noted that despite the paper being published in 2006, most guidelines that the authors applied in the study have since been updated and they differ from those included in the analysis. In addition, the risk threshold for eligibility for treatment differs in different guidelines. Lowering the risk threshold for eligibility for treatment means that more individuals will be prescribed a preventive medicine. However, this will also increase the associated costs to an extent dependent on the particular cut-points adopted.

Regarding potential lipid target with treatment, although there are some inconsistencies between different sets of guidelines, most suggest that people with high risk should have a TC <4.5 mmol/l or preferably <4.0 mmol/l and LDL-C level <2.5 mmol/l, or as low as 2.0 or 1.8 mmol/l if feasible [22, 57, 86, 110, 111]. Some guidelines state HDL-C or triglyceride levels that should also be targeted [86]. Interestingly, the New Zealand guidelines do not present an exact value for lipid control and suggest that the aim of CVD prevention is to reduce 5-year CVD risk to less than 15% [112], which might better reflect the fact that the CVD risk and its reduction represents a continuum and results from the synergistic effect of different risk factors.

CARDIOVASCULAR RISK PREDICTION IN THE FUTURE

To improve risk assessment, contemporary population-specific risk prediction tools for future CVD or CHD events may be further developed and refined by incorporating other risk factors, such as anthropometric measures [53, 91], family history of premature CHD [69] or measures of socioeconomic position [69, 104]. Considerable research also centres on the potential value of inflammatory and other biomarkers, alleles identified from genome-wide association studies [115] and imaging techniques [116], particularly in individuals considered to be at intermediate risk.

Over more than 30 years of development of CVD risk prediction models, several types of statistical methods have been applied, such as logistic regression, Weibull accelerated failure time and Cox proportional hazards regression models. Voss and colleagues [104] have also applied another neural network technique using data from the Prospective Cardiovascular Munster project. They found that the multilayer perceptron neural network was superior to the logistic regression model in identifying people with 10-year CHD risk >20%. Using the neural network approach, it was possible to identify about 8% of men aged 35–65 years who were responsible for 74.5% of CVD events over the next 10 years. However, prediction tools are based on analysis of data from large cohorts. As discussed, new statistical approaches could address the important question as to how improved risk prediction at an individual level may be quantified.

CONCLUSIONS

1. CVD is a multifactorial disease and is highly preventable.
2. To inform the most cost-effective CVD prevention strategies, those who are at higher risk and have the most to benefit need to be identified.
3. Consideration of multiple risk factors in determining an individual's absolute risk is the most efficient and cost-effective strategy.
4. In addition to the Framingham risk prediction equations or Framingham risk scores, other prediction tools have been developed and validated.
5. Treatment decisions should be based primarily on absolute estimates of cardiovascular risk rather than a single risk factor.
6. Many clinical practice guidelines have incorporated absolute risk assessment approaches and recommend initiation of drug therapy based on this.

REFERENCES

1. World Health Organization. Preventing chronic diseases: a vital investment. World Health Organization, Geneva, Switzerland, 2005.
2. World Health Organization. The world health report 2004 – changing history. World Health Organization, Geneva, Switzerland, 2004.
3. Access Economics. The shifting burden of cardiovascular disease. Report for National Heart Foundation of Australia. National Heart Foundation of Australia, Canberra, 2005.
4. Rosamond W, Flegal K, Furie K *et al.* Heart Disease and Stroke Statistics – 2008 Update: A report from the American Heart Association Statistics Committee and Stroke Statistics Subcommittee. *Circulation* 2008; 117:e25–e146.
5. Leal J, Luengo-Fernandez R, Gray A, Petersen S, Rayner M. Economic burden of cardiovascular diseases in the enlarged European Union. *Eur Heart J* 2006; 27:1610–1619.
6. Myerburg RJ, Kessler KM, Castellanos A. Sudden cardiac death: epidemiology, transient risk, and intervention assessment. *Ann Intern Med* 1993; 119:1187–1197.
7. Feigin VL, Lawes CMM, Bennett DA, Anderson CS. Stroke epidemiology: a review of population-based studies of incidence, prevalence, and case-fatality in the late 20th century. *Lancet Neurol* 2003; 2:43–53.
8. Strong JP, Malcom GT, Oalmann MC, Wissler RW. The PDAY Study: natural history, risk factors, and pathobiology. Pathobiological Determinants of Atherosclerosis in Youth. *Ann N Y Acad Sci* 1997; 811:226–237.
9. Tonkin AM. Future challenges. In: Tonkin AM (ed.) *Atherosclerosis and heart disease.* Martin Dunitz, London, 2003, pp 203–212.

10. Yusuf S, Reddy S, Ounpuu S, Anand S. Global burden of cardiovascular diseases: Part II: variations in cardiovascular disease by specific ethnic groups and geographic regions and prevention strategies. *Circulation* 2001; 104:2855–2864.

11. Law MR, Wald NJ. Risk factor thresholds: their existence under scrutiny. *Br Med J* 2002; 324:1570–1576.

12. Kannel WB, D'Agostino RB, Sullivan L, Wilson PWF. Concept and usefulness of cardiovascular risk profiles. *Am Heart J* 2004; 148:16–26.

13. Neaton JD, Wentworth D. Serum cholesterol, blood pressure, cigarette smoking, and death from coronary heart disease. Overall findings and differences by age for 316,099 white men. Multiple Risk Factor Intervention Trial Research Group. *Arch Intern Med* 1992; 152:56–64.

14. Stratton IM, Adler AI, Neil HA *et al.* Association of glycaemia with macrovascular and microvascular complications of type 2 diabetes (UKPDS 35): prospective observational study. *Br Med J* 2000; 321:405–412.

15. Baigent C, Keech A, Kearney PM *et al.* Efficacy and safety of cholesterol-lowering treatment: prospective meta-analysis of data from 90 056 participants in 14 randomised trials of statins. *Lancet* 2005; 366:1267–1278.

16. Thavendiranathan P, Bagai A, Brookhart M, Choudhry NK. Primary prevention of cardiovascular diseases with statin therapy: a meta-analysis of randomized controlled trials. *Arch Intern Med* 2006; 166:2307–2313.

17. Yusuf S, Hawken S, Ounpuu S *et al.* Effect of potentially modifiable risk factors associated with myocardial infarction in 52 countries (the INTERHEART study): case-control study. *Lancet* 2004; 364:937–952.

18. Stampfer MJ, Hu FB, Manson JE, Rimm EB, Willett WC. Primary prevention of coronary heart disease in women through diet and lifestyle. *N Engl J Med* 2000; 343:16–22.

19. Taylor R, Dobson A, Mirzaei M. Contribution of changes in risk factors to the decline of coronary heart disease mortality in Australia over three decades. *Eur J Cardiovasc Prev Rehabil* 2006; 13:760–768.

20. Ford ES, Ajani UA, Croft JB *et al.* Explaining the decrease in U.S. deaths from coronary disease, 1980–2000. *N Engl J Med* 2007; 356:2388–2398.

21. Grundy SM, Bazzarre T, Cleeman J *et al.* Prevention Conference V: Beyond secondary prevention: identifying the high-risk patient for primary prevention: medical office assessment: Writing Group I. *Circulation* 2000; 101:E3–E11.

22. Graham I, Atar D, Borch-Johnsen K *et al.* European guidelines on cardiovascular disease prevention in clinical practice: executive summary. Fourth Joint Task Force of the European Society of Cardiology and other societies on cardiovascular disease prevention in clinical practice (constituted by representatives of nine societies and by invited experts). *Eur J Cardiovasc Prev Rehabil* 2007; 14(suppl 2):E1–E40.

23. Barratt A, Wyer PC, Hatala R *et al.* Tips for learners of evidence-based medicine: 1. Relative risk reduction, absolute risk reduction and number needed to treat. *CMAJ* 2004; 171:353–358.

24. Scandinavian Simvastatin Survival Study Group. Randomised trial of cholesterol lowering in 4444 patients with coronary heart disease: the Scandinavian Simvastatin Survival Study (4S). *Lancet* 1994; 344:1383–1389.

25. Shepherd J, Cobbe SM, Ford I *et al.* Prevention of coronary heart disease with pravastatin in men with hypercholesterolemia. *N Engl J Med* 1995; 333:1301–1307.

26. Sacks FM, Pfeffer MA, Moye LA *et al.* The effect of pravastatin on coronary events after myocardial infarction in patients with average cholesterol levels. Cholesterol and Recurrent Events Trial investigators. *N Engl J Med* 1996; 335:1001–1009.

27. The Long-Term Intervention with Pravastatin in Ischaemic Disease (LIPID) Study Group. Prevention of cardiovascular events and death with pravastatin in patients with coronary heart disease and a broad range of initial cholesterol levels. *N Engl J Med* 1998; 339:1349–1357.

28. Downs JR, Clearfield M, Weis S *et al.* Primary prevention of acute coronary events with lovastatin in men and women with average cholesterol levels: results of AFCAPS/TexCAPS. Air Force/Texas Coronary Atherosclerosis Prevention Study. *JAMA* 1998; 279:1615–1622.

29. The ALLHAT Officers and Coordinators for the ALLHAT collaborative Research Group. Major outcomes in moderately hypercholesterolemic, hypertensive patients randomized to pravastatin vs usual care: The Antihypertensive and Lipid-Lowering Treatment to Prevent Heart Attack Trial (ALLHAT-LLT). *JAMA* 2002; 288:2998–3007.

30. Heart Protection Study Collaborative Group. MRC/BHF Heart Protection Study of cholesterol lowering with simvastatin in 20,536 high-risk individuals: a randomised placebo-controlled trial. *Lancet* 2002; 360:7–22.

31. Shepherd J, Blauw GJ, Murphy MB *et al.* Pravastatin in elderly individuals at risk of vascular disease (PROSPER): a randomised controlled trial. *Lancet* 2002; 360:1623–1630.

32. Sever PS, Dahlof B, Poulter NR *et al.* Prevention of coronary and stroke events with atorvastatin in hypertensive patients who have average or lower-than-average cholesterol concentrations, in the Anglo-Scandinavian Cardiac Outcomes Trial–Lipid Lowering Arm (ASCOT-LLA): a multicentre randomised controlled trial. *Lancet* 2003;361:1149–1158.

33. Colhoun HM, Betteridge DJ, Durrington PN, *et al.* Primary prevention of cardiovascular disease with atorvastatin in type 2 diabetes in the Collaborative Atorvastatin Diabetes Study (CARDS): multicentre randomised placebo-controlled trial. *Lancet* 2004; 364:685–696.

34. Knopp RH, d'Emden M, Smilde JG, Pocock SJ. Efficacy and safety of atorvastatin in the prevention of cardiovascular end points in subjects with type 2 diabetes: the Atorvastatin Study for Prevention of Coronary Heart Disease Endpoints in non-insulin-dependent diabetes mellitus (ASPEN). *Diabetes Care* 2006; 29:1478–1485.

35. Nakamura H, Arakawa K, Itakura H *et al.* Primary prevention of cardiovascular disease with pravastatin in Japan (MEGA Study): a prospective randomised controlled trial. *Lancet* 2006; 368:1155–1163.

36. Ridker PM, Danielson E, Fonseca FAH *et al.* Rosuvastatin to Prevent Vascular Events in Men and Women with Elevated C-Reactive Protein. *N Engl J Med* 2008; 359:2195–2207.

37. Jackson R. Guidelines on preventing cardiovascular disease in clinical practice. *BMJ* 2000; 320:659–661.

38. Truett J, Cornfield J, Kannel W. A multivariate analysis of the risk of coronary heart disease in Framingham. *J Chronic Dis* 1967; 20:511–524.

39. Kannel WB, McGee D, Gordon T. A general cardiovascular risk profile: the Framingham Study. *Am J Cardiol* 1976; 38:46–51.

40. Wilson PW, Castelli WP, Kannel WB. Coronary risk prediction in adults (the Framingham Heart Study). *Am J Cardiol* 1987; 59:91G–94G.

41. Levy D, Wilson PW, Anderson KM, Castelli WP. Stratifying the patient at risk from coronary disease: new insights from the Framingham Heart Study. *Am Heart J* 1990; 119:712–717 (discussion 717).

42. Anderson KM, Odell PM, Wilson PW, Kannel WB. Cardiovascular disease risk profiles. *Am Heart J* 1991; 121:293–298.

43. Anderson KM, Wilson PW, Odell PM, Kannel WB. An updated coronary risk profile. A statement for health professionals. *Circulation* 1991; 83:356–362.

44. Wolf PA, D'Agostino RB, Belanger AJ, Kannel WB. Probability of stroke: a risk profile from the Framingham Study. *Stroke* 1991; 22:312–318.

45. D'Agostino RB, Wolf PA, Belanger AJ, Kannel WB. Stroke risk profile: adjustment for antihypertensive medication. The Framingham Study. *Stroke* 1994; 25:40–43.

46. Murabito JM, D'Agostino RB, Silbershatz H, Wilson WF. Intermittent claudication. A risk profile from The Framingham Heart Study. *Circulation* 1997; 96:44–49.

47. Wilson PW, D'Agostino RB, Levy D *et al.* Prediction of coronary heart disease using risk factor categories. *Circulation* 1998; 97:1837–1847.

48. Kannel WB, D'Agostino RB, Silbershatz H *et al.* Profile for estimating risk of heart failure. *Arch Intern Med* 1999; 159:1197–1204.

49. D'Agostino RB, Russell MW, Huse DM *et al.* Primary and subsequent coronary risk appraisal: new results from the Framingham study. *Am Heart J* 2000; 139:272–281.

50. D'Agostino RB Sr, Grundy S, Sullivan LM, Wilson P; CHD Risk Prediction Group. Validation of the Framingham coronary heart disease prediction scores: results of a multiple ethnic groups investigation. *JAMA* 2001; 286:180–187.

51. Wang TJ, Massaro JM, Levy D *et al.* A risk score for predicting stroke or death in individuals with new-onset atrial fibrillation in the community: the Framingham Heart Study. *JAMA* 2003; 290:1049–1056.

52. D'Agostino RB Sr, Vasan RS, Pencina MJ *et al.* General cardiovascular risk profile for use in primary care: The Framingham Heart Study. *Circulation* 2008; 117:743–753.

53. Wilson PWF, Bozeman SR, Burton TM *et al.* Prediction of first events of coronary heart disease and stroke with consideration of adiposity. *Circulation* 2008; 118:124–130.

54. National Cholesterol Education Program Expert Panel. Third Report of the National Cholesterol Education Program (NCEP) Expert Panel on Detection, Evaluation, and Treatment of High Blood Cholesterol in Adults (Adult Treatment Panel III) final report. *Circulation* 2002; 106:3143–3421.

55. Jackson R, Barham P, Bills J *et al.* Management of raised blood pressure in New Zealand: a discussion document. *Br Med J* 1993; 307:107–110.

56. Jackson R. Updated New Zealand cardiovascular disease risk-benefit prediction guide. *Br Med J* 2000; 320:709–710.

57. British Cardiac Society; British Hypertension Society; Diabetes UK *et al.* JBS 2: Joint British Societies' guidelines on prevention of cardiovascular disease in clinical practice. *Heart* 2005; 91(suppl 5):v1–v52.

58. Ramsay LE, Haq IU, Jackson PR *et al.* Targeting lipid-lowering drug therapy for primary prevention of coronary disease: an updated Sheffield table. *Lancet* 1996; 348:387–388.

59. McCormack JP, Levine M, Rangno RE. Primary prevention of heart disease and stroke: a simplified approach to estimating risk of events and making drug treatment decisions. *CMAJ* 1997; 157:422–428.

60. Knuiman MW, Vu HT. Prediction of coronary heart disease mortality in Busselton, Western Australia: an evaluation of the Framingham, national health epidemiologic follow up study, and WHO ERICA risk scores. *J Epidemiol Community Health* 1997; 51:515–519.

61. Simons LA, Simons J, Friedlander Y, McCallum J, Palaniappan L. Risk functions for prediction of cardiovascular disease in elderly Australians: the Dubbo Study. *Med J Aust* 2003; 178:113–116.

62. Milne R, Gamble G, Whitlock G, Jackson R. Framingham Heart Study risk equation predicts first cardiovascular event rates in New Zealanders at the population level. *N Z Med J* 2003; 116:U662.

63. Brindle P, Beswick A, Fahey T, Ebrahim S. Accuracy and impact of risk assessment in the primary prevention of cardiovascular disease: a systematic review. *Heart* 2006; 92:1752–1759.

64. Eichler K, Puhan MA, Steurer J, Bachmann LM. Prediction of first coronary events with the Framingham score: a systematic review. *Am Heart J* 2007; 153:722–731.

65. Brindle PM, McConnachie A, Upton MN *et al.* The accuracy of the Framingham risk-score in different socioeconomic groups: a prospective study. *Br J Gen Pract* 2005; 55:838–845.

66. Wang Z, Hoy WE. Is the Framingham coronary heart disease absolute risk function applicable to Aboriginal people? *Med J Aust* 2005; 182:66–69.

67. Lee ET, Howard BV, Wang W *et al.* Prediction of coronary heart disease in a population with high prevalence of diabetes and albuminuria: the Strong Heart Study. *Circulation* 2006; 113:2897–2905.

68. Hippisley-Cox J, Coupland C, Vinogradova Y *et al.* Derivation and validation of QRISK, a new cardiovascular disease risk score for the United Kingdom: prospective open cohort study. *Br Med J* 2007; 335:136.

69. Hippisley-Cox J, Coupland C, Vinogradova Y *et al.* Predicting cardiovascular risk in England and Wales: prospective derivation and validation of QRISK2. *Br Med J* 2008; 336:1475–1482.

70. Conroy RM, Pyörälä K, Fitzgerald AP *et al.* Estimation of ten-year risk of fatal cardiovascular disease in Europe: the SCORE project. *Eur Heart J* 2003; 24:987–1003.

71. Lindman AS, Selmer R, Tverdal A *et al.* The SCORE risk model applied to recent population surveys in Norway compared to observed mortality in the general population. *Eur J Cardiovasc Prev Rehabil* 2006; 13:731–737.

72. Neuhauser HK, Ellert U, Kurth BM. A comparison of Framingham and SCORE-based cardiovascular risk estimates in participants of the German National Health Interview and Examination Survey 1998. *Eur J Cardiovasc Prev Rehabil* 2005; 12:442–450.

73. Ulmer H, Kollerits B, Kelleher C, Diem G, Concin H. Predictive accuracy of the SCORE risk function for cardiovascular disease in clinical practice: a prospective evaluation of 44 649 Austrian men and women. *Eur J Cardiovasc Prev Rehabil* 2005; 12:433–441.

74. Aspelund T, Thorgeirsson G, Sigurdsson G, Gudnason V. Estimation of 10-year risk of fatal cardiovascular disease and coronary heart disease in Iceland with results comparable with those of the Systematic Coronary Risk Evaluation project. *Eur J Cardiovasc Prev Rehabil* 2007; 14:761–768.

75. Menotti A, Lanti M, Agabiti-Rosei E *et al.* Riskard 2005. New tools for prediction of cardiovascular disease risk derived from Italian population studies. *Nutr Metab Cardiovasc Dis* 2005; 15:426–440.

76. Ferrario M, Chiodini P, Chambless LE *et al.* Prediction of coronary events in a low incidence population. Assessing accuracy of the CUORE Cohort Study prediction equation. *Int J Epidemiol* 2005; 34:413–421.

77. Zhang XF, Attia J, D'Este C, Yu XH, Wu XG. A risk score predicted coronary heart disease and stroke in a Chinese cohort. *J Clin Epidemiol* 2005; 58:951–958.

78. Wu Y, Liu X, Li X et al. Estimation of 10-year risk of fatal and nonfatal ischemic cardiovascular diseases in Chinese adults. *Circulation* 2006; 114:2217–2225.

79. Nippon Data Research Group. Risk assessment chart for death from cardiovascular disease based on a 19-year follow-up study of a Japanese representative population. *Circ J* 2006; 70:1249–1255.

80. Asia Pacific Cohort Studies Collaboration. Cardiovascular risk prediction tools for populations in Asia. *J Epidemiol Community Health* 2007; 61:115–121.

81. Berry JD, Lloyd-Jones DM, Garside DB, Greenland P. Framingham risk score and prediction of coronary heart disease death in young men. *Am Heart J* 2007; 154:80–86.

82. McMahan CA, Gidding SS, Fayad ZA et al. Risk scores predict atherosclerotic lesions in young people. *Arch Intern Med* 2005; 165:883–890.

83. Lloyd-Jones DM. Short-term versus long-term risk for coronary artery disease: implications for lipid guidelines. *Curr Opin Lipidol* 2006; 17:619–625.

84. Ridker PM, Buring JE, Rifai N, Cook NR. Development and validation of improved algorithms for the assessment of global cardiovascular risk in women: the Reynolds Risk Score. *JAMA* 2007; 297:611–619.

85. Cook NR, Buring JE, Ridker PM. The effect of including C-reactive protein in cardiovascular risk prediction models for women. *Ann Intern Med* 2006; 145:21–29.

86. Tonkin A, Barter P, Best J et al. National Heart Foundation of Australia and the Cardiac Society of Australia and New Zealand: position statement on lipid management – 2005. *Heart Lung Circ* 2005; 14:275–291.

87. Genest J, Frohlich J, Fodor G, McPherson R. Recommendations for the management of dyslipidemia and the prevention of cardiovascular disease: summary of the 2003 update. *CMAJ* 2003; 169:921–924.

88. Kothari V, Stevens RJ, Adler AI et al. UKPDS 60: risk of stroke in type 2 diabetes estimated by the UK Prospective Diabetes Study risk engine. *Stroke* 2002; 33:1776–1781.

89. Stevens RJ, Kothari V, Adler AI, Stratton IM; United Kingdom Prospective Diabetes Study Group. The UKPDS risk engine: a model for the risk of coronary heart disease in Type II diabetes (UKPDS 56). *Clin Sci (Colch)* 2001; 101:671–679.

90. Donnan PT, Donnelly L, New JP, Morris AD. Derivation and validation of a prediction score for major coronary heart disease events in a U.K. type 2 diabetic population. *Diabetes Care* 2006; 29: 1231–1236.

91. Folsom AR, Chambless LE, Duncan BB, Gilbert AC, Pankow JS. Prediction of coronary heart disease in middle-aged adults with diabetes. *Diabetes Care* 2003; 26:2777–2784.

92. Yang X, So WY, Kong AP et al. Development and validation of a total coronary heart disease risk score in type 2 diabetes mellitus. *Am J Cardiol* 2008; 101:596–601.

93. Yang X, So WY, Kong AP et al. Development and validation of stroke risk equation for Hong Kong Chinese patients with type 2 diabetes: the Hong Kong Diabetes Registry. *Diabetes Care* 2007; 30:65–70.

94. Lewis S, MacLeod M, McKnight J et al. Predicting vascular risk in Type 1 diabetes: stratification in a hospital based population in Scotland. *Diabet Med* 2005; 22:164–171.

95. Asia Pacific Cohort Studies Collaboration. Coronary risk prediction for those with and without diabetes. *Eur J Cardiovasc Prev Rehabil* 2006; 13:30–36.

96. Balkau B, Hu G, Qiao Q et al. Prediction of the risk of cardiovascular mortality using a score that includes glucose as a risk factor. The DECODE Study. *Diabetologia* 2004; 47:2118–2128.

97. Bhopal R, Fischbacher C, Vartiainen E et al. Predicted and observed cardiovascular disease in South Asians: application of FINRISK, Framingham and SCORE models to Newcastle Heart Project data. *J Public Health (Oxf)* 2005; 27:93–100.

98. Thomsen TF, Davidsen M, Ibsen H et al. A new method for CHD prediction and prevention based on regional risk scores and randomized clinical trials; PRECARD and the Copenhagen Risk Score. *J Cardiovasc Risk* 2001; 8:291–297.

99. Assmann G, Schulte H, Cullen P, Seedorf U. Assessing risk of myocardial infarction and stroke: new data from the Prospective Cardiovascular Munster (PROCAM) study. *Eur J Clin Invest* 2007; 37:925–932.

100. Danesh J, Wheeler JG, Hirschfield GM et al. C-reactive protein and other circulating markers of inflammation in the prediction of coronary heart disease. *N Engl J Med* 2004; 350:1387–1397.

101. Shah T, Casas JP, Cooper JA et al. Critical appraisal of CRP measurement for the prediction of coronary heart disease events: new data and systematic review of 31 prospective cohorts. *Int J Epidemiol* 2008; Oct 17 [Epub ahead of print]

102. Cook NR. Use and misuse of the receiver operating characteristic curve in risk prediction. *Circulation* 2007; 115:928–935.

103. Pencina MJ, D' Agostino RB Sr, D'Agostino RB Jr, Vasan RS. Evaluating the added predictive ability of a new marker: From area under the ROC curve to reclassification and beyond. *Stat Med* 2008; 27:157–172.

104. Woodward M, Brindle P, Tunstall-Pedoe H; for the SIGN group on risk estimation. Adding social deprivation and family history to cardiovascular risk assessment: the ASSIGN score from the Scottish Heart Health Extended Cohort (SHHEC). *Heart* 2007; 93:172–176.

105. Hippisley-Cox J, Coupland C, Vinogradova Y, Robson J, Brindle P. Performance of the QRISK cardiovascular risk prediction algorithm in an independent UK sample of patients from general practice: a validation study. *Heart* 2008; 94:34–39.

106. Guilbert JJ. The world health report 2002 – reducing risks, promoting healthy life. *Educ Health* 2003; 16:230.

107. Manuel DG, Lim J, Tanuseputro P *et al*. Revisiting Rose: strategies for reducing coronary heart disease. *Br Med J* 2006; 332:659–662.

108. Murray CJ, Lauer JA, Hutubessy RC *et al*. Effectiveness and costs of interventions to lower systolic blood pressure and cholesterol: a global and regional analysis on reduction of cardiovascular-disease risk. *Lancet* 2003; 361:717–725.

109. Franco OH, Peeters A, Looman CW, Bonneux L. Cost effectiveness of statins in coronary heart disease. *J Epidemiol Community Health* 2005; 59:927–933.

110. Grundy SM, Cleeman JI, Merz CN *et al*. Implications of recent clinical trials for the National Cholesterol Education Program Adult Treatment Panel III guidelines. *Circulation* 2004; 110:227–239.

111. McPherson R, Frohlich J, Fodor G, Genest J, Canadian Cardiovascular Society. Canadian Cardiovascular Society position statement – recommendations for the diagnosis and treatment of dyslipidemia and prevention of cardiovascular disease. *Can J Cardiol* 2006; 22:913–927.

112. New Zealand Guidelines Group. The assessment and management of cardiovascular risk. Wellington: New Zealand Guidelines Group. 2003; www.nzgg.org.nz/guidelines/0035/CVD_Risk_Full.pdf

113. Manuel DG, Kwong K, Tanuseputro P *et al*. Effectiveness and efficiency of different guidelines on statin treatment for preventing deaths from coronary heart disease: modelling study. *Br Med J* 2006; 332:1419.

114. Ridker PM, Paynter NP, Rifai N, Gaziano JM, Cook NR. C-reactive protein and parental history improve global cardiovascular risk prediction. The Reynolds Risk Score for men. *Circulation* 2008; 118:2243–2251.

115. Humphries SE, Cooper JA, Talmud PJ, Miller GJ. Candidate Gene Genotypes, Along with Conventional Risk Factor Assessment, Improve Estimation of Coronary Heart Disease Risk in Healthy UK Men. *Clin Chem* 2007; 53:8–16.

116. Greenland P, LaBree L, Azen SP, Doherty TM, Detrano RC. Coronary artery calcium score combined with Framingham score for risk prediction in asymptomatic individuals. *JAMA* 2004; 291:210–215.

117. Voss R, Cullen P, Schulte H, Assmann G. Prediction of risk of coronary events in middle-aged men in the Prospective Cardiovascular Munster Study (PROCAM) using neural networks. *Int J Epidemiol* 2002; 31:1253–1262 (discussion 1262–1264).

13

Pleiotropic effects of statins and potential new indications

J. Davignon, H. Wassef

INTRODUCTION

A key attribute of biological molecules is that they have multiple biochemical and physiological (i.e. pleiotropic) effects. A case in point is clusterin, also known as apolipoprotein J, whose multiple effects explain why it has more than 14 different names, as it was rediscovered many times by different scientists working in widely different fields [1]. Advances in molecular biology have provided insight into the mechanisms underlying the multiple effects of a single molecule [2]. In the last decade, much attention has been given to pleiotropic effects of drugs, with 3-hydroxy-3-methylglutaryl coenzyme A (HMG-CoA) reductase inhibitors (statins) standing out as one of the most widely studied in this respect.

In addition to their well-established lipid-modulating abilities, statins influence many signalling pathways that are involved in inflammation, immunomodulation, vasoactive and angiogenic processes, oxidative stress, and coagulation [3–6]. In the cardiovascular area, animal experimentation has proven that the majority of these pleiotropic effects are beneficial and cardioprotective. In humans, the pleiotropic effects are deemed responsible in part for the well-established ability of statins to reduce coronary heart disease (CHD) risk and mortality. It is difficult, however, to dissociate the relative contribution of pleiotropic effects from those directly attributable to low-density lipoprotein cholesterol (LDL-C) lowering. Some have questioned their importance on the basis that risk reduction correlated with LDL-C reduction with sufficient strength to dispel the importance that other effects might have [7]. This position was echoed by the observation that new biomarkers of atherosclerosis, such as markers of inflammation, have added very little to the impact of standard CHD risk factors on risk prediction in receiver operating characteristic analyses [8]. Others, in contrast, emphasise the fact that interrupting the cholesterol synthesis pathway at the mevalonate step by statins not only prevents cholesterol synthesis from squalene but also the formation of isoprenes such as farnesyl-pyrophosphate and geranylgeranyl-pyrophosphate necessary for isoprenylation of regulatory proteins (Figure 13.1). Statins could therefore impair the isoprenylation of small G proteins such as Ras, Rac and RhoA, preventing these molecular switches from turning on pro-inflammatory, pro-oxidant, pro-proliferative and prothrombotic molecules [5]. Since these major metabolic effects (i.e. cholesterol synthesis and isoprene synthesis) occur downstream from mevalonate and are presumably of the

Jean Davignon, OC, GOQ, MD, MSc, FRCP(C), FACP, FACN, FAHA, FRSC, Professor of Medicine, University of Montreal; Director, Hyperlipidemia and Atherosclerosis Group, Clinical Research Institute of Montreal, Montreal, Quebec, Canada

Hanny Wassef, MSc, PhD Candidate, McGill University, Hyperlipidemia and Atherosclerosis Group, Clinical Research Institute of Montreal, Montreal, Quebec, Canada

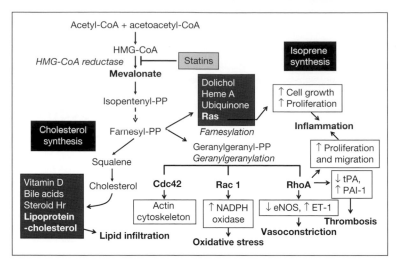

Figure 13.1 Statin effects: importance of pathways downstream from mevalonate. Cholesterol is an important constituent of cell membranes and is an essential element for synthesis of vitamins, steroid hormones, bile acids and lipoprotein molecules. The rate-limiting step in cholesterol synthesis is the conversion of hydroxy-methyl-glutaryl-coenzyme A (HMG-CoA) to mevalonate via HMG-CoA reductase. Statins act as HMG-CoA reductase inhibitors by competitively binding this enzyme's active site and blocking the interaction with its natural substrate HMG-CoA. There are two equally important pathways downstream from mevalonate, one leading to cholesterol synthesis, the other to isoprene synthesis. The isoprene synthesis pathway accounts for the less obvious pleiotropic effects of statin therapy. The isoprenoid intermediate, farnesyl-pyrophosphate (FPP) leads to the formation of dolichol (a multi-isoprene unit that anchors sugars to membranes), heme A (a transporter of iron), ubiquinone (also known as coenzyme Q10 used by the mitochondria to help generate ATP), and another isoprene geranylgeranyl-pyrophosphate (GPP). The isoprenes act as lipid attachments for small G-proteins such as Ras, Cdc42, Rac1 and RhoA. Isoprenylation of these molecules allows their translocation from the cytosol where they are in the inactive form (GDP-bound) to the cell membrane where they become attached and activated (GTP-bound). Ras activation is dependent on farnesylation and can activate cell cycle progression through the MAP-kinase pathway which can induce reactive oxygen species (ROS) production and lead to oxidative stress causing smooth muscle cell and cardiac hypertrophy, and endothelial dysfunction [114]. Activation of the Rho GTPase members Cdc42, Rac 1 and RhoA is dependent on geranylgeranylation. Cdc42 can rearrange the actin cytoskeleton leading to altered cell morphogenesis [114]. Rac 1 will catalyse superoxide formation from nicotinamide adenine dinucleotide phosphate (NADPH) and oxygen [115] leading to oxidative stress. RhoA is implied in many pathways. It can decrease endothelial nitric oxide synthase (eNOS) mRNA stability, which leads to altered vascular tone, platelet aggregation and smooth muscle cell proliferation. It can also increase the production of vasoconstriction substrates such as endothelin-1 (ET-1) and angiotensin II [6]. RhoA can induce prothrombotic plasminogen activator inhibitor-1 (PAI-1) expression and activity [116] and impede the expression and activity of tissue plasminogen activator (tPA) in endothelial cells and vascular smooth muscle cells as well as in monocytes/macrophages [117].

same magnitude, it is not surprising that their impact can be closely correlated in some circumstances [9, 10] and not in others [11, 12].

The pleiotropic properties of statins can account for effects observed beyond the prediction of risk by the Framingham equations in clinical trials and effects on event rates that were independent of LDL-C in overlap analysis of placebo- and statin-treated patients [13]. They could also account for the early separation of survival curves between placebo and treatment groups such as in ASCOT (Anglo-Scandinavian Cardiac Outcomes Trial) [14] and CARDS (Collaborative Atorvastatin Diabetes Study) [15] which contrasts to the late separation in the POSCH (Program on the Surgical Control of the Hyperlipidemias) [16] trial in which LDL-C was lowered by partial ileal bypass surgery, not by statin use. Similarly, endothelial dysfunction was improved by simvastatin and not by ezetimibe, a cholesterol absorption inhibitor, in spite of identical reduction in LDL-C [17]. Statins also had a beneficial effect on stroke recurrence in SPARCL (Stroke Prevention by Aggressive Reduction in Cholesterol Levels) [18] even if total cholesterol is not a major risk factor for all causes of stroke. In addition, statins were found to have direct anti-inflammatory effects in the absence of inhibition of HMG-CoA reductase by selectively blocking the interaction between a cell surface integrin (αLβ2) and its corresponding adhesion molecule (ICAM-1) [19]; a purely pleiotropic effect unrelated to cholesterol synthesis or isoprenylation.

Recent advances have revealed beneficial properties in diseases in which cholesterol has little or no contribution to the aetiology. Animal studies have opened the door to potentially new indications for statin use in humans. This chapter addresses some of the emergent clinical indications, focusing in particular on bioprosthetic valve protection, aortic stenosis, arthritis, and sepsis.

CARDIOVASCULAR DISEASE

BIOPROSTHETIC VALVE PROTECTION

Compared to mechanical devices, bioprosthetic valves have low thrombogenicity, do not usually require anticoagulant use and have excellent haemodynamic performance [20]. However, they have limited durability because of structural degeneration. This is presumably due to a combination of mechanical stress, calcification, inflammation, pannus overgrowth and possibly hypercholesterolaemia. There are several manifestations of bioprosthetic valve degeneration including cuspal tears, crescentic tears at the base of the sinus, irregular central tears of the cusp and multiple small perforations. In one report, degeneration of the aortic valve bioprosthetic of a 77-year-old man was caused by marked deposition of cholesterol crystals and a severe foreign body giant cell reaction, 21.5 years after replacement. This observation seemed unrelated to hypercholesterolaemia since his lipoprotein profile had been in the low normal range over the years [21]. Tissue valves are preferred in the elderly and represent up to 70% of all valve replacement devices used in patients $\geqslant$70 years of age [20]. A safe drug that would reduce this degenerative process is highly desirable.

In a systematic retrospective analysis of the echocardiographic database of adults with a bioprosthetic valve (porcine valve or pericardial xenograft) stenosis, Antonini-Canterin and colleagues [22] have shown that degeneration of prosthetic valves is delayed with statin administration. Statin treatment (22 treated compared to 145 untreated patients) significantly decreased the annual rate of increase in peak velocity across the aortic prosthetic valve (m/s/yr) and annual rate of change in indexed effective orifice area (cm^2/m^2/yr) (P <0.001 for both). Age $\geqslant$70 years, presence of diabetes, hypertension, CHD, hypercholesterolaemia >220 mg/dl or body mass index (BMI) $\geqslant$25 kg/m^2 had no effect on these measures. The effects of statins on inflammation, calcification, immune response and dyslipidaemia are likely to account for this beneficial effect. Recently, Skowash and co-workers [23] found a 3.7-fold larger amount of resident C-reactive protein (CRP) in degenerative aortic prosthetic valves than in native cusps. This correlated with serum CRP levels. Both were reduced by statin treatment. Whether statins are used or not, plasma cholesterol measurement is not a useful predictor of bioprosthetic aortic valve structural deterioration according to a prospective study of 7150 patients (mean age 68 ± 12 years) conducted at the Cleveland Clinic [24]. In multivariable analysis, only younger age (P <0.0001), greater body weight (P <0.0001), elevated serum creatinine level (P = 0.0004) and use of a pericardial valve (P = 0.04) predicted structural valve degeneration.

At this time, statin use should be considered in elderly patients undergoing heart valve replacement with a bioprosthesis. However, a sufficiently-powered, prospective, randomised placebo-controlled trial is needed to firmly establish this interesting original observation that is likely to lead to a new indication for statins.

AORTIC VALVE STENOSIS AND SCLEROSIS

Calcific aortic stenosis is the third most common cause of cardiac disease in developed countries and is present in 2–4% of adults over 65 years of age [25]. Due to similarities between atherosclerosis and aortic valve stenosis (AVS), including chronic inflammatory changes (foam-cell macrophages and T-lymphocytes), lipid deposition, calcification and basement membrane disruption (Figure 13.2), it has been suggested that this condition would respond to statin therapy. Like atherosclerosis, AVS is an active inflammatory process [26] and it is likely that pleiotropic effects of statins beyond LDL-C reduction such as anti-inflammatory properties might be beneficial.

This contention is supported by the demonstration in several studies that the progression of aortic stenosis showed no trend of association with LDL-C levels despite statin treatment being associated with slowed progression [12]. Similarly, statin-treated patients have a reduced rate of bioprosthetic valve degeneration in spite of higher cholesterol levels as compared to untreated subjects, a phenomenon attributed to their anti-inflammatory effect [22]. Experimental evidence also supports a multifaceted mechanism of action. In the aortic valve of a cholesterol-fed rabbit model as compared to chow-fed controls, Rajamannan and colleagues [27] found an increase in macrophages, evidence of active myofibroblast proliferation (also referred to as valve interstitial cells, VIC) and increases in bone matrix proteins and markers of enhanced osteoblastic activity (alkaline phosphatase, osteopontin, and the osteoblast lineage-specific transcription factor *Cbfa-1*) (Figure 13.2). All of these early manifestations of aortic valve stenosis were reduced by atorvastatin.

Calcification is an important component of aortic stenosis since it is directly related to the degree of stenosis, while stiffening is the basis for haemodynamic deterioration [28]. In cultured myofibroblasts from porcine aortic valves, Wu and colleagues [29] demonstrated that the effects of statins on bone formation *in vitro* can be dissociated from the effect on cholesterol concentration, and that this action is mediated through inhibition of the cholesterol biosynthetic pathway (i.e. partially reversed by mevalonate but unexpectedly not by Manumycin A, an inhibitor of farnesyl transferase seemingly excluding isoprenylation). Primary cultures of human aortic valve interstitial cells can differentiate into osteoblast-like cells when exposed to an osteogenic medium that results in increased activity and expression of alkaline phosphatase. Osman and colleagues [30] demonstrated that atorvastatin treatment causes a downregulation in the activity of bone morphogenetic protein (BMP) 2 and 6 (stimulators of osteoblastic activity), of transforming growth factor (TGF) β2 and β3 and a significant reduction in alkaline phosphatase activity. Rajamannan and colleagues [31], in another experiment with cholesterol-fed rabbits, showed that atorvastatin inhibited calcification via down-regulation of endothelial nitric oxide synthase (eNOS). Therefore, the osteoblastic differentiation of aortic valve interstitial cells, presumably responsible for valve calcification, can be prevented by a statin. Using electron-beam computed tomography (EBCT) at least 6 months apart, Shavelle and co-workers [32] showed in a retrospective cohort study ($n = 65$) that patients treated by statins ($n = 28$) had a 62–63% lower rate of calcium deposition in the aortic valve and fewer treated patients had progression of aortic valve calcium accumulation ($P < 0.006$). Finally, low-grade inflammation manifested by increased serum vascular cell adhesion molecule 1 (VCAM-1) and by increased valvular and serum CRP has been reported in patients with aortic stenosis, and both VCAM-1 and CRP can be reduced by statin therapy [23, 33].

Several retrospective cohort studies involving a relatively small number of subjects have consistently shown a beneficial effect of statin therapy on the progression of aortic stenosis.

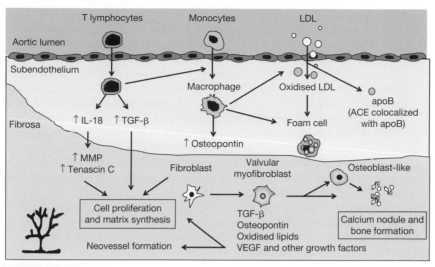

Figure 13.2 Pathways leading to aortic valve stenosis. As in atherosclerosis, infiltration of the endothelium by T lymphocytes, macrophages and LDL takes place. T cells release pro-inflammatory cytokines such as interleukin-18 (IL-18) and transforming growth factor-β (TGF-β). These act on valvular fibroblasts to promote cellular proliferation and extracellular matrix remodelling by matrix metalloproteinases (MMPs) and tenascin C. The latter is a molecule involved in growth promotion, stimulation of bone formation, and mineralisation. It is both co-expressed and overexpressed with MMPs in calcified aortic leaflets. A subset of valvular fibroblasts within the fibrosa layer differentiates into myofibroblasts that have characteristics of smooth muscle cells. They are also called valve interstitial cells (VICs). They maintain the integrity and stability of normal valves and regulate repair processes during disease and following valve injury. They secrete many inflammatory cytokines and chemokines, especially upon activation. These include: TGF-β1, TGF-β3, TNF-α, platelet-derived growth factor-BB, monocyte chemoattractant protein-4 (MCP-4), bone morphogenetic protein-4 (BMP-4), and insulin-like growth factor-4 (IGF-4). Five cell types have been reported: embryonic progenitor endothelial/mesenchymal, quiescent (qVIC), activated (aVIC), progenitor (pVIC), and osteoblastic (obVIC) cells [49]. A subset of valvular myofibroblasts differentiates into an osteoblast phenotype (obVIC) that is capable of promoting calcium nodule and bone formation. They secrete alkaline phosphatase, osteocalcin, osteopontin, bone sialoprotein, chondromodulin-1 and bone morphogenetic proteins (BMP). Macrophages also release osteopontin, a protein needed for bone formation. The avascularity of the heart valves maintained by the expression of chondromodulin-1 is abrogated in aortic stenosis [116, 117]. Chondromodulin-1, a natural anti-angiogenic factor, is downregulated, vascular endothelial growth factor (VEGF) is secreted and new vessels are formed which are most abundant in moderate valve stenosis and in the presence of inflammation. Neovascularisation is reduced by statins. LDL and the apolipoprotein B (apoB) they contain, infiltrating the subendothelial layer, are oxidised and engulfed by macrophages to form foam cells. Angiotensin converting enzyme (ACE) colocalises with apoB and facilitates conversion of angiotensin I to angiotensin II (AngII), which acts on angiotensin-1 receptors (AT-1R), expressed on valvular myofibroblasts (modified with permission from [115]).

Aronow and colleagues [34] studied subjects ⩾60 years of age (mean 82 ± 5 years) with mild aortic stenosis and serum LDL-C ⩾125 mg/dl who were residing in a long-term healthcare institution. Of the 180 subjects followed for 2 or more years, 62 were treated with a statin. By stepwise multiple linear regression analysis, the independent predictors of the peak systolic gradient across the aortic valve were male gender, smoking, arterial hypertension, diabetes mellitus, high LDL-C, low high-density lipoprotein cholesterol (HDL-C) and the use of a statin (an inverse association). Novaro and co-workers [35] evaluated the progression of mild–moderate calcific aortic stenosis over an average of 21 months in high cardiovascular risk subjects with a mean age of 68 ± 12 years (*n* = 174; 57 on a statin). On multivariate analysis, they found that statin usage was a significant independent predictor of a smaller decrease in valve area ($P = 0.01$) and a lesser increase in peak gradient ($P = 0.02$). The community-based study of Bellamy and colleagues [36] involved subjects with a mean age of 77 $\pm$ 12 years and a mean interval of 3.7 years between echocardiographic evaluations ($n = 156$; 38 on statin). The gradient and area across the aortic valve deteriorated in the untreated and improved in the statin-treated subjects. Stenosis progression showed no association with cholesterol levels. The odds ratio of AVS progression with statin treatment was 0.46 (95% confidence interval [CI] 0.21–0.96). Similarly, in 211 consecutive patients (50 on statin) in Austria (70 $\pm$ 10 years of age), Rosenhek and colleagues [37] showed a significant reduction in the progression of mild-to-moderate as well as severe aortic stenosis as measured by peak jet velocity over a 6-month interval. No effect of angiotensin converting enzyme (ACE) inhibitors ($n = 102$) was observed. One other observational retrospective study could not demonstrate any improvement of mild and moderate aortic stenosis on statin treatment although statins did improve aortic sclerosis [38].

In 2005, the Scottish Aortic Stenosis Lipid Lowering Trial, Impact on Regression (SALTIRE), the first randomised, placebo-controlled prospective study, was published [39]. One hundred and fifty-five patients with calcific aortic stenosis were randomised to placebo ($n = 78$; 68 $\pm$ 11 years of age) or atorvastatin 80 mg ($n = 77$; 68 $\pm$ 10 years of age) and followed for a median of 25 months. There were no beneficial effects of statin therapy on aortic stenosis progression, measured by Doppler-echocardiography, or on aortic valve calcium score, measured by helical computed tomography. In this cohort, baseline plasma LDL-C was relatively low (130 $\pm$ 30 mg/dl) and reduced in the statin group to 63 $\pm$ 23 mg/dl. Statins neither halted progression nor induced regression of AVS. There was no relationship between LDL-C levels and progression of aortic stenosis, nor any demonstrable effect of high-dose atorvastatin on clinical endpoints.

More recently, Moura and colleagues [40] demonstrated benefit in the Rosuvastatin Affecting Aortic Valve Endothelium (RAAVE) study, an open-label prospective trial of 121 consecutive patients (mean age 73.7 $\pm$ 8.9 years) with asymptomatic moderate–severe AVS. Sixty-one subjects with an elevated LDL-C receiving 20 mg/day of rosuvastatin were compared with 60 normocholesterolaemic, non statin-treated subjects. They were evaluated by echocardiography every 6 months for 18 months. After a mean follow-up of 73 $\pm$ 24 weeks, the change in aortic valve area in the untreated group was -0.10 ± 0.09 cm^2/year versus -0.05 ± 0.12 cm^2/year in those receiving rosuvastatin ($P = 0.014$). The increase in aortic valve velocity was 0.24 $\pm$ 0.30 m/s/year and 0.04 $\pm$ 0.38 m/s/year in the control and rosuvastatin groups, respectively ($P = 0.007$). There were significant improvements in serum lipid and echocardiographic measures of AVS in the statin group.

The large Simvastatin and Ezetimibe in Aortic Stenosis (SEAS) study has also been published [41]. A total of 1873 patients with mild–moderate aortic stenosis without symptoms and with no indications for statin therapy were randomised to receive simvastatin 40 mg and ezetimibe 10 mg daily or placebo. Despite a reduction in LDL-C of 61% to a mean of 53 mg/dl, treatment with simvastatin and ezetimibe failed to reduce the primary endpoints, a composite of aortic valve disease events and ischaemic events (hazard ratio [HR] 0.96; $P = 0.59$). Nor was there a significant reduction in aortic valve disease events alone, a secondary endpoint (HR 0.97; $P = 0.73$). These events included surgical aortic valve replacement, hospitalisation because of heart failure and cardiovascular death.

Possible explanations for these discordant findings have been reviewed [42]. Major obstacles to contend with in clinical trials of the effects of statins on aortic stenosis include interindividual variation in disease progression [43], unequal distribution of CVD risk factors [44], differences in concomitant medication, limitations in assessment of valvular calcification [45], extent of calcification, severity of valvular disease, inclusion of patients with very severe stenosis, the dose and duration of statin administration, differences among statins, small numbers or loss of power with drop-outs, and exclusion of hyperlipidaemic subjects. Among CHD risk factors that could influence progression of AVS, it is interesting to note that in one study, total cholesterol to HDL-C (TC/HDL-C) ratio (a surrogate predictor of the metabolic syndrome) was an independent predictor of progression of stenosis along with smoking and CHD [46].

The final answer concerning AVS as an indication for statin therapy will also be informed by the results of other ongoing trials. The Aortic Stenosis Progression Observation: Measuring the Effect of Rosuvastatin (ASTRONOMER) study is comparing rosuvastatin 40 mg/day versus placebo in 272 AVS patients not needing statin therapy, who are being recruited from 23 Canadian centres. Changes in severity of AVS are being measured by aortic transvalvular gradient and valve areas, and the rate of cardiac death and aortic valve replacement is the secondary endpoint [47]. Ancillary studies are included to assess the pleiotropic effects of statin beyond cholesterol lowering. Finally, the Italian Society of Cardiovascular Echography (SIEC) is organising a large, observational, multicentre study involving a large network of echo-laboratories, called the Asymptomatic aortic Sclerosis/ Stenosis: Influence of Statins (ASSIST) study [43]. It is designed to follow at least 3000 patients with asymptomatic aortic valve disease for 3–5 years and the proportion of patients that will be taking statin therapy is estimated to range from 20–40%.

Older persons with valvular aortic stenosis have a higher prevalence of CHD risk factors, a higher prevalence of CHD and a higher incidence of new coronary events [34]. This also applies to aortic sclerosis, presumed to be a milder early phase of aortic stenosis. In a cohort of 816 patients from the prospective Heart and Soul Study [48] aortic sclerosis (but not stenosis) was present in 40% of patients with CHD and was independently associated with a 2.4-fold increased rate of subsequent myocardial infarction. In subjects not administered statins ($n = 289$), the adjusted HR was 4.1 (95% CI 1.1–15.7; $P = 0.04$), but in those administered statins ($n = 525$) it was 1.7 (95% CI 0.8–3.9; $P = 0.18$). In this condition where the valve is thickened but the leaflet mobility is preserved, statin treatment still has a beneficial effect. CHD is an indication for statin therapy from the standpoint of secondary prevention alone. It is also noteworthy that in the SEAS study [41], there was a significant reduction in ischaemic events, including non-fatal myocardial infarction, coronary revascularisation, hospitalisation because of unstable angina, non-haemorrhagic stroke and cardiovascular death with simvastatin/ezetimibe (HR 0.78; $P = 0.02$).

There is an increasing prevalence of AVS in ageing adults [33], therefore an effective medical treatment that would avoid surgical management in the frail elderly at high risk of CHD would be particularly worthwhile. Statins may still become indicated in such subjects with aortic sclerosis for preventive purposes. The aortic valve interstitial cells are central to the progression of aortic stenosis, are abundant and exist in five different types (Figure 13.2). The activated type (aVIC) contributes to disease via TGF-β release and other effects on cell migration and proliferation, osteoblast transformation, stimulation of collagen, elastin, proteoglycans and matrix protein alteration [49]. It is encouraging that statins can inhibit osteoblastic differentiation. It will be important in the future to learn more about the effect of statins on specific cell types and on VIC activation.

NON-VASCULAR INFLAMMATORY DISEASES

ARTHRITIS

Because of their anti-inflammatory effects [50] and immunomodulatory properties [51] statins have been tested in many animal models of inflammatory and autoimmune diseases. Beneficial effects have been observed in conditions as diverse as chronic and relapsing autoimmune encephalomyelitis, a model of multiple sclerosis [52–55], other neuroinflammatory disorders [56, 57], spinal cord injury [58], myocarditis [59], cardiac allograft rejection [60, 61], aortic aneurysm [62], nephropathy [63], glomerulonephritis [64], acute peritoneal inflammation [65], colitis [66], allergic asthma [67], and systemic lupus erythematosus [68].

Autoimmune retinal disease was also found to be suppressed by lovastatin [69] but statins had little effect in experimental uveitis [70]. The early demonstration that simvastatin was comparable to indomethacin in reducing the inflammation associated with carrageenan-induced foot pad oedema in mice [71] prompted studies in experimental arthritis models. These met with some success [72–74] and encouraged further studies in humans.

SYSTEMIC JUVENILE IDIOPATHIC ARTHRITIS

The anecdotal but spectacular result of statin therapy in a case of therapy-refractory juvenile idiopathic arthritis (sJIA, Still's disease) stands as a proof of concept that the anti-inflammatory effect of a statin is potent and potentially applicable to cases of severe inflammatory arthritis. Ten Cate and colleagues [75] reported the history of a boy diagnosed with sJIA at the age of 2 years. After a 4-year remission following a varicella infection, a relapse was triggered by a mild respiratory infection. A protracted course ensued, characterised by uncontrolled inflammation, spiking fever, rash, serositis and polyarthralgia refractory to multiple immunomodulatory strategies that included steroids, non-steroidal anti-inflammatory drugs, methotrexate and cyclosporin (Figure 13.3). At the age of 9 years he developed osteoporosis and joint destruction and was soon confined to a wheelchair. There was a temporary relief of 7 weeks after autologous stem cell transplantation and immunosuppression. After that, he again became steroid-dependent, received intra-articular steroids, a treatment with anti-TNF (tumour necrosis factor) agents (infliximab and etanercept) that was stopped because of inefficacy, and a short course of thalidomide that induced acute renal failure. Primarily because of its anti-inflammatory and immunomodulatory properties, atorvastatin was then given in progressively increasing doses from 10 to 30 mg/day. Serum cholesterol had been normal. After atorvastatin was commenced, the disease parameters improved gradually, erythrocyte sedimentation rate and CRP normalised, and prednisone could be tapered and stopped. The improvement was dramatic on atorvastatin 30 mg/day such that after a few months he was no longer wheelchair-dependent and became an active and fully normal child. Until a controlled trial is undertaken to firmly establish a new therapeutic indication, this anecdotal success in a protracted case, resistant to other therapy, warrants other attempts in similar instances in view of the safety profile of the drug and the debilitating effects of the disease.

RHEUMATOID ARTHRITIS

Rheumatoid arthritis is a chronic systemic inflammatory disease affecting multiple joints and leading to deterioration of quality of life and crippling disability. It is associated with accelerated atherosclerosis and increased cardiovascular risk and mortality [76–78]. It also represents a major economic burden on health resources. Autoimmune diseases such as rheumatoid arthritis (RA) and systemic lupus erythematosus (SLE) share many features and pathogenic determinants with atherosclerosis. These include inflammation, immune injury and oxidative stress [79]. Both diseases are major independent risk factors for atherosclerotic vascular disease. Chronic inflammation over time may induce endothelial dysfunction, insulin resistance and a dyslipidaemic lipoprotein profile [76]. Endothelial dysfunction may be present even in young to middle-aged RA patients free from cardiovascular risk factors and with only low disease activity [80]. These findings, and the positive results of animal experimentation, have prompted the use of statin therapy in severely affected patients and the performance of clinical trials [81].

Since 2002, several small-scale pilot studies have indicated the clinical benefit of statins in RA and/or SLE [82–84], while others have demonstrated specific positive effects on endothelial dysfunction [85] and/or systemic arterial stiffness [86].

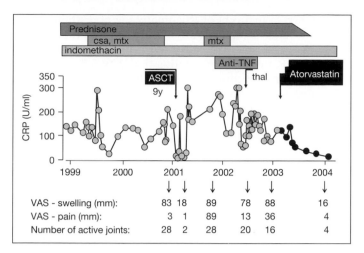

Figure 13.3 A case of refractory juvenile idiopathic arthritis responding to a statin. The protracted course of a patient as reported in [75]. The upper panel shows the time course of CRP and therapeutic interventions, i.e. prednisone, cyclosporin A (csa), methotrexate (mtx), indomethacin (NSAID), infliximab and etanercept infusions (anti-TNF-α), thalidomide (thal) and autologous stem cell transplantation (ASCT). In the lower panel, three PRINTO (Paediatric Rheumatology International Trial Organisation) variables are given: visual analogue scale (VAS, range 0–100 mm) by the paediatrician, VAS by the patient and the number of active joints. A complete list of PRINTO variables is available as supplementary data at Rheumatology Online. After the start of atorvastatin, the disease parameters improved gradually, eosinophil sedimentation rate (ESR) and C-reactive protein (CRP) normalised, and steroids could be tapered and stopped (modified with permission from [75]).

The Trial of Atorvastatin in Rheumatoid Arthritis (TARA) conducted in Glasgow by McCarey and colleagues [87] was the first double-blind, randomised, placebo-controlled trial in RA. Atorvastatin 40 mg daily was administered for 6 months as an adjunct to anti-rheumatic drug therapy to half of 116 subjects who had a median age of 56 years and median disease duration of 11.5 years. The primary outcome measure was disease activity, assessed by a 28-joint Disease Activity Score (DAS28), and the proportion of subjects meeting EULAR (European League Against Rheumatism)–DAS28 binary response criteria. DAS28 improved significantly on atorvastatin (-0.52; 95% CI -0.87– -0.17; $P = 0.004$). The EULAR response was achieved in 31% of patients on atorvastatin compared with 10% in those receiving a placebo (odds ratio [OR] 3.9; 95% CI 1.42–10.72; $P = 0.006$). The count of swollen joints was also reduced by 24% ($P = 0.0058$). More patients on atorvastatin remained on treatment to completion. The primary outcome measure remained significant after adjustment for differences in use of methotrexate. Secondary outcome measures included surrogate markers of vascular risk. There were significant reductions in CRP (-50%; $P <0.0001$) and erythrocyte sedimentation rate (-28%; $P <0.005$), even after adjustment for potential confounders. Plasma viscosity, fibrinogen, sICAM-1 and interleukin (IL)-6 also declined in the atorvastatin group but not in the placebo group. The expected changes in plasma lipoproteins with atorvastatin 40 mg occurred but there was no correlation between changes in LDL-C and disease score changes or other measured variables. Two patients on oral prednisolone at baseline were clinical non-responders. There was no effect of atorvastatin on the health assessment questionnaire. This study showed that statins can mediate clinically significant, albeit modest, anti-inflammatory effects and beneficial modification of cardiovascular risk factors despite the presence of high-grade inflammation in an autoimmune disease.

Recently, a cross-sectional study carried out in Tokyo by Okamoto and colleagues [88] in 4152 patients (83.5% women) from a single-institute-based prospective observational cohort of 7512 RA patients (IORRA; Institute of Rheumatology and Rheumatoid Arthritis) confirmed the beneficial effects of statins in daily rheumatology practice. RA disease activity was measured by patient's assessment of pain, physician evaluation (visual analogue scale), and swollen joint counts. Patients taking statins ($n = 279$; 6.7%) had significantly lower plasma CRP levels and lower joint counts after adjustments for a slightly more frequent use of corticosteroids in subjects not using a statin.

Mechanisms responsible for the favourable impact of statins in RA have recently been reviewed [78, 89, 90]. They include the well-established cardioprotective properties of statins [91], their anti-inflammatory, immunomodulating and anti-oxidant effects, but also effects, that directly affect synovial inflammation. In one study, fluvastatin and pitavastatin, but not pravastatin, induced apoptosis of synoviocytes from RA patients *in vitro*. This occurred via a mitochondrial-and caspase 3-dependent pathway, and by inhibition of geranylgeranylation of RhoA which is needed for synoviocyte attachment to the membrane where they are activated [92]. This effect on RA cells was not observed with synoviocytes obtained from patients with non-RA osteoarthropathy. This is an important finding since the activation and proliferation of synovial cells is thought to be a key step in the destruction of cartilaginous and bony tissues in RA joints. In a 12-week placebo-controlled trial in patients with active RA without dyslipidaemia ($n = 20$), Charles-Schoeman and colleagues [93] demonstrated that high doses of atorvastatin rendered HDL more anti-inflammatory. This is interesting since it has been reported that in non-RA patients with CHD, HDL may become pro-inflammatory and pro-atherogenic and that this can be improved with simvastatin treatment [94].

A new indication for statin therapy in RA as an add-on to disease-modifying antirheumatic drugs (DMARD) may be established on the following grounds:

1. The frequency, severity and protracted course of RA.
2. Similarities with atherosclerosis and the associated increased incidence of cardiovascular disease.
3. Refractoriness or intolerance in many patients to the current therapeutic approaches.
4. The strength of the experimental evidence in models of autoimmune arthritis.
5. The established cardio-and vasculoprotective effects of statins via their pleiotropic effects.
6. The established long-term safety of statin administration.
7. The evidence of specific effects on RA synovitis.
8. The evidence of anti-inflammatory and immunomodulatory effects additive to DMARD translated into significant clinical benefit in several pilot studies, in a controlled clinical trial and in an observational study.

Caution should be exercised for potential drug interactions, however, and future studies must address:

■ Potential differences in efficacy according to the stage of the disease, the particular statin and dose administered, and possible interaction with concomitant medications.
■ Whether long-term administration will improve cardiovascular outcomes in RA.

SEPSIS

Sepsis is a devastating systemic response to infection and is characterised by systemic inflammation involving many signalling pathways that result in widespread tissue injury [95]. Its incidence is rising and the mortality rate is high. Since the strategy of blocking a single element of the many inflammatory pathways involved has neither been entirely successful nor necessarily affordable, approaches that target many mediators of inflammation have been considered. Among these, statins became promising candidates because of the benefit they exerted in diseases involving vascular inflammation and injury [96]. A series of animal and human studies have tested this hypothesis.

Cerivastatin was found to dramatically improve survival (73% vs. 27% at 7 days; P = 0.016) in lipopolysaccharide-induced manifestations of sepsis in mice, resulting in significant reductions in markers of sepsis (TNF-α and IL-1β peak at 2 hours and nitric oxide increase at 8 hours) [97]. In another study in a mouse model of sepsis (caecal ligation and perforation [CLP]), treatment with simvastatin increased survival time nearly 4-fold with complete preservation of cardiac and haemodynamic function as compared to untreated mice [98]. Later, the improvement in survival in the model was shown to take place even when statin treatment was initiated *after* the onset of sepsis [99]. Acute kidney injury occurs in 51% of septic shock patients with positive blood culture and is associated with 70% mortality [100]. In elderly CLP mice with kidney injury, simvastatin improved mortality, attenuated tubular damage and reversed CLP-induced reduction of intrarenal microvascular perfusion, renal tubular hypoxia at 24 hours, and restored towards normal CLP-induced renal vascular protein leak and serum TNF-α [101]. The improved sepsis-induced acute kidney injury with simvastatin was attributed to direct actions on the renal vasculature, reversal of tubular hypoxia and a systemic anti-inflammatory effect. In summary, much insight has been gained over the past few years into the mechanisms whereby statins could be contributing to a beneficial effect in sepsis (Figure 13.4).

In parallel, several observations in patients with sepsis have indicated a protective effect of statins. In a retrospective review of 388 bacteraemic infections due to aerobic Gram-negative bacilli or *Staphylococcus aureus*, Liappis and co-workers [102] reported a significant reduction in both overall (6% vs. 28%; P = 0.002) and attributable (3% vs. 20%; P = 0.010) mortality among patients taking statins compared with patients not taking statins. In a prospective observational cohort of 361 patients admitted for presumed or documented bacterial infections (pneumonia, cellulitis or urinary tract infection) studied by Almog and colleagues [103], only 2.4% of 82 patients treated with statins before their admission developed severe sepsis as compared to 19% of the 279 non-statin treated subjects. Statin treatment was associated with a relative risk (RR) of developing severe sepsis of 0.13 (95% CI 0.03–0.52), reflecting an absolute risk reduction of 16.6%. In addition, the overall rate of admission to the intensive care unit was significantly reduced (3.7% vs. 12.2%; P = 0.025; RR 0.30; 95% CI 0.1–0.95). In both studies, statin-users had significantly higher rates of major comorbidities than did non-users, suggesting that coexisting illness was not responsible for the findings. One Danish observational study based on prospective registration of episodes of bacteraemia and mortality over a 6-year period reported by Thomsen and colleagues [104] did not find a difference in 30-day mortality after a positive blood culture between statin-users (n = 176) and non-users (n = 5177). This is in contrast with the report of Liappis and colleagues [102] and that of Mortensen and co-workers [105]. However, Thomsen and colleagues observed a substantial reduction in mortality up to 180 days after diagnosed bacteremia (8.4% vs. 17.5%; adjusted mortality rate ratio 0.44; 95% CI 0.24–0.80). A very large observational study using linked administrative databases was carried out in Ontario, Canada, by Hackam and colleagues [106] in 2006 to evaluate the impact of statin treatment on sepsis. These investigators identified 141 487 patients older than 65 years of age admitted between 1997 and 2002 with cardiovascular disease who survived for at least 3 months after discharge. After propensity-based matching and careful adjustment for confounders, the study yielded a well-paired and homogeneous cohort of 69 168 patients, half of whom had received statin within 90 days of discharge. There was a 19% reduction in the incidence of sepsis with statin use that was maintained after adjustment for demographic characteristics, sepsis risk factors, comorbidities and aspects of healthcare (HR 0.81; 95% CI 0.72–0.90). The protection afforded by statins persisted in high-risk subgroups, such as in patients with diabetes, chronic renal failure, or a history of infections. It also included reductions in severe (-16%) as well as in fatal sepsis (-25%). No protection was observed

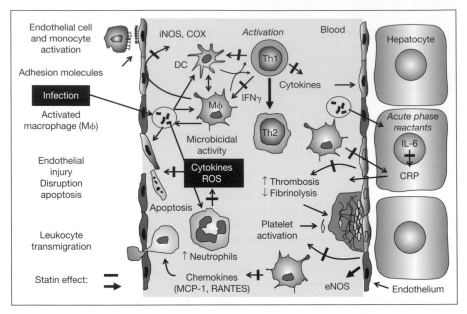

Figure 13.4 Pleiotropic effects of statins in sepsis. Sepsis may initially be characterised by increases in inflammatory mediators (*the uncontrolled inflammatory response*) but as it persists there is a shift towards an anti-inflammatory immunosuppressive state, therefore treatment effects may be different depending on the stage of evolution [118]. Sepsis induces activation of the inflammatory cascade, cytokine release and endothelial dysfunction and leads to tissue injury and organ dysfunction. A positive effect of statin is indicated by a thick arrow, a negative or inhibitory effect by a thick line crossing a thin arrow. Infection represented by pathogens (circle) induces direct activation of neutrophils, macrophages (Mφ) and dendritic cells (DC) by ingestion of bacteria or indirect activation by pro-inflammatory helper T cells (Th1) via interferon-gamma (IFNγ). *Statins tend to shift naive T cells toward formation of Th2 cells that release anti-inflammatory cytokines such as IL-10 which suppresses macrophage activation. Statins also suppress Th1 cell activity and therefore cytokine release.* The infectious process also induces endothelial cell activation through the concerted action of the pathogens (lipopolysaccharide [LPS], endotoxin), CRP released by macrophages or by acute phase reactants (IL-6, IL-1β) in the liver (cells on the right), and other cytokines released by T cells, macrophages and neutrophils, their count being increased by the infection. Endothelial activation results in surface expression of adhesion molecules (VCAM-1, ICAM-1, selectins), interaction of endothelium with leucocytes (expression of monocyte cell surface integrins) and release of chemokines (such as monocyte chemoattractant protein-1 (MCP-1) and 'regulated upon activation normal T cells expressed and secreted' (RANTES)) that attract leucocytes to site of infection or tissue damage and favour their transmigration. There is a reduction of endothelial nitric oxide synthase (eNOS) and an increase of inducible NOS (iNOS) and of the inflammatory molecule cyclooxygenase (COX), leading to endothelial vasoreactive dysfunction to which release of reactive oxygen species (ROS) by the various activated cells contributes. *Statins inhibit chemokine (MCP-1, RANTES) and cytokine (IL-8) expression and reduce expression of adhesion molecules. They increase nitric oxide production by eNOS and improve endothelial dysfunction.* Sepsis is also associated with a procoagulant state (lower right). Macrophages and activated endothelium produce tissue factor (TF), the main activator of coagulation; thrombomodulin is downregulated and low, which renders the anticoagulant protein C ineffective; the endothelium releases prothrombotic (PAI-1) and antifibrinolytic molecules (tPA). Platelets are activated by endotoxins or by the platelet activation factor (PAF). *Statins abrogate this procoagulant state by blunting monocyte TF expression, increasing thrombomodulin expression and function (therefore improving the relative protein C deficiency), and increasing endothelial cell-derived tissue plasminogen activator (tPA)* (modified with permission from [113]).

with lipid-lowering agents other than statins. Recently, in 11 362 patients with atherosclerosis followed for 3 years, Almog and colleagues [107] reported that mortality due to infection was reduced by 78% in subjects using a statin during the last month of follow-up as compared to non-users, even though statin-users had more cardiovascular comorbidities including obesity, dyslipidaemia and hypertension. However, the Charlson index, which computes the burden of as many as 19 comorbid conditions, was equal among the two groups, and after adjusting for all known possible confounders using stepwise Cox proportional hazard survival analysis, including a propensity score for receiving statins, the protective effect of statins remained highly significant (HR 0.37; 95% CI 0.27–0.52). The protective effect appeared to dissipate upon discontinuation of the statin. In patients with chronic kidney disease (n = 1041), Gupta and co-workers [108] in a multicentre study of a cohort followed for 3.4 years demonstrated that rates of hospitalisation for sepsis (n = 303) were significantly reduced in statin-users (41/1000 patient-years; n = 143) as compared to non-users (110/1000 patient-years; n = 898; P <0.001). This effect persisted after adjusting for demographics, dialysis modality, comorbidities and laboratory values (incidence rate ratio 0.38; 95% CI 0.21–0.67) and in a propensity-matched subcohort, statin use was even more protective (incidence rate ratio 0.24; 95% CI 0.11–0.49).

Therefore, the results of the available observational studies consistently support a protective effect of statins in patients with sepsis. These are not randomised comparisons. However, the congruence of the findings in observational studies suggest that statin administration is associated with reduced incidence and severity of sepsis, improvement in vascular complications, a reduction in mortality which is perhaps greater in the long term than in the short term, and a consistent trend for a reduced admission to intensive care units. Discrepancies between studies [105, 109, 110] may be explained partly by differences in the statin and dose used (not always mentioned) and the duration of administration, age of subjects, gender distribution, clinical setting, type of associated comorbidities and medication, the study design (sample size, number of centres, database used), possible withdrawal of statins (which was not accounted for), and the primary source of infection. Mechanisms evoked for this beneficial effect of statins are largely related to their pleiotropic effects, particularly their anti-inflammatory and immunomodulatory properties and their ability to improve endothelial dysfunction. In one small retrospective cohort study, which showed a 30% lower rate of severe sepsis but no reduction in in-hospital mortality on a statin, the rate of cardiovascular dysfunction defined as hypotension requiring vasopressor therapy was significantly lower in those treated with a statin (38% vs. 73%; P <0.02) [111]. Statins do not have direct antibacterial activity but they do influence a broad array of pathogenic micro-organisms (see [96] for review).

The early and profound protection observed in animals with sepsis, the evidence gathered from observational studies in humans, the magnitude of such effects and the established safety of statin therapy suggest that statins may be used in the future for the prevention of complications of bacteraemia or sepsis, especially in the elderly and in extreme cases such as in the presence of kidney injury where there is virtually no effective therapy. It is noteworthy that the one effective treatment for severe sepsis in patients who are at high risk of death, recombinant activated protein C, is expensive, can cause serious bleeding, and is reserved for those who have multiple organ failure, a high risk of death and a low risk for bleeding [96].

However, prospective, randomised, placebo-controlled trials (if deemed ethical) may need to be done to definitely establish sepsis as an indication for statin use and to optimise doses, timing and duration of treatment. One of the first steps towards establishing this indication would be to change the current prescribing guidelines in some countries recommending that statins be discontinued in critically ill patients since sepsis is a leading cause of death in such patients [112]. It is certain that it would be ill-advised to discontinue statins in those being treated appropriately for dyslipidaemia or for secondary prevention of CHD when life-threatening infections occur, given the deleterious cardiovascular consequences that might then develop [113].

CONCLUSIONS

We have discussed here but a few of the conditions that are evolving towards new indications for statin therapy. In considering these, one must distinguish between prevention and treatment, between use as monotherapy or typically in combination with other proven therapies and whether there already exists another indication to prescribe a statin (e.g. secondary prevention of CHD, atherogenic dyslipoproteinaemia). Concomitant medication must be appraised because of the possibility of drug interactions. Potential side-effects, effectiveness and the cost of standard therapy must also be considered. The congruence and strength of the evidence are both important. These considerations can enlighten the decision of the physician to prevent, heal and do no harm, taking each case individually and maximizing the results of his or her intervention with full knowledge of the clinical context. This is crucial for most of the conditions we have selected, in which hard evidence for benefit is either still to be obtained, is forthcoming, or cannot be obtained for ethical reasons or because of the rarity of the disease.

REFERENCES

1. Rosenberg ME, Silkensen J. Clusterin: physiologic and pathophysiologic considerations. *Int J Biochem Cell Biol* 1995; 27:633–645.
2. Berger J, Moller DE. The mechanisms of action of PPARs. *Annu Rev Med* 2002; 53:409–435.
3. Liao JK. Isoprenoids as mediators of the biological effects of statins. *J Clin Invest* 2002; 110:285–288.
4. Davignon J. Beneficial cardiovascular pleiotropic effects of statins. *Circulation* 2004; 109:39–43.
5. Liao JK, Laufs U. Pleiotropic effects of statins. *Annu Rev Pharmacol Toxicol* 2005; 45:89–118.
6. Noma K, Oyama N, Liao JK. Physiological role of ROCKs in the cardiovascular system. *Am J Physiol Cell Physiol* 2006; 290:C661–C668.
7. Robinson JG, Smith B, Maheshwari N, Schrott H. Pleiotropic effects of statins: Benefit beyond cholesterol reduction? A meta-regression analysis. *J Am Coll Cardiol* 2005; 46:1855–1862.
8. Wang TJ, Gona P, Larson MG *et al*. Multiple biomarkers for the prediction of first major cardiovascular events and death. *N Engl J Med* 2006; 355:2631–2639.
9. Kohno M, Murakawa K, Yasunari K *et al*. Improvement of erythrocyte deformability by cholesterol-lowering therapy with pravastatin in hypercholesterolemic patients. *Metabolism* 1997; 46:287–291.
10. De Caterina R, Cipollone F, Filardo FP *et al*. Low-density lipoprotein level reduction by the 3-hydroxy-3-methylglutaryl coenzyme-A inhibitor simvastatin is accompanied by a related reduction of F_2-isoprostane formation in hypercholesterolemic subjects: no further effect of vitamin E. *Circulation* 2002; 106:2543–2549.
11. Ridker PM, Cannon CP, Morrow D *et al*. C-reactive protein levels and outcomes after statin therapy. *N Engl J Med* 2005; 352:20–28.
12. Chua D, Kalb K. Statins and progression of calcified aortic stenosis. *Ann Pharmacother* 2006; 40:2195–2199.
13. Packard CJ, Shepherd J, Cobbe SM *et al*. Influence of pravastatin and plasma lipids on clinical events in the West of Scotland Coronary Prevention Study (WOSCOPS). *Circulation* 1998; 97:1440–1445.
14. Sever PS, Dahlöf B, Poulter NR *et al*. Prevention of coronary and stroke events with atorvastatin in hypertensive patients who have average or lower-than-average cholesterol concentrations, in the Anglo-Scandinavian Cardiac Outcomes Trial-Lipid Lowering Arm (ASCOT-LLA): a multicentre randomised controlled trial. *Lancet* 2003; 361:1149–1158.
15. Colhoun HM, Betteridge DJ, Durrington PN *et al*. Primary prevention of cardiovascular disease with atorvastatin in type 2 diabetes in the Collaborative Atorvastatin Diabetes Study (CARDS): multicentre randomised placebo-controlled trial. *Lancet* 2004; 364:685–696.
16. Buchwald H, Varco RL, Matts JP *et al*. Effect of partial ileal bypass surgery on mortality and morbidity from coronary heart disease in patients with hypercholesterolemia. report of the Program on the Surgical Control of the Hyperlipidemias (POSCH). *N Engl J Med* 1990; 323:946–955.
17. Landmesser U, Bahlmann F, Mueller M *et al*. Simvastatin versus ezetimibe: pleiotropic and lipid-lowering effects on endothelial function in humans. *Circulation* 2005; 111:2356–2363.

18. Amarenco P, Bogousslavsky J, Callahan A *et al.* High-dose atorvastatin after stroke or transient ischemic attack. *N Engl J Med* 2006; 355:549–559.

19. Weitz-Schmidt G, Welzenbach K, Brinkmann V *et al.* Statins selectively inhibit leukocyte function antigen-1 by binding to a novel regulatory integrin site. *Nat Med* 2001; 7:687–692.

20. Colli A, Gherli T, Mestres CA, Pomar JL. Degeneration of native and tissue prosthetic valve in aortic position: do statins play an effective role in prevention? *Int J Cardiol* 2007; 116:144–152.

21. Price L, Sniderman A, Omerglu A, Lachapelle K. Bioprosthetic valve degeneration due to cholesterol deposition in a patient with normal lipid profile. *Can J Cardiol* 2007; 23:233–234.

22. Antonini-Canterin F, Zuppiroli A, Popescu BA *et al.* Effect of statins on the progression of bioprosthetic aortic valve degeneration. *Am J Cardiol* 2003; 92:1479–1482.

23. Skowasch D, Schrempf S, Preusse CJ *et al.* Tissue resident C reactive protein in degenerative aortic valves: correlation with serum C reactive protein concentrations and modification by statins. *Heart* 2006; 92:495–498.

24. Gring CN, Houghtaling P, Novaro GM *et al.* Preoperative cholesterol levels do not predict explant for structural valve deterioration in patients undergoing bioprosthetic aortic valve replacement. *J Heart Valve Dis* 2006; 15:261–268.

25. Rajamannan NM, Gersh B, Bonow RO. Calcific aortic stenosis: from bench to the bedside – emerging clinical and cellular concepts. *Heart* 2003; 89:801–805.

26. Helske S, Kupari M, Lindstedt KA, Kovanen PT. Aortic valve stenosis: an active atheroinflammatory process. *Curr Opin Lipidol* 2007; 18:483–491.

27. Rajamannan NM, Subramaniam M, Springett M *et al.* Atorvastatin inhibits hypercholesterolemia-induced cellular proliferation and bone matrix production in the rabbit aortic valve. *Circulation* 2002; 105:2660–2665.

28. Borer JS. Aortic stenosis and statins: more evidence of 'pleotropy'? *Arterioscler Thromb Vasc Biol* 2005; 25:476–477.

29. Wu B, Elmariah S, Kaplan FS, Cheng GJ, Mohler ER III. Paradoxical effects of statins on aortic valve myofibroblasts and osteoblasts: implications for end-stage valvular heart disease. *Arterioscler Thromb Vasc Biol* 2005; 25:592–597.

30. Osman L, Yacoub MH, Latif N, Amrani M, Chester AH. Role of human valve interstitial cells in valve calcification and their response to atorvastatin. *Circulation* 2006; 114:I547–I552.

31. Rajamannan NM, Subramaniam M, Stock SR *et al.* Atorvastatin inhibits calcification and enhances nitric oxide synthase production in the hypercholesterolaemic aortic valve. *Heart* 2005; 91:806–810.

32. Shavelle DM, Takasu J, Budoff MJ, Mao SS, Zhao XQ, O'Brien KD. HMG CoA reductase inhibitor (statin) and aortic valve calcium. *Lancet* 2002; 359:1125–1126.

33. Pate GE, Tahir MN, Murphy RT, Foley JB. Anti-inflammatory effects of statins in patients with aortic stenosis. *J Cardiovasc Pharmacol Ther* 2003; 8:201–206.

34. Aronow WS, Ahn C, Kronzon I, Goldman ME. Association of coronary risk factors and use of statins with progression of mild valvular aortic stenosis in older persons. *Am J Cardiol* 2001; 88:693–695.

35. Novaro GM, Tiong IY, Pearce GL, Lauer MS, Sprecher DL, Griffin BP. Effect of hydroxymethylglutaryl coenzyme A reductase inhibitors on the progression of calcific aortic stenosis. *Circulation* 2001; 104:2205–2209.

36. Bellamy MF, Pellikka PA, Klarich KW, Tajik AJ, Enriquez-Sarano M. Association of cholesterol levels, hydroxymethylglutaryl coenzyme-A reductase inhibitor treatment, and progression of aortic stenosis in the community. *J Am Coll Cardiol* 2002; 40:1723–1730.

37. Rosenhek R, Rader F, Loho N *et al.* Statins but not angiotensin-converting enzyme inhibitors delay progression of aortic stenosis. *Circulation* 2004; 110:1291–1295.

38. Antonini-Canterin F, Popescu BA, Huang G *et al.* Progression of aortic valve sclerosis and aortic valve stenosis: what is the role of statin treatment? *Ital Heart J* 2005; 6:119–124.

39. Cowell SJ, Newby DE, Prescott RJ *et al.* A randomized trial of intensive lipid-lowering therapy in calcific aortic stenosis. *N Engl J Med* 2005; 352:2389–2397.

40. Moura LM, Ramos SF, Zamorano JL *et al.* Rosuvastatin affecting aortic valve endothelium to slow the progression of aortic stenosis. *J Am Coll Cardiol* 2007; 49:554–561.

41. Rossebo AB, Pedersen TR, Boman K *et al.* Intensive lipid lowering with simvastatin and ezetimibe in aortic stenosis. *N Engl J Med* 2008; 359:1343–1356.

42. Newby DE, Cowell SJ, Boon NA. Emerging medical treatments for aortic stenosis: statins, angiotensin converting enzyme inhibitors, or both? *Heart* 2006; 92:729–734.

43. Antonini-Canterin F, Corrado G, Faggiano P et al. A medical therapy for aortic valve sclerosis and aortic valve stenosis? Rationale of the ASSIST study (Asymptomatic aortic Sclerosis/Stenosis: Influence of STatins): a large, observational, prospective, multicenter study of the Italian Society of Cardiovascular Echography. J Cardiovasc Med (Hagerstown) 2006; 7:464–469.

44. Aronow WS, Schwartz KS, Koenigsberg M. Correlation of serum lipids, calcium, and phosphorus, diabetes mellitus and history of systemic hypertension with presence or absence of calcified or thickened aortic cusps or root in elderly patients. Am J Cardiol 1987; 59:998–999.

45. Melina G, Rubens MB, Yacoub MH. Statins, electron-beam CT, and aortic-valve calcification. Lancet 2002; 360:258.

46. Yilmaz MB, Guray U, Guray Y et al. Lipid profile of patients with aortic stenosis might be predictive of rate of progression. Am Heart J 2004; 147:915–918.

47. Chan KL, Teo K, Tam J, Dumesnil JG. Rationale, design, and baseline characteristics of a randomized trial to assess the effect of cholesterol lowering on the progression of aortic stenosis: the Aortic Stenosis Progression Observation: Measuring Effects of Rosuvastatin (ASTRONOMER) trial. Am Heart J 2007; 153:925–931.

48. Shah SJ, Ristow B, Ali S, Na BY, Schiller NB, Whooley MA. Acute myocardial infarction in patients with versus without aortic valve sclerosis and effect of statin therapy (from the Heart and Soul Study). Am J Cardiol 2007; 99:1128–1133.

49. Liu AC, Joag VR, Gotlieb AI. The emerging role of valve interstitial cell phenotypes in regulating heart valve pathobiology. Am J Pathol 2007; 171:1407–1418.

50. Abeles AM, Pillinger MH. Statins as anti-inflammatory and immunomodulatory agents: a future in rheumatologic therapy? Arthritis Rheum 2006; 54:393–407.

51. Kwak B, Mulhaupt F, Myit S, Mach F. Statins as a newly recognized type of immunomodulator. Nat Med 2000; 6:1399–1402.

52. Stanislaus R, Pahan K, Singh AK, Singh I. Amelioration of experimental allergic encephalomyelitis in Lewis rats by lovastatin. Neurosci Lett 1999; 269:71–74.

53. Youssef S, Stüve O, Patarroyo JC et al. The HMG-CoA reductase inhibitor, atorvastatin, promotes a Th2 bias and reverses paralysis in central nervous system autoimmune disease. Nature 2002; 420:78–84.

54. Aktas O, Waiczies S, Smorodchenko A et al. Treatment of relapsing paralysis in experimental encephalomyelitis by targeting Th1 cells through atorvastatin. J Exp Med 2003; 197:725–733.

55. Paintlia AS, Paintlia MK, Singh AK et al. Regulation of gene expression associated with acute experimental autoimmune encephalomyelitis by Lovastatin. J Neurosci Res 2004; 77:63–81.

56. Stüve O, Youssef S, Steinman L, Zamvil SS. Statins as potential therapeutic agents in neuroinflammatory disorders. Curr Opin Neurol 2003; 16:393–401.

57. Turowski P, Adamson P, Greenwood J. Pharmacological targeting of ICAM-1 signaling in brain endothelial cells: potential for treating neuroinflammation. Cell Mol Neurobiol 2005; 25:153–170.

58. Pannu R, Barbosa E, Singh AK, Singh I. Attenuation of acute inflammatory response by atorvastatin after spinal cord injury in rats. J Neurosci Res 2005; 79:340–350.

59. Azuma RW, Suzuki J, Ogawa M et al. HMG-CoA reductase inhibitor attenuates experimental autoimmune myocarditis through inhibition of T cell activation. Cardiovasc Res 2004; 64:412–420.

60. Maggard MA, Ke BB, Wang T et al. Effects of pravastatin on chronic rejection of rat cardiac allografts. Transplantation 1998; 65:149–155.

61. Shimizu K, Aikawa M, Takayama K, Libby P, Mitchell RN. Direct anti-inflammatory mechanisms contribute to attenuation of experimental allograft arteriosclerosis by statins. Circulation 2003; 108:2113–2120.

62. Steinmetz EF, Buckley C, Shames ML et al. Treatment with simvastatin suppresses the development of experimental abdominal aortic aneurysms in normal and hypercholesterolemic mice. Ann Surg 2005; 241:92–101.

63. Li C, Yang CW, Park JH et al. Pravastatin treatment attenuates interstitial inflammation and fibrosis in a rat model of chronic cyclosporine-induced nephropathy. Am J Physiol Renal Physiol 2004; 286:F46–F57.

64. Christensen M, Su AW, Snyder RW, Greco A, Lipschutz JH, Madaio MP. Simvastatin protection against acute immune-mediated glomerulonephritis in mice. Kidney Int 2006; 69:457–463.

65. Fischetti F, Carretta R, Borotto G et al. Fluvastatin treatment inhibits leucocyte adhesion and extravasation in models of complement-mediated acute inflammation. Clin Exp Immunol 2004; 135:186–193.

66. Naito Y, Katada K, Takagi T et al. Rosuvastatin, a new HMG-CoA reductase inhibitor, reduces the colonic inflammatory response in dextran sulfate sodium-induced colitis in mice. Int J Mol Med 2006; 17:997–1004.

67. McKay A, Leung BP, McInnes IB, Thomson NC, Liew FY. A novel anti-inflammatory role of simvastatin in a murine model of allergic asthma. *J Immunol* 2004; 172:2903–2908.

68. Lawman S, Mauri C, Jury EC, Cook HT, Ehrenstein MR. Atorvastatin inhibits autoreactive B cell activation and delays lupus development in New Zealand black/white F₁ mice. *J Immunol* 2004; 173:7641–7646.

69. Gegg ME, Harry R, Hankey D *et al.* Suppression of autoimmune retinal disease by lovastatin does not require Th2 cytokine induction. *J Immunol* 2005; 174:2327–2335.

70. Thomas PB, Albini T, Giri RK, See RF, Evans M, Rao NA. The effects of atorvastatin in experimental autoimmune uveitis. *Br J Ophthalmol* 2005; 89:275–279.

71. Sparrow CP, Burton CA, Hernandez M *et al.* Simvastatin has anti-inflammatory and antiatherosclerotic activities independent of plasma cholesterol lowering. *Arterioscler Thromb Vasc Biol* 2001; 21:115–121.

72. Barsante MM, Roffê E, Yokoro CM *et al.* Anti-inflammatory and analgesic effects of atorvastatin in a rat model of adjuvant-induced arthritis. *Eur J Pharmacol* 2005; 516:282–289.

73. Palmer G, Chobaz V, Talabot-Ayer D *et al.* Assessment of the efficacy of different statins in murine collagen-induced arthritis. *Arthritis Rheum* 2004; 50:4051–4059.

74. Yamagata T, Kinoshita K, Nozaki Y, Sugiyama M, Ikoma S, Funauchi M. Effects of pravastatin in murine collagen-induced arthritis. *Rheumatol Int* 2007; 27:631–639.

75. Ten Cate R, Nibbering PH, Bredius RGM. Therapy-refractory systemic juvenile idiopathic arthritis successfully treated with statins. *Rheumatology* 2004; 43:934–935.

76. Gonzalez-Gay MA, Gonzalez-Juanatey C, Martin J. Rheumatoid arthritis: a disease associated with accelerated atherogenesis. *Semin Arthritis Rheum* 2005; 35:8–17.

77. Watson DJ, Rhodes T, Guess HA. All-cause mortality and vascular events among patients with rheumatoid arthritis, osteoarthritis, or no arthritis in the UK General Practice Research Database. *J Rheumatol* 2003; 30:1196–1202.

78. Paraskevas KI. Statin treatment for rheumatoid arthritis: a promising novel indication. *Clin Rheumatol* 2008; 27:281–287.

79. Abou-Raya A, Abou-Raya S. Inflammation: a pivotal link between autoimmune diseases and atherosclerosis. *Autoimmun Rev* 2006; 5:331–337.

80. Vaudo G, Marchesi S, Gerli R *et al.* Endothelial dysfunction in young patients with rheumatoid arthritis and low disease activity. *Ann Rheum Dis* 2004; 63:31–35.

81. Gazi IF, Boumpas DT, Mikhailidis DP, Ganotakis ES. Clustering of cardiovascular risk factors in rheumatoid arthritis: the rationale for using statins. *Clin Exp Rheumatol* 2007; 25:102–111.

82. Kanda H, Hamasaki K, Kubo K *et al.* Antiinflammatory effect of simvastatin in patients with rheumatoid arthritis. *J Rheumatol* 2002; 29:2024–2026.

83. Abud-Mendoza C, de la Fuente H, Cuevas-Orta E, Baranda L, Cruz-Rizo J, Gonzalez-Amaro R. Therapy with statins in patients with refractory rheumatic diseases: a preliminary study. *Lupus* 2003; 12:607–611.

84. Maki-Petaja KM, Booth AD, Hall FC *et al.* Ezetimibe and simvastatin reduce inflammation, disease activity, and aortic stiffness and improve endothelial function in rheumatoid arthritis. *J Am Coll Cardiol* 2007; 50:852–858.

85. Hermann F, Forster A, Chenevard R *et al.* Simvastatin improves endothelial function in patients with rheumatoid arthritis. *J Am Coll Cardiol* 2005; 45:461–464.

86. Van Doornum S, McColl G, Wicks IP. Atorvastatin reduces arterial stiffness in patients with rheumatoid arthritis. *Ann Rheum Dis* 2004; 63:1571–1575.

87. McCarey DW, McInnes LB, Madhok R *et al.* Trial of Atorvastatin in Rheumatoid Arthritis (TARA): double-blind, randomised placebo-controlled trial. *Lancet* 2004; 363:2015–2021.

88. Okamoto H, Koizumi K, Kamitsuji S *et al.* Beneficial action of statins in patients with rheumatoid arthritis in a large observational cohort. *J Rheumatol* 2007; 34:964–968.

89. Abeles AM, Marjanovic N, Park J *et al.* Protein isoprenylation regulates secretion of matrix metalloproteinase 1 from rheumatoid synovial fibroblasts: effects of statins and farnesyl and geranylgeranyl transferase inhibitors. *Arthritis Rheum* 2007; 56:2840–2853.

90. Tristano AG, Fuller K. Immunomodulatory effects of statins and autoimmune rheumatic diseases: novel intracellular mechanism involved. *Int Immunopharmacol* 2006; 6:1833–1846.

91. Davignon J. The cardioprotective effects of statins. *Curr Atheroscler Rep* 2004; 6:27–35.

92. Nagashima T, Okazaki H, Yudoh K, Matsuno H, Minota S. Apoptosis of rheumatoid synovial cells by statins through the blocking of protein geranylgeranylation – a potential therapeutic approach to rheumatoid arthritis. *Arthritis Rheum* 2006; 54:579–586.

93. Charles-Schoeman C, Khanna D, Furst DE *et al*. Effects of high-dose atorvastatin on antiinflammatory properties of high density lipoprotein in patients with rheumatoid arthritis: a pilot study. *J Rheumatol* 2007; 34:1459–1464.

94. Ansell BJ, Navab M, Hama S *et al*. Inflammatory/antiinflammatory properties of high-density lipoprotein distinguish patients from control subjects better than high-density lipoprotein cholesterol levels and are favorably affected by simvastatin treatment. *Circulation* 2003; 108:2751–2756.

95. Marshall JC. Sepsis: current status, future prospects. *Curr Opin Crit Care* 2004; 10:250–264.

96. Terblanche M, Almog Y, Rosenson RS, Smith TS, Hackam DG. Statins: panacea for sepsis? *Lancet Infect Dis* 2006; 6:242–248.

97. Ando H, Takamura T, Ota T, Nagai Y, Kobayashi K. Cerivastatin improves survival of mice with lipopolysaccharide-induced sepsis. *J Pharmacol Exp Ther* 2000; 294:1043–1046.

98. Merx MW, Liehn EA, Janssens U *et al*. HMG-CoA reductase inhibitor simvastatin profoundly improves survival in a murine model of sepsis. *Circulation* 2004; 109:2560–2565.

99. Merx MW, Liehn EA, Graf J *et al*. Statin treatment after onset of sepsis in a murine model improves survival. *Circulation* 2005; 112:117–124.

100. Schrier RW, Wang W. Mechanisms of disease: acute renal failure and sepsis. *N Engl J Med* 2004; 351:159–169.

101. Yasuda H, Yuen PST, Hu X, Zhou H, Star RA. Simvastatin improves sepsis-induced mortality and acute kidney injury via renal vascular effects. *Kidney Int* 2006; 69:1535–1542.

102. Liappis AP, Kan VL, Rochester CG, Simon GL. The effect of statins on mortality in patients with bacteremia. *Clin Infect Dis* 2001; 33:1352–1357.

103. Almog Y, Shefer A, Novack V *et al*. Prior statin therapy is associated with a decreased rate of severe sepsis. *Circulation* 2004; 110:880–885.

104. Thomsen RW, Hundborg HH, Johnsen SP *et al*. Statin use and mortality within 180 days after bacteremia: a population-based cohort study. *Crit Care Med* 2006; 34:1080–1086.

105. Mortensen EM, Restrepo MI, Anzueto A, Pugh J. The effect of prior statin use on 30-day mortality for patients hospitalized with community-acquired pneumonia. *Respir Res* 2005; 6:82.

106. Hackam DG, Mamdani M, Li P, Redelmeier DA. Statins and sepsis in patients with cardiovascular disease: a population-based cohort analysis. *Lancet* 2006; 367:413–418.

107. Almog Y, Novack V, Eisinger M, Porath A, Novack L, Gilutz H. The effect of statin therapy on infection-related mortality in patients with atherosclerotic diseases. *Crit Care Med* 2007; 35:372–378.

108. Gupta R, Plantinga LC, Fink NE *et al*. Statin use and hospitalization for sepsis in patients with chronic kidney disease. *JAMA* 2007; 297:1455–1464.

109. Chua D, Tsang RS, Kuo IF. The role of statin therapy in sepsis. *Ann Pharmacother* 2007; 41:647–652.

110. Majumdar SR, McAlister FA, Eurich DT, Padwal RS, Marrie TJ. Statins and outcomes in patients admitted to hospital with community acquired pneumonia: population based prospective cohort study. *Br Med J* 2006; 333:999.

111. Martin CP, Talbert RL, Burgess DS, Peters JI. Effectiveness of statins in reducing the rate of severe sepsis: a retrospective evaluation. *Pharmacotherapy* 2007; 27:20–26.

112. Bromilow J, Schuster Bruce MJ. The use of statins in intensive care unit patients with sepsis. *Anaesth Intensive Care* 2007; 35:256–258.

113. Terblanche M, Almog Y, Rosenson RS, Smith TS, Hackam DG. Statins and sepsis: multiple modifications at multiple levels. *Lancet Infect Dis* 2007; 7:358–368.

114. Yung LM, Leung FP, Yao X, Chen ZY, Huang Y. Reactive oxygen species in vascular wall. *Cardiovasc Hematol Disord Drug Targets* 2006; 6:1–19.

115. Freeman RV, Otto CM. Spectrum of calcific aortic valve disease: pathogenesis, disease progression, and treatment strategies. *Circulation* 2005; 111:3316–3326.

116. Soini Y, Salo T, Satta J. Angiogenesis is involved in the pathogenesis of nonrheumatic aortic valve stenosis. *Hum Pathol* 2003; 34:756–763.

117. Yoshioka M, Yuasa S, Matsumura K *et al*. Chondromodulin-I maintains cardiac valvular function by preventing angiogenesis. *Nat Med* 2006; 12:1151–1159.

118. Hotchkiss RS, Karl IE. The pathophysiology and treatment of sepsis. *N Engl J Med* 2003; 348:138–150.

14

The role of imaging endpoints in clinical trials

S. J. Nicholls

INTRODUCTION

For more than 100 years, cholesterol has been proposed to play a pivotal role in the development of atherosclerotic cardiovascular disease. Numerous randomised controlled trials have demonstrated that medical therapies that lower levels of low-density lipoprotein cholesterol (LDL-C) are associated with a reduction in cardiovascular events [1–6]. Accordingly, lowering LDL-C has become a cornerstone of therapeutic guidelines for cardiovascular prevention [7]. However, despite the use of established medical therapies, event rates are reduced by no more than 40% in clinical trials, suggesting that the majority of clinical events continue to occur. As a result, there is an ongoing need to develop new therapeutic approaches in order to achieve more effective prevention of cardiovascular disease.

Increasing use of concomitant medical therapies presents a major challenge for the development of new anti-atherosclerotic strategies. Declining placebo event rates create a scenario in which future clinical trials will require to follow larger numbers of patients (>10 000) for increasing periods of time (>7 years) to demonstrate clinical efficacy. Given the prohibitive resources that would be required to subject all promising agents to this approach, increasing attention has focused on the role of surrogate markers of efficacy to triage those therapies with the greatest likelihood of success to advanced stages of clinical development. In particular, imaging modalities that visualise the extent of atherosclerosis have been increasingly employed in clinical trials of lipid-modifying therapies.

CORONARY ANGIOGRAPHY

During the fifty years since it was first performed, coronary angiography has been widely used to diagnose and determine the extent of coronary artery disease (CAD). This has enabled the appropriate triage of patients to a range of medical and revascularisation strategies. Angiography has been widely used in randomised clinical trials to evaluate the impact of medical therapies on the rate of progression of obstructive disease. Specifically, these studies have demonstrated a beneficial impact of medical therapies that lower LDL-C and raise high-density lipoprotein cholesterol (HDL-C).

Early studies revealed that cholesterol-lowering interventions slowed the progression of angiographic disease. In the National Heart, Lung and Blood Institute Type II Coronary Intervention Study, patients treated with cholestyramine (6 g four times daily) demonstrated a 26% lowering of LDL-C and were less likely to undergo disease progression (32 vs. 49%)

Stephen J. Nicholls, MBBS, PhD, Cardiologist, Department of Cardiovascular Medicine and Cell Biology, Cleveland Clinic, Cleveland, USA

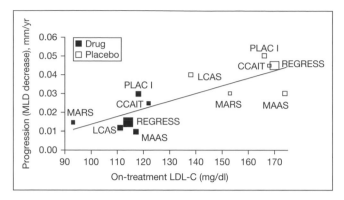

Figure 14.1 Relationship between on-treatment levels of low-density lipoprotein cholesterol (LDL-C) and progression of minimum lumen diameter (MLD) in clinical studies that employ serial evaluation by quantitative coronary angiography (with permission from [18]).

than placebo-treated patients [8]. The St Thomas' Atherosclerosis Regression Study (STARS) similarly found that the use of cholestyramine in combination with dietary intervention not only slowed progression of disease, but was also associated with a greater rate of progression and increase in coronary lumen diameter [9]. The Program on the Surgical Control of the Hyperlipidemias (POSCH) was a randomised controlled clinical trial of partial ileal bypass in 838 survivors of myocardial infarction. Lowering LDL-C by 38% with surgery resulted in a 35% reduction in the combination of coronary heart disease (CHD) death and non-fatal myocardial infarction. This was associated with less disease progression when angiograms were followed for up to 10 years [10].

A number of groups subsequently reported that LDL apheresis resulted in angiographic regression in patients with familial hypercholesterolaemia [11, 12]. However, while disease progression was halted in clinical trials of LDL apheresis, net regression was not observed. Combination therapy with simvastatin 40 mg in addition to either LDL apheresis or colestipol in the Familial Hypercholesterolemia Regression Study was associated with halting of progression in both treatment groups [13]. A similar result was observed in the LDL-Apheresis Atherosclerosis Regression Study (LAARS), in which use of apheresis in simvastatin-treated patients had no greater effect on angiographic disease progression than statin treatment alone [14].

A large number of studies have subsequently investigated the impact of LDL-C lowering with statins on the rate of progression of angiographic disease. In an early study of statin therapy, lowering LDL-C by 38% with lovastatin 80 mg daily in the Monitored Atherosclerosis Regression Study (MARS) retarded progression of the global extent of angiographic disease and was associated with a 2-fold greater proportion of patients who underwent disease regression [15]. These findings were supported in studies of subsequent generations of statins. Use of pravastatin for 3 years in the Pravastatin Limitation of Atherosclerosis in the Coronary Arteries (PLAC-1) study lowered LDL-C by 28% and slowed disease progression by 40% compared with placebo-treated patients [16]. Similarly, the use of simvastatin 20 mg/day lowered LDL-C by 31% and resulted in less progression and more regression of disease in the Multicentre Anti-Atherosclerosis Study (MAAS) [17]. A subsequent pooled meta-analysis of clinical trials of LDL-C lowering therapies demonstrated a direct relationship between the achieved level of LDL-C and the rate of progression of obstructive disease. Extrapolation of this relationship suggests that the greatest degree of LDL lowering can actually promote plaque regression [18] (Figure 14.1).

Group	n	Myocardial infarction or coronary death		Any coronary event*	
		Relative risk (95% CI)	P value**	Relative risk (95% CI)	P value**
Total sample		1.4 (1.1–1.8)	0.02	1.4 (1.2–1.7)	0.002
IMT <0.566 mm**	36	1.0		1.0	
IMT 0.566–0.635 mm	35	5.5 (1.2–25.2)		3.6 (1.5–8.6)	
IMT 0.636–0.732 mm	38	6.7 (1.5–30.1)		2.7 (1.1–6.7)	
IMT ≥0.733 mm	37	7.7 (1.7–34.7)		4.9 (2.1–11.6)	
Placebo group		1.2 (0.9–1.7)	>0.2	1.2 (0.9–1.5)	>0.2
IMT <0.566 mm**	11	1.0		1.0	
IMT 0.566–0.635 mm	19	5.0 (0.6–40.3)		5.5 (1.3–24.2)	
IMT 0.636–0.732 mm	22	6.2 (0.8– 48.8)		3.8 (0.9–17.1)	
IMT ≥0.733 mm	21	5.7 (0.7– 46.6)		4.5 (1.0–20.6)	
Drug group		1.9 (1.2–3.0)	0.009	2.0 (1.4–2.9)	<0.001
IMT <0.566 mm**	25	1.0		1.0	
IMT 0.566–0.635 mm	16	5.6 (0.6–54.3)		2.2 (0.7–7.3)	
IMT 0.636–0.732 mm	16	6.5 (0.7–63.2)		1.7 (0.4–6.2)	
IMT ≥0.733 mm	16	11.8 (1.3–104.5)		6.0 (2.0–18.4)	

Absolute intima–media thickness measured 2 years after treatment and expressed per SD equal to a 0.13-mm increase. Quartiles were based on the distribution of carotid arterial intima-media thickness at baseline. The event rates in the first quartile for myocardial infarction or coronary death and for any clinical coronary event were 0.6 per 100 person-years and 2.1 events per 100 person-years, respectively. Event rates for any other quartile may be estimated by multiplying the rate for the first quartile by the relative risk

IMT = intima-media thickness.

* Non-fatal myocardial infarction, coronary death, or coronary artery revasularisation.

** Chi-square likelihood ratio test for trend. Adjusted for treatment group (for analyses of total sample) and whether the patient continued into the extension of the trial.

Figure 14.2 Absolute common carotid intimal-medial thickness and risk of coronary events (with permission from [25]).

Medical therapies that target lipids in addition to LDL-C have demonstrated a beneficial effect on progression of angiographic disease. Lowering triglycerides and raising HDL-C with the fibric-acid derivative, bezafibrate, reduced the rate of decrease of minimum lumen diameter by 65% in middle-aged dyslipidaemic male survivors of myocardial infarction in the Bezafibrate Coronary Atherosclerosis Intervention Trial (BECAIT) [19]. The benefit of fibrate therapy on disease progression was also observed in the Diabetes Atherosclerosis Intervention Study (DAIS), in which micronised fenofibrate 200 mg daily slowed disease progression in a group of patients with diffuse CAD [20]. The potential beneficial impact of raising HDL-C in addition to LDL-C lowering was further highlighted by the demonstration of benefit of combining nicotinic acid and simvastatin in the HDL-Atherosclerosis Treatment Study (HATS). Lowering LDL-C by 42% and HDL-C elevation by 26% after three years of treatment was associated with 0.4% disease regression, a finding that was no longer observed in patients who were also treated with a cocktail of multi-vitamins [21]. These findings suggest that the combination of effective LDL-C lowering, in addition to promoting HDL activity, might have the greatest chance of promoting disease regression.

CAROTID INTIMAL-MEDIAL THICKNESS

Despite its clinical utility, angiographic techniques are limited in the information that they provide regarding the natural history of disease. Given that angiography generates a two-dimensional silhouette of the lumen it does not visualise the vessel wall, the site in which plaque accumulates [22]. This has stimulated the development of imaging modalities that visualise the artery wall in order to permit a more complete evaluation of the disease process. Non-invasive B-mode ultrasonic imaging of the carotid and femoral arteries visualises the artery wall in high resolution, which enables measurement of the thickness of the intimal-medial layer. Increasing degrees of carotid intima-media thickness (cIMT) have been reported in population studies to be associated with a greater prevalence of risk factors and established atherosclerotic disease in other vascular territories [23]. Furthermore, increasing cIMT is associated with an adverse cardiovascular outcome [24, 25] (Figure 14.2). Given that cIMT can be measured non-invasively at different time-points, it has provided an ideal tool to evaluate the impact of lipid-modifying therapies on early changes in the artery wall that precede formation of macroscopic plaque.

A large number of studies, using different research protocols, have demonstrated that lowering LDL-C with statins slows the progression of cIMT on serial evaluation [26]. This benefit has been demonstrated in both the primary and secondary prevention settings. Treatment with lovastatin 20–40 mg/day for 3 years in the Asymptomatic Carotid Artery Progression Study (ACAPS) was associated with regression of disease at the most diseased segment [27]. Similarly, pravastatin 40 mg/day for 3 years slowed overall cIMT progression in asymptomatic subjects with hypercholesterolaemia who participated in the Kuopio Atherosclerosis Prevention Study [28]. These benefits have also been demonstrated in patients with established CAD on coronary angiography. Treatment with lovastatin 80 mg/day in the MARS [29] and with pravastatin 40 mg/day in the Regression Growth Evaluation Statin Substudy (REGRESS) [30] retarded cIMT progression compared with placebo in patients with CAD and hypercholesterolaemia.

Serial evaluation of cIMT was the initial modality employed to evaluate the impact of use of an intensive compared with a moderate lipid-lowering strategy. The Atorvastatin versus Simvastatin Atherosclerosis Progression (ASAP) study randomised patients with heterozygous familial hypercholesterolaemia to treatment with intensive (atorvastatin 80 mg/day) or moderate (simvastatin 40 mg/day) lipid-lowering regimens for 2 years. Greater lowering of LDL-C was associated with cIMT regression (−0.031 mm) in intensively treated patients, as opposed to evidence of disease progression by 0.036 mm in the moderately treated patients [31]. This finding was extended to a cohort of middle-aged males with hypercholesterolemia in the Arterial Biology for the Investigation of Treatment Effects of Reducing Cholesterol (ARBITER) study. Treatment with an intensive lipid-lowering strategy (atorvastatin 80 mg/day) resulted in a decrease in cIMT (−0.034 mm), while moderate lipid lowering (pravastatin 40 mg daily) was associated with disease progression (+0.025 mm) [32]. Meta-analysis of studies that evaluated the impact of LDL-C lowering on serial cIMT confirmed the observation from angiographic studies that there was a direct inverse relationship between the LDL-C level achieved and the rate of disease progression [26]. Furthermore, more recent controlled studies which demonstrated an incremental benefit of intensive lipid lowering, have suggested that lowering LDL-C to very low levels might have a dramatic clinical impact.

Recent findings have suggested that statin therapy can have an impact on the disease process in low-risk patients. In the Measuring Effects on Intima-Media Thickness: an Evaluation of Rosuvastatin (METEOR) study, asymptomatic patients with modest hypercholesterolaemia and low risk as estimated from the Framingham equations were treated with rosuvastatin 20 mg/day or placebo for 24 months. LDL-C lowering was associated with halting of cIMT progression, suggesting that statin therapy could have a benefit in low-risk patients, who would not typically be considered candidates for lipid-lowering therapy [33]. The findings also suggest that arterial wall imaging may identify appropriate patients for use of medical therapies. More recently, the impact of incremental LDL-C lowering achieved by inhibition of cholesterol absorption was investigated in the Ezetimibe and Simvastatin in Hypercholesterolemia Enhances Atherosclerosis Regression (ENHANCE) study. Despite greater lowering of LDL-C (58 vs. 41%), addition of ezetimibe 10 mg to simvastatin 80 mg did not slow progression of cIMT compared with use of simvastatin 80 mg alone in patients with familial hypercholesterolaemia [34]. While the reasons for the lack of an observed benefit are uncertain, it is possible that different therapeutic approaches to LDL-C lowering have varying influences on the arterial wall.

Serial evaluation of cIMT has also been employed to assess the impact of therapies which have significant impact on lipids other than LDL-C alone. In the ARBITER 2 study, patients with established atherosclerotic disease and low levels of HDL-C were treated with extended-release niacin or placebo, on a background of statin therapy. Raising HDL-C with niacin was associated with halting cIMT progression, providing further evidence of an incremental benefit of promoting HDL activity in addition to lowering LDL-C [35]. In a follow-up investigation of patients continuing treatment with extended-release niacin, cIMT regression was observed after 24 months. This suggests that more prolonged therapy could have a more substantial impact on very early changes in the artery wall [36]. The benefit of raising HDL-C on cIMT progression was further supported by use of the peroxisome proliferator-activated receptor-gamma (PPAR-γ) agonist, pioglitazone, in people with diabetes. In the Carotid Intima-Media Thickness in Atherosclerosis Using Pioglitazone (CHICAGO) study, people with diabetes were treated with pioglitazone 15–45 mg/day or glimeparide 1–4 mg/day for 72 weeks. Treatment with pioglitazone arrested the cIMT progression that was observed in glimeparide-treated patients [37]. More recent analysis revealed that the 15% increase in HDL-C independently predicted the benefit of pioglitazone on cIMT progression [38].

Considerable interest subsequently focused on whether a benefit would be observed by substantially raising HDL-C with pharmacological inhibitors of cholesteryl ester transfer protein (CETP). In the Rating Atherosclerotic Disease Changes by Imaging with a New Cholesteryl Ester Transfer Protein Inhibitor (RADIANCE) 1 and 2 studies, patients with familial hypercholesterolaemia and atherogenic dyslipidaemia, respectively, were treated with the CETP inhibitor, torcetrapib 60 mg/day or placebo, in addition to background therapy with atorvastatin [39, 40]. Despite raising HDL-C by 50% and promoting an incremental lowering of LDL-C by 20%, treatment with torcetrapib did not slow cIMT progression. Given the recent reports that torcetrapib activates the rennin–angiotensin–aldosterone axis and raises blood pressure [41], it is possible that other CETP inhibitors without vascular toxicity may have a beneficial influence on changes in cIMT.

INTRAVASCULAR ULTRASOUND

Intravascular ultrasound (IVUS) was developed on the basis that high-frequency ultrasound transducers within arterial lumens, in close proximity to the endothelial surface, would generate high-resolution imaging of the entire thickness of the vessel wall. As a result, ultrasonic imaging can visualise the full extent of atherosclerotic plaque. The ability of IVUS to demonstrate substantial atherosclerosis in segments which appear normal on angiography [42], reflects the ability of the artery wall to remodel in response to plaque accumulation [43]. Given that artery walls typically expand in the early stages of atherosclerosis, there is often a substantial amount of disease by the time abnormalities are detected on angiography of the lumen [43]. Serial imaging with IVUS within an arterial segment permits the opportunity to evaluate the impact of lipid-modifying therapies on the precise volumetric extent of established atherosclerosis in the coronary artery wall.

Despite early case reports of angiographic disease regression [11, 12], subsequent clinical trials failed to demonstrate a consistent benefit of combining LDL apheresis with medical therapy in patients with familial hypercholesterolaemia [13, 14]. More recent clinical trials that employed IVUS have demonstrated a beneficial effect of LDL apheresis on plaque burden. Eighteen patients with familial hypercholesterolaemia in the Low Density Lipoprotein-Apheresis Coronary Morphology and Reserve Trial (LACMART) were treated with medical therapy alone or in combination with apheresis for 12 months. Greater LDL-C lowering with apheresis was associated with a reduction in plaque area and an increase in the minimum lumen diameter, consistent with disease regression [44].

Several investigators have subsequently employed IVUS to determine whether intensive LDL-C lowering with statin therapy has a beneficial impact on changes in atheroma volume. In the earliest report, in the German Atorvastatin Investigation (GAIN) study, serial IVUS was used to monitor coronary atherosclerosis progression of patients treated in an open-labelled comparison of atorvastatin or usual care for 12 months. Despite greater LDL-C lowering with atorvastatin (86 vs. 140 mg/dl), the rate of plaque progression did not differ between the groups. In contrast, an increase in echogenicity of plaque was observed in ator-vastatin-treated patients, suggesting that the intensive lipid-lowering approach had a beneficial influence on the composition of coronary plaque [45].

In the Reversal of Atherosclerosis with Aggressive Lipid Lowering (REVERSAL) study, 502 patients with angiographic coronary artery disease and a LDL-C between 125 and 210 mg/dl were treated for 18 months with either an intensive (atorvastatin 80 mg/day) or moderate (pravastatin 40 mg/day) lipid-lowering strategy. Intensive LDL-C lowering (79 vs. 110 mg/dl) was accompanied by slowing in disease progression. Atheroma volume increased in moderately treated patients, but did not change in patients given the intensive regimen [46]. This suggested that lowering LDL-C below 80 mg/dl could halt the natural history of plaque progression. Further analysis revealed a direct relationship between the degree of LDL-C lowering and the change in atheroma volume [46]. However, patients treated with pravastatin were required to result in greater lowering of LDL-C to achieve the same impact on atheroma volume as observed in atorvastatin-treated patients. This suggested that additional differences between the agents, beyond LDL-C lowering, were likely to be relevant to the greater effect of atorvastatin. Greater lowering of C-reactive protein (CRP) (36 vs. 5%), in addition to the observation of a direct relationship between changes in CRP and atheroma volume, suggested that anti-inflammatory properties may have contributed to the impact of high-dose atorvastatin on plaque progression [47].

The findings of REVERSAL complemented the results of the Pravastatin or Atorvastatin Evaluation and Infection Therapy (PROVE IT-TIMI 22) study, in which atorvastatin 80 mg/day treatment resulted in a reduction in clinical events compared with pravastatin 40 mg/day in patients with an acute coronary syndrome [48]. In particular, patients with the greatest lowering of both LDL-C and CRP demonstrated the lowest rates of clinical events [49] and plaque progression [47]. These findings were particularly evident in obese patients, in whom a greater reduction in CRP, consistent with greater anti-inflammatory activity, had the largest influence in slowing plaque progression [50]. These findings suggested that pleiotropic properties of statin therapy were likely to contribute to their benefit and provided an important demonstration that effects of medical therapies on disease in the artery wall and clinical outcome were complementary.

A Study to Evaluate the Effect of Rosuvastatin on Intravascular Ultrasound-Derived Coronary Atheroma Burden (ASTEROID) explored whether more intensive lowering of LDL-C to very low levels could promote plaque regression. Lowering LDL-C by 53% to 60.8 mg/dl and raising HDL-C by 14.7% to 49 mg/dl with rosuvastatin 40 mg/day was associated with statistically significant reductions in all parameters of atheroma burden, consistent with regression. A total of 63–78% of patients demonstrated plaque regression, depending on the particular measure of atheroma burden. Statistically significant regression was only observed in those patients who achieved a LDL-C below 70 mg/dl with therapy. This finding suggested that driving LDL-C to very low levels could promote regression of coronary atherosclerosis [51] (Figure 14.3).

The findings of ASTEROID support observations of regression with statin therapy in short arterial segments of small cohorts of subjects. In the ESTABLISH study [52], patients with an acute coronary syndrome were treated with atorvastatin 20 mg/day or placebo for 6 months. Lowering LDL-C by 41.7% was associated with plaque regression. Similar findings were reported in a cohort of middle-aged Danish males, in whom lowering LDL-C with simvastatin was associated with a reduction in atheroma volume [53].

The potential contribution of raising HDL-C to the observed benefit in ASTEROID remained to be elucidated. In a pooled analysis of four clinical trials that employed serial evaluation of coronary atherosclerosis by IVUS, raising HDL-C by a mean of 7.5% was a strong independent predictor of the beneficial effect of statin therapy on plaque progression. Raising HDL-C by more than 7.5% had an incremental effect in addition to lowering LDL-C below 87.5 mg/dl, the most profound regression being observed in these patients in whom

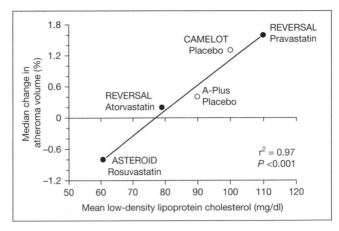

Figure 14.3 Relationship between achieved levels of low-density lipoprotein cholesterol and median changes in percent atheroma volume in clinical trials that employed serial evaluation of plaque burden by intravascular ultrasound (with permission from [51]).

both effects occurred [54]. This observation strongly supports the proposition that raising HDL-C contributes to the beneficial effects of statins. Furthermore, the finding that the greatest lipid predictor of benefit was the change in the apolipoprotein B/AI ratio supports the concept that therapeutic strategies that target both pro-atherogenic and protective lipoproteins are likely to have the greatest impact in patients with CAD.

The beneficial effects of HDL on coronary atherosclerosis have been demonstrated in small cohorts studied with IVUS. In a seminal study of 57 patients with a recent acute coronary syndrome, weekly infusions of reconstituted HDL containing recombinant human apolipoprotein AI_{Milano} for five weeks promoted rapid plaque regression, with no changes in systemic HDL-C levels [55] (Figure 14.4). This finding suggested that infusing lipid-depleted forms of HDL is able to rapidly mobilise cholesterol out of the artery wall. This is supported by the subsequent finding that the greatest regression was observed in the 10 mm segments containing the greatest amount of plaque at baseline, regions which are likely to contain more lipid [56]. The observation that regression was accompanied by shrinkage of the vessel wall, with no change in lumen dimensions, further underscores the need to visualise the entire vessel wall in order to accurately demonstrate regression in response to medical therapies [56]. A similar benefit has been recently reported for infusions of reconstituted HDL containing wild-type apolipoprotein AI. When infused weekly for 4 weeks, a strong trend toward regression and increase in plaque echogenicity, a surrogate of stabilisation, was observed [57]. These findings suggest that HDL has a profound impact on the artery wall in humans.

Considerable interest has focused on the potential impact of substantially raising HDL-C levels with pharmacological CETP inhibitors. In the Investigation of Lipid Level Management Using Coronary Ultrasound to Assess Reduction of Atherosclerosis by CETP Inhibition and HDL Elevation (ILLUSTRATE) study, patients were treated with torcetrapib 60 mg/day or placebo, on a background of treatment with atorvastatin. Despite raising HDL-C by 61% and an incremental lowering of LDL-C by 21% in addition to statin therapy, administration of torcetrapib did not slow the progression of coronary atherosclerosis [58] (Figure 14.5). This result is consistent with the lack of efficacy of this therapeutic approach on progression of cIMT [39, 40] and clinical events [59]. Subsequent analysis revealed an inverse relationship between levels of HDL-C on therapy and the rate of plaque progression, with marked regression observed in those patients achieving the highest HDL-C levels. The benefit of raising

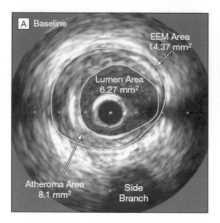
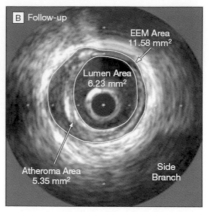

Figure 14.4 Images at baseline (left panel) and follow-up (right panel) at a matched coronary artery site illustrating atheroma regression in response to treatment with reconstituted HDL particles containing recombinant human apoAI$_{Milano}$ (with permission from [55]). EEM = external elastic membrane.

HDL-C on plaque progression was not observed in those patients with the lowest potassium levels, a surrogate of increased activation of the rennin–angiotensin–aldosterone axis [60]. This is consistent with preliminary reports that the highest HDL-C levels were associated with lower event rates and that torcetrapib promotes release of aldosterone from adrenocortical cells [61]. These findings suggest that use of an alternative CETP inhibitor with no impact on mineralocorticoids could still be beneficial in patients with established CAD.

Uptake of esterified cholesterol by macrophages, forming foam cells, is a pivotal stage in plaque formation and propagation. While inhibition of acyl-coenzyme A:cholesterol acyltransferase (ACAT), a factor involved in esterification of cholesterol, has a profound influence on lesion formation in animal models of atherosclerosis [62], no benefit is observed in humans. In the Avasimibe and Progression of coronary Lesions assessed by intravascular Ultrasound (A-PLUS) study [63], the ACAT inhibitor avasimibe had no impact on plaque progression. However, avasimibe induces statin metabolism, resulting in higher LDL-C levels, which may have mitigated against any potential benefit of ACAT inhibition. The placebo-controlled ACAT Intravascular Atherosclerosis Treatment Evaluation (ACTIVATE) study tested the efficacy of pactimibe, an ACAT inhibitor without any influence on statin metabolism. Greater progression of coronary atherosclerosis was observed in pactimibe-treated patients suggesting that ACAT inhibition may be pro-atherogenic in humans [64]. Cytotoxicity in response to increased intracellular levels of free cholesterol has been proposed as a potential mechanism contributing to the potential detrimental effect of ACAT inhibitors [64].

While IVUS has provided an important opportunity to assess the impact of medical therapies on progression of established coronary atherosclerosis, a number of important caveats should be noted. Given that IVUS requires invasive cardiac catheterisation, all patients have symptomatic CHD. It is therefore uncertain whether the findings can be applied to the setting of primary prevention. Conventional ultrasonic imaging provides a very limited characterisation of plaque composition. While it is likely that plaque regression is accompanied by removal of lipid, necrotic and inflammatory material from the artery wall, this remains to be established. Preliminary analysis of the radiofrequency backscatter signal generates a tissue map, which bears a strong correlation with histological findings [65]. In a pilot backscatter analysis of patients with an acute coronary syndrome, treatment with a statin for 6 months resulted in plaque containing more fibrotic and less lipidic material [66]. Further

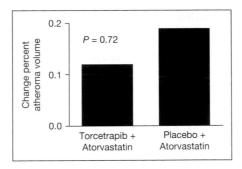

Figure 14.5 Impact of therapy with torcetrapib or placebo, in addition to background atorvastatin, on the change in percent atheroma volume, determined by intravascular ultrasound (with permission from [58]).

studies will provide the opportunity to elucidate the value of this technique for studying the impact of medical therapies that target pro-atherogenic and protective lipids in the artery wall.

Considerable interest has focused on the clinical implications of the findings of regression–progression studies. The application of cIMT and coronary angiography in large numbers of patients with a broad range of cardiovascular risk has demonstrated a direct relationship between the extent of disease and clinical outcome [24, 67]. In an early IVUS study, progression of plaque area in the left main coronary artery was reported to be greater in patients who had a clinical event [68]. These findings have been confirmed by analysis of combined treatment groups in the ILLUSTRATE trial in which patients who experienced a clinical event had a greater percentage atheroma volume at baseline and progression on serial evaluation [69]. In addition, complementary effects of intensive lipid lowering [46–49], antihypertensive agents [70] and anti-immunodulatory agents [71] on disease progression and clinical outcome have been observed. As a result, monitoring changes in disease progression with IVUS has been incorporated into the clinical development of experimental anti-atherosclerotic therapies.

COMPUTED TOMOGRAPHY

Considerable interest has focused on the development of imaging modalities that visualise the coronary arteries in a non-invasive fashion. Quantitation of coronary calcification has been reported to predict the presence and extent of CAD and the likelihood of clinical events in population studies [72, 73]. Several groups have investigated the impact of lipid lowering on progression of coronary calcification. While an initial report demonstrated that treatment with cerivastatin slowed the progression of coronary calcification [74], this could not be confirmed by two subsequent studies, in which there was no difference in findings between intensive and moderate lipid-lowering strategies [75, 76]. These observations contrast with the observation from IVUS that intensive lipid lowering has a beneficial impact on the extent of coronary atherosclerosis [46]. The potential limitation of studying the impact of medical therapies on calcification is further highlighted by the observation from IVUS that calcified lesions are less likely to regress or progress with medical therapies [77]. Increasing resolution permits the visualisation of lumen stenoses and plaque within the artery wall using computed tomography angiographic techniques [78]. However, this imaging approach currently lacks the precision required to accurately assess the impact of medical therapies on disease. Use of molecular-targeted contrast may permit more definitive imaging of atherosclerosis within the coronary arteries [79].

19. Ericsson CG, Hamsten A, Nilsson J, Grip L, Svane B, de Faire U. Angiographic assessment of effects of bezafibrate on progression of coronary artery disease in young male postinfarction patients. *Lancet* 1996; 347:849–853.

20. Effect of fenofibrate on progression of coronary-artery disease in type 2 diabetes: the Diabetes Atherosclerosis Intervention Study, a randomised study. *Lancet* 2001; 357:905–910.

21. Brown BG, Zhao X-Q, Chait A *et al*. Simvastatin and niacin, antioxidant vitamins, or the combination for the prevention of coronary disease. *N Engl J Med* 2001; 345:1583–1592.

22. Topol EJ, Nissen SE. Our preoccupation with coronary luminology. The dissociation between clinical and angiographic findings in ischemic heart disease. *Circulation* 1995; 92:2333–2342.

23. Chambless LE, Heiss G, Folsom AR *et al*. Association of coronary heart disease incidence with carotid arterial wall thickness and major risk factors: the Atherosclerosis Risk in Communities (ARIC) Study, 1987–1993. *Am J Epidemiol* 1997; 146:483–494.

24. Lorenz MW, Markus HS, Bots ML, Rosvall M, Sitzer M. Prediction of clinical cardiovascular events with carotid intima-media thickness: a systematic review and meta-analysis. *Circulation* 2007; 115:459–467.

25. Hodis HN, Mack WJ, LaBree L *et al*. The role of carotid arterial intima-media thickness in predicting clinical coronary events. *Ann Intern Med* 1998; 128:262–269.

26. Kang S, Wu Y, Li X. Effects of statin therapy on the progression of carotid atherosclerosis: a systematic review and meta-analysis. *Atherosclerosis* 2004; 177:433–442.

27. Furberg CD, Adams HP Jr, Applegate WB *et al*. Effect of lovastatin on early carotid atherosclerosis and cardiovascular events. Asymptomatic Carotid Artery Progression Study (ACAPS) Research Group. *Circulation* 1994; 90:1679–1687.

28. Salonen R, Nyyssönen K, Porkkala E *et al*. Kuopio Atherosclerosis Prevention Study (KAPS). A population-based primary preventive trial of the effect of LDL lowering on atherosclerotic progression in carotid and femoral arteries. *Circulation* 1995; 92:1758–1764.

29. Hodis HN, Mack WJ, LaBree L *et al*. Reduction in carotid arterial wall thickness using lovastatin and dietary therapy: a randomized controlled clinical trial. *Ann Intern Med* 1996; 124:548–556.

30. de Groot E, Jukema JW, Montauban van Swijndregt AD *et al*. B-mode ultrasound assessment of pravastatin treatment effect on carotid and femoral artery walls and its correlations with coronary arteriographic findings: a report of the Regression Growth Evaluation Statin Study (REGRESS). *J Am Coll Cardiol* 1998; 31:1561–1567.

31. Smilde TJ, van Wissen S, Wollersheim H, Trip MD, Kastelein JJ, Stalenhoef AF. Effect of aggressive versus conventional lipid lowering on atherosclerosis progression in familial hypercholesterolaemia (ASAP): a prospective, randomised, double-blind trial. *Lancet* 2001; 357:577–581.

32. Taylor AJ, Kent SM, Flaherty PJ, Coyle LC, Markwood TT, Vernalis MN. ARBITER: Arterial Biology for the Investigation of the Treatment Effects of Reducing Cholesterol: a randomized trial comparing the effects of atorvastatin and pravastatin on carotid intima medial thickness. *Circulation* 2002; 106:2055–2060.

33. Crouse JR, 3rd, Raichlen JS, Riley WA *et al*. Effect of rosuvastatin on progression of carotid intima-media thickness in low-risk individuals with subclinical atherosclerosis: the METEOR Trial. *JAMA* 2007; 297:1344–1353.

34. http://www.theheart.org/article/837243.do

35. Taylor AJ, Sullenberger LE, Lee HJ, Lee JK, Grace KA. Arterial Biology for the Investigation of the Treatment Effects of Reducing Cholesterol (ARBITER) 2: a double-blind, placebo-controlled study of extended-release niacin on atherosclerosis progression in secondary prevention patients treated with statins. *Circulation* 2004; 110:3512–3517.

36. Taylor AJ, Lee HJ, Sullenberger LE. The effect of 24 months of combination statin and extended-release niacin on carotid intima-media thickness: ARBITER 3. *Curr Med Res Opin* 2006; 22:2243–2250.

37. Mazzone T, Meyer PM, Feinstein SB *et al*. Effect of pioglitazone compared with glimepiride on carotid intima-media thickness in type 2 diabetes: a randomized trial. *JAMA* 2006; 296:2572–2581.

38. Davidson MH, Meyer PM, Haffner SM *et al*. Increases in HDL-C in the CHICAGO study explain the benefits of pioglitazone in reducing CIMT progression in patients with type 2 diabetes. *Circulation* 2007; 116:II_824.

39. Kastelein JJ, van Leuven SI, Burgess L *et al*. Effect of torcetrapib on carotid atherosclerosis in familial hypercholesterolemia. *N Engl J Med* 2007; 356:1620–1630.

40. Bots ML, Visseren FL, Evans GW *et al*. Torcetrapib and carotid intima-media thickness in mixed dyslipidaemia (RADIANCE 2 study): a randomised, double-blind trial. *Lancet* 2007; 370:153–160.

41. Davidson MH, McKenney JM, Shear CL, Revkin JH. Efficacy and safety of torcetrapib, a novel cholesteryl ester transfer protein inhibitor, in individuals with below-average high-density lipoprotein cholesterol levels. *J Am Coll Cardiol* 2006; 48:1774–1781.

42. Mintz GS, Painter JA, Pichard AD *et al*. Atherosclerosis in angiographically 'normal' coronary artery reference segments: an intravascular ultrasound study with clinical correlations. *J Am Coll Cardiol* 1995; 25:1479–1485.

43. Glagov S, Weisenberg E, Zarins CK, Stankunavicius R, Kolettis GJ. Compensatory enlargement of human atherosclerotic coronary arteries. *N Engl J Med* 1987; 316:1371–1375.

44. Matsuzaki M, Hiramori K, Imaizumi T *et al*. Intravascular ultrasound evaluation of coronary plaque regression by low density lipoprotein-apheresis in familial hypercholesterolemia: the Low Density Lipoprotein-Apheresis Coronary Morphology and Reserve Trial (LACMART). *J Am Coll Cardiol* 2002; 40:220–227.

45. Schartl M, Bocksch W, Koschyk DH *et al*.Use of intravascular ultrasound to compare effects of different strategies of lipid-lowering therapy on plaque volume and composition in patients with coronary artery disease. *Circulation* 2001; 104:387–392.

46. Nissen SE, Tuzcu EM, Schoenhagen P *et al*. Effect of intensive compared with moderate lipid-lowering therapy on progression of coronary atherosclerosis: a randomized controlled trial. *JAMA* 2004; 291:1071–1080.

47. Nissen SE, Tuzcu EM, Schoenhagen P *et al*. Statin therapy, LDL cholesterol, C-reactive protein, and coronary artery disease. *N Engl J Med* 2005; 352:29–38.

48. Cannon CP, Braunwald E, McCabe CH *et al*. Intensive versus moderate lipid lowering with statins after acute coronary syndromes. *N Engl J Med* 2004; 350:1495–1504.

49. Ridker PM, Cannon CP, Morrow D *et al*. C-reactive protein levels and outcomes after statin therapy. *N Engl J Med* 2005; 352:20–28.

50. Nicholls SJ, Tuzcu EM, Sipahi I *et al*. Effects of obesity on lipid-lowering, anti-inflammatory, and antiatherosclerotic benefits of atorvastatin or pravastatin in patients with coronary artery disease (from the REVERSAL Study). *Am J Cardiol* 2006; 97:1553–1557.

51. Nissen SE, Nicholls SJ, Sipahi I *et al*. Effect of very high-intensity statin therapy on regression of coronary atherosclerosis: the ASTEROID trial. *JAMA* 2006; 295:1556–1565.

52. Okazaki S, Yokoyama T, Miyauchi K *et al*. Early statin treatment in patients with acute coronary syndrome: demonstration of the beneficial effect on atherosclerotic lesions by serial volumetric intravascular ultrasound analysis during half a year after coronary event: the ESTABLISH Study. *Circulation* 2004; 110:1061–1068.

53. Jensen LO, Thayssen P, Pedersen KE, Stender S, Haghfelt T. Regression of coronary atherosclerosis by simvastatin: a serial intravascular ultrasound study. *Circulation* 2004; 110:265–270.

54. Nicholls SJ, Tuzcu EM, Sipahi I *et al*. Statins, high-density lipoprotein cholesterol, and regression of coronary atherosclerosis. *JAMA* 2007; 297:499–508.

55. Nissen SE, Tsunoda T, Tuzcu EM *et al*. Effect of recombinant ApoA-I Milano on coronary atherosclerosis in patients with acute coronary syndromes: a randomized controlled trial. *JAMA* 2003; 290:2292–2300.

56. Nicholls SJ, Tuzcu EM, Sipahi I *et al*. Relationship between atheroma regression and change in lumen size after infusion of apolipoprotein A-I Milano. *J Am Coll Cardiol* 2006; 47:992–997.

57. Tardif JC, Gregoire J, L'Allier PL *et al*. Effects of reconstituted high-density lipoprotein infusions on coronary atherosclerosis: a randomized controlled trial. *JAMA* 2007; 297:1675–1682.

58. Nissen SE, Tardif JC, Nicholls SJ *et al*. Effect of torcetrapib on the progression of coronary atherosclerosis. *N Engl J Med* 2007; 356:1304–1316.

59. Barter PJ, Caulfield M, Eriksson M *et al*. Effects of torcetrapib in patients at high risk for coronary events. *N Engl J Med* 2007; 357:2109–2122.

60. Nicholls SJ, Brennan DM, Wolski K *et al*. Changes in levels of high-density lipoprotein cholesterol predict the impact of torcetrapib on progression of coronary atherosclerosis: insights from ILLUSTRATE. *Circulation* 2007; 116:II_127.

61. http://www.medscape.com/viewarticle/565393

62. Delsing DJ, Offerman EH, van Duyvenvoorde W *et al*. Acyl-CoA:cholesterol acyltransferase inhibitor avasimibe reduces atherosclerosis in addition to its cholesterol-lowering effect in ApoE*3-Leiden mice. *Circulation* 2001; 103:1778–1786.

63. Tardif JC, Grégoire J, L'Allier PL *et al*. Effects of the acyl coenzyme A:cholesterol acyltransferase inhibitor avasimibe on human atherosclerotic lesions. *Circulation* 2004; 110:3372–3377.

64. Nissen SE, Tuzcu EM, Brewer HB *et al.* Effect of ACAT inhibition on the progression of coronary atherosclerosis. *N Engl J Med* 2006; 354:1253–1263.

65. Nair A, Kuban BD, Tuzcu EM, Schoenhagen P, Nissen SE, Vince DG. Coronary plaque classification with intravascular ultrasound radiofrequency data analysis. *Circulation* 2002; 106:2200–2206.

66. Kawasaki M, Sano K, Okubo M *et al.* Volumetric quantitative analysis of tissue characteristics of coronary plaques after statin therapy using three-dimensional integrated backscatter intravascular ultrasound. *J Am Coll Cardiol* 2005; 45:1946–1953.

67. Mock MB, Ringqvist I, Fisher LD *et al.* Survival of medically treated patients in the coronary artery surgery study (CASS) registry. *Circulation* 1982; 66:562–568.

68. von Birgelen C, Hartmann M, Mintz GS, Baumgart D, Schmermund A, Erbel R. Relation between progression and regression of atherosclerotic left main coronary artery disease and serum cholesterol levels as assessed with serial long-term (> or =12 months) follow-up intravascular ultrasound. *Circulation* 2003; 108:2757–2762.

69. Nicholls SJ, Hsu A, Brennan DM *et al.* Baseline and changes in atheroma volume predict clinical outcome in patients with coronary artery disease: insights from ILLUSTRATE. *Circulation* 2007; 116:II_750.

70. Nissen SE, Tuzcu EM, Libby P *et al.* Effect of antihypertensive agents on cardiovascular events in patients with coronary disease and normal blood pressure: the CAMELOT study: a randomized controlled trial. *JAMA* 2004; 292:2217–2225.

71. Eisen HJ, Tuzcu EM, Dorent R *et al.* Everolimus for the prevention of allograft rejection and vasculopathy in cardiac-transplant recipients. *N Engl J Med* 2003; 349:847–858.

72. Greenland P, LaBree L, Azen SP, Doherty TM, Detrano RC. Coronary artery calcium score combined with Framingham score for risk prediction in asymptomatic individuals. *JAMA* 2004; 291:210–215.

73. Pletcher MJ, Tice JA, Pignone M, Browner WS. Using the coronary artery calcium score to predict coronary heart disease events: a systematic review and meta-analysis. *Arch Intern Med* 2004; 164:1285–1292.

74. Achenbach S, Ropers D, Pohle K *et al.* Influence of lipid-lowering therapy on the progression of coronary artery calcification: a prospective evaluation. *Circulation* 2002; 106:1077–1082.

75. Raggi P, Davidson M, Callister TQ *et al.* Aggressive versus moderate lipid-lowering therapy in hypercholesterolemic postmenopausal women: Beyond Endorsed Lipid Lowering with EBT Scanning (BELLES). *Circulation* 2005; 112:563–571.

76. Schmermund A, Achenbach S, Budde T *et al.* Effect of intensive versus standard lipid-lowering treatment with atorvastatin on the progression of calcified coronary atherosclerosis over 12 months: a multicenter, randomized, double-blind trial. *Circulation* 2006; 113:427–437.

77. Nicholls SJ, Tuzcu EM, Wolski K *et al.* Coronary artery calcification and changes in atheroma burden in response to established medical therapies. *J Am Coll Cardiol* 2007; 49:263–270.

78. Achenbach S, Daniel WG. Imaging of coronary atherosclerosis using computed tomography: current status and future directions. *Curr Atheroscler Rep* 2004; 6:213–218.

79. Hyafil F, Cornily JC, Feig JE *et al.* Noninvasive detection of macrophages using a nanoparticulate contrast agent for computed tomography. *Nat Med* 2007; 13:636–641.

80. Corti R, Fayad ZA, Fuster V *et al.* Effects of lipid-lowering by simvastatin on human atherosclerotic lesions: a longitudinal study by high-resolution, noninvasive magnetic resonance imaging. *Circulation* 2001; 104:249–252.

81. Corti R, Fuster V, Fayad ZA *et al.* Lipid lowering by simvastatin induces regression of human atherosclerotic lesions: two years' follow-up by high-resolution noninvasive magnetic resonance imaging. *Circulation* 2002; 106:2884–2887.

82. Corti R, Fuster V, Fayad ZA *et al.* Effects of aggressive versus conventional lipid-lowering therapy by simvastatin on human atherosclerotic lesions: a prospective, randomized, double-blind trial with high-resolution magnetic resonance imaging. *J Am Coll Cardiol* 2005; 46:106–112.

83. Hatsukami T, Zhao X-Q, Krauss LW. Assessment of rosuvastatin treatment on carotid atherosclerosis in moderately hypercholesterolemic subjects using high-resolution magnetic resonance imaging. *Eur Heart J* 2005; 26:626.

84. Viles-Gonzalez JF, Fuster V, Corti R *et al.* Atherosclerosis regression and TP receptor inhibition: effect of S18886 on plaque size and composition – a magnetic resonance imaging study. *Eur Heart J* 2005; 26:1557–1561.

85. Corti R, Osende J, Hutter R *et al.* Fenofibrate induces plaque regression in hypercholesterolemic atherosclerotic rabbits: in vivo demonstration by high-resolution MRI. *Atherosclerosis* 2007; 190:106–113.

86. Stamper D, Weissman NJ, Brezinski M. Plaque characterization with optical coherence tomography. *J Am Coll Cardiol* 2006; 47:C69–C79.

87. Schaar JA, Mastik F, Regar E *et al.* Current diagnostic modalities for vulnerable plaque detection. *Curr Pharm Des* 2007; 13:995–1001.

88. Rocha R, Silveira L Jr, Villaverde AB *et al.* Use of near-infrared Raman spectroscopy for identification of atherosclerotic plaques in the carotid artery. *Photomed Laser Surg* 2007; 25:482–486.

89. O'Malley SM, Vavuranakis M, Naghavi M, Kakadiaris IA. Intravascular ultrasound-based imaging of vasa vasorum for the detection of vulnerable atherosclerotic plaque. *Med Image Comput Comput Assist Interv Int Conf Med Image Comput Comput Assist Interv* 2005; 8:343–351.

90. Jaffer FA, Libby P, Weissleder R. Molecular imaging of cardiovascular disease. *Circulation* 2007; 116:1052–1061.

15

Biomarkers in cardiovascular disease

S. Blankenberg, R. B. Schnabel

INTRODUCTION

Clinical evaluation is the cornerstone of the diagnosis and management of cardiovascular diseases. Atherosclerotic coronary disease is the most common cause of death in the western world. Its clinical presentation may be with stable angina or an acute coronary syndrome (ACS), either unstable angina or acute myocardial infarction. Clinical manifestation of the disease is associated with a significantly increased risk of recurrent events, morbidity and mortality. To help early diagnosis and risk assessment, risk tools such as the Framingham risk score have been developed to guide physicians and patients. However, none of the scores comprising the classical, easily available risk factors reach the diagnostic accuracy observed in the original Framingham publication. This, at least partly, is because, owing to these pioneering efforts to identify risk indicators, a broad awareness in the general population has been achieved and they are a target of (often insufficient) intervention.

With advances in technology and an increased understanding of the pathophysiological pathways leading to cardiovascular disease, biological markers have become an attractive tool, leading to countless attempts to improve existing risk scores and to gain additional information beyond known risk factors. Among numerous definitions of a biological marker (biomarker), the one proposed by the National Institutes of Health Biomarkers Working Group has gained broad recognition. In 2001 they defined a biomarker as: *'a characteristic that is objectively measured and evaluated as an indicator of normal biological processes, pathogenic processes, or pharmacological responses to a therapeutic intervention'* [1]. Biomarkers comprise biological samples (e.g. blood, urine, tissue), as well as measurements or imaging obtained from a person (e.g. blood pressure, electrocardiogram [ECG], ultrasound). Most attractive are those biomarkers that can be obtained non-invasively or with minimally invasive measures. Recent scientific efforts in large-scale studies have been devoted to blood and urinary biomarkers and are the focus of this chapter. They are relatively easily available and intriguing because of the notion that they may closely mirror pathophysiological processes, although often there is no linear relationship between tissue concentrations and circulating biomarkers. However, tissue samples are more difficult to acquire, especially in a case-control study setting involving healthy individuals. As long as a biomarker is correlated with a disease process even if it is not on the causal pathway, it remains a risk marker. If it is bio-

Stefan Blankenberg, MD, Professor of Medicine, Deputy Director, Department of Medicine II, Johannes Gutenberg-University, Mainz, Germany

Renate B. Schnabel, MD, MSc, Physician and Epidemiologist, Department of Medicine II, Johannes Gutenberg-University, Mainz, Germany

Table 15.1 General biomarker characteristics

Pre-analytic requirements	▪ Intra-individual stability ▪ No relevant correlation with age, sex, race/ethnicity ▪ Stable at different temperatures over a long time period ▪ Stable against environmental influences ▪ Point-of-care testing possible
Laboratory analysis	▪ Measurable in easily available samples (plasma, serum, urine) ▪ Accuracy and precision; intra-/inter-assay coefficients of variation <10% ▪ Cost-effective measurement method ▪ Standardised measurement ▪ Instantaneous results
Clinical evaluation	▪ Decisions based on biomarker intervention, change management of patients ▪ Acceptable to patient ▪ Related to diagnosis or prognosis ▪ Little overlap between normal population (high sensitivity/specificity) and diseased ▪ Cut-off available ▪ Cost-and time-effective determination ▪ Modifiable ▪ Strong correlation with disease process, changes in biomarker closely reflect disease state ▪ Useful for therapy monitoring ▪ Adds information to known risk factors: good calibration, discrimination and meaningful reclassification

logically plausible and central to the pathophysiology of the disease or symptoms – and thus predictive of the disease endpoint of interest – it can serve as a surrogate marker. A biomarker becomes a risk factor if it is a causal agent in the disease process. In this case, interventions targeting this factor should reduce the risk of disease outcomes.

Table 15.1 indicates important characteristics of biomarkers. They have different strengths along the cardiovascular disease continuum. They may:

▪ Indicate susceptibility for disease before disease-specific characteristics can be identified.
▪ Indicate subclinical disease.
▪ Assist in the diagnosis of manifest asymptomatic and symptomatic disease.
▪ Inform assessment of the prognosis or stage of clinically overt disease.
▪ Help with disease monitoring and therapy titration.

On the other hand, a biomarker may be informative concerning pathways implicated in a disease and its underlying disease mechanisms but provide little information that is of use in clinical decision-making.

RISK STRATIFICATION IN PRIMARY PREVENTION

The INTERHEART [2] study was one of the larger trials to quantify the population-attributable risk of the traditional cardiovascular risk factors that were first identified in the early

1960s [3]. The INTERHEART investigators found that the combined population-attributable risk for acute myocardial infarction explained by modifiable, classical and behavioural risk factors was around 90%. Such data help to formulate targets for public health interventions because known risk factors can be controlled, but it also leaves room for further improvement in risk assessment. The key here is the better understanding of the pathophysiology of disease, which may help to unmask some of the classical risk factors as surrogate indicators of underlying pathophysiological processes.

Accurate risk assessment is the first step in risk management. For cardiovascular disease, the Framingham risk profile is widely used to assess the 10-year (or sometimes 5-year) risk of a first major cardiovascular event, based on traditional risk factors [4]. The observation of a strong experimental and clinical relationship between hypercholesterolaemia and atheroma [5], led to the first community-based investigation of blood lipid variables of pro-atherogenic low-density lipoprotein cholesterol (LDL-C) and protective high-density lipoprotein cholesterol (HDL-C). Since then, they have been incorporated in risk scores for the prediction of incident cardiovascular events in the broad population [6, 7], and for the titration of treatment in manifest disease [8, 9]. LDL-C and HDL-C thus constitute biomarkers which have found successful implementation in clinical practice and typify the concept that sound pathophysiological evidence of the actions of candidate systems may ultimately translate into routine clinical practice. Whether more novel lipoproteins like apolipoprotein A1, apolipoprotein B100 or apolipoprotein E help to refine risk prediction is the subject of considerable research and debate.

Two major novel concepts in the pathophysiology of atherosclerosis have emerged in recent decades:

1. The observation that all stages of the atherosclerotic process are accompanied by substantial local and systemic inflammatory activity.
2. The role of oxidant stress in the initiation and perpetuation of atherosclerotic vascular wall changes leading to arterial wall remodelling.

Emerging from these concepts, countless circulating biomarkers relating to the respective pathophysiological processes have been evaluated for their ability to provide diagnostically or prognostically useful information.

INFLAMMATION

Intriguingly, hyperlipidaemia could be directly linked to endothelial damage and vascular wall inflammation [10]. Innate and adaptive immunity perpetuate local inflammatory processes. Beyond the plaque area and its direct neighbourhood, inflammatory cytokines such as tumour necrosis factor-alpha (TNF-α), interferon-gamma (IFN-γ), and interleukin-1 (IL-1) produced by immunoactive cells in the plaque region induce a systemic inflammatory response. The exact role of inflammatory markers at all stages of the inflammatory cascade is still under investigation. The amplification of the pro-inflammatory signals along the cascade results in a measurable increase in acute-phase reactants mainly produced in the liver, such as C-reactive protein (CRP), serum amyloid A and fibrinogen. Meanwhile, standardised measurements for all three proteins exist. Fibrinogen was the first marker to be examined in relation to incident cardiovascular disease in large-scale studies [11]. In the late 1990s, with the availability of high sensitivity assays, CRP became a target of close scrutiny as a biomarker for cardiovascular risk prediction in primary prevention. It is easy and comparatively inexpensive to measure. It has been proposed that measurement of CRP may add information beyond that obtained from the Framingham risk score and at different concentrations of LDL-C [12, 13].

However, as an acute phase reactant, CRP is a relatively non-specific marker of inflammatory activity and underlying metabolic conditions. In this respect, CRP is related to overall mortality and may not be a sufficiently specific marker for cardiovascular disease despite a high correlation with the atherosclerotic process.

Compared to the classical risk factors [14] and across the whole range of risk [15], the prognostic ability of CRP is only modest and might not add information for risk stratification beyond that obtained from classical risk models. Whether it merits broad application in community screening programmes remains controversial. A second beguiling aspect of CRP is that it might not only be a surrogate marker of ongoing inflammation, but also a causal agent. This fact would imply that a therapy targeted to reduce CRP concentrations would improve event-free survival. The pleiotropic vasculoprotective effects of statins comprise anti-inflammatory activities and seem to have beneficial effects on inflammatory biomarkers [16].

The JUPITER (Justification for the Use of statins in Primary prevention: an Intervention Trial Evaluating Rosuvastatin) trial investigated the effect of statin treatment in initially healthy individuals with moderate to low LDL concentrations and low-grade inflammation reflected by CRP concentrations ≥ 2 mg/l [17]. The trial was terminated prematurely on the recommendation of its Data and Safety Monitoring Committee with clear evidence that apparently healthy persons without hyperlipidaemia, but with mildly elevated CRP protein concentrations, benefit from rosuvastatin by showing a reduction of the incidence of major cardiovascular events. The study thus confirmed that statins are potent in reducing CRP and this suggests that any decrease in inflammatory activity, even at mild CRP elevations, is beneficial for cardiovascular outcome. The investigation lacked the treatment arm without CRP measurements and the trial design does not permit us to answer the question as to whether CRP is a causal factor in atherothrombotic disease. Consequently, the recommendations of the American Heart Association — that CRP is an independent marker of risk — remain, but the benefits of a therapy based on CRP concentrations in intermediate risk groups and the use of CRP as part of a global coronary risk assessment, or as a motivation for patients to improve their lifestyle behaviours, remain uncertain and require further evaluation [18].

OXIDATIVE STRESS

Emerging evidence demonstrates that oxidative stress is one of the most potent inductors of endothelial dysfunction and by repeat or continuous exposure is responsible for chronic changes and remodelling in the arterial wall [19]. Oxidation is involved at all stages of atherosclerotic plaque development from the fatty streak to the devastating event of plaque rupture or erosion and fits well into the model of observed chronic subclinical inflammation [20].

Experimental and animal models provide a clear association between the amount of oxidative challenge and reversible vascular dysfunction that can be observed before permanent alterations of the vessel wall occur.

Dominant sources of oxidants in mammals are reactive oxygen species (ROS) and nitrosating agents. As antioxidative defence cannot be completely efficient; an excess of free-radical formation is likely to induce damage in the form of oxidative stress which acts at both molecular and cellular levels. Of importance for cardiovascular biology is the consumption of nitric oxide (NO). Endothelium relaxant factor is a central molecule in vascular homeostasis as a modulator of endothelial tone and reactivity [21]. It is produced by NO synthases and exerts positive pleiotropic effects on the cardiovascular system. Oxidative modification of NO not only leads to reduced bioavailability but also produces the toxic oxidant, peroxynitrite which further aggravates the imbalance of protective and aggressive factors.

Since oxidative stress is central in atherosclerosis, many efforts have been undertaken to translate this knowledge into the characterisation and identification of biomarkers that will enable the detection of oxidative stress and allow improved cardiovascular risk stratification by integration into conventional risk models.

The problem that protagonists of oxidative stress have in common is that they are highly active, short-lived agents which almost immediately react with surrounding molecules at their site of formation and are therefore not suitable as biomarkers for clinical application.

However, oxidative species leave a detectable trace of modified oxidative products as is known for oxidised low-density lipoprotein at the site of atherosclerotic lesions. Oxidised low-density lipoprotein can be measured from blood samples, and has been shown to be elevated in cardiovascular disease and to correlate with endothelial performance [22–24]. The concern is the high plasma clearance capacity, which results in low blood concentrations that do not necessarily reflect tissue levels.

Among the short-lived indirect molecular indicators that undergo changes in response to oxidative stress at the site of non-specific radical attack, F_2-isoprostanes have been the focus of much interest [25]. In contrast to enzymatically produced prostaglandins, they are diverse regioisomers derived from oxidative assault on cell membrane arachidonic acid. As a marker of lipid peroxidation, they are correlated with the burden of cardiovascular risk factors and the severity of disease [26]. Methods are available to measure isoprostanes in the urine and other body fluids, but as these products are active and therefore unstable agents, subject preparation and pre-analytic conditions have to be highly standardised to allow comparability.

Another detectable source of oxidatively modified products after free radical attack is nitrosated tyrosine residues which result from hydrogen peroxide oxidation of NO including peroxynitrite or a hemoperoxidase-catalysed pathway. Similar pathways lead to the formation of bromo-and chlorotyrosines. The majority of data in the cardiovascular field are available for nitrotyrosines. They are elevated in coronary artery disease and may be targeted by statin therapy [27, 28]. Large-scale investigations have so far been prevented by the lack of a suitable method for inexpensive and reliable measurement.

To assess the capacity of anti-oxidative defence, concentrations of glutathione, especially its ratio to oxidised glutathione have been suggested as indicators of oxidative imbalance [29]. Erythrocyte glutathione-peroxidase-1 (GPx-1) has also been of interest as it can be measured from washed erythrocytes following a simple protocol and has been shown to be predictive of future cardiovascular events in patients with manifest coronary artery disease [30].

A vast body of literature is available concerning homocysteine and its relevance in the cardiovascular system and to atherosclerosis [31, 32]. Since the first description of cerebrovascular disorders in individuals with homocystinuria in 1962 [33], multiple pathways have been examined which may be responsible for an increased risk of atherosclerosis due to hyperhomocysteinaemia, even in individuals with mild- to moderately-elevated homocysteine. One of the major characteristics is the potential to directly or indirectly produce ROS [34]. Disappointingly, intervention trials with folic acid and vitamin B_{12}, which are catalytically involved in homocysteine metabolism, have demonstrated a reduction in circulating homocysteine concentration and improvement in endothelial function, but no benefit for long-term survival [35–39]. Among the possible explanations might be that endogenous anti-oxidative defence capacity in individuals enrolled was not taken into consideration. This may confound the overall association. In addition, there might be a non-linear risk association with a threshold for adverse effects of homocysteine.

Finally, myeloperoxidase recently joined the list of proposed biomarkers of oxidative stress. Myeloperoxidase is produced by neutrophils and monocytes/macrophages and was first identified in host defence and innate immunity. The enzyme sets free highly reactive substances such as hypochlorus acid and nitrogen dioxides which are useful during the oxidative burst in antimicrobial defence but become deleterious to the host at sites of chronic exposure such as the damaged arterial wall. An association with endothelial function and also long-term cardiovascular outcome has been observed [40], but needs further investigation.

Asymmetric dimethylarginine (ADMA) is another systemically measurable biomarker. It is the product of endogenous L-arginine residue methylation of proteins. Because of the similarity of its structure with L-arginine, the natural precursor for NO formation, it may act as a competitive inhibitor of endothelial NO synthase (eNOS), and thus reduces NO generation. It has also been shown to interfere with the biological effects of NO and may finally lead to uncoupling of eNOS. The reasons for elevated ADMA concentrations are not well established. Interestingly, it is oxidant-sensitive at its catalytic site and conditions that lead to oxidative challenge such as homocysteine or oxidised low-density lipoprotein (oxLDL) application are related to elevated ADMA concentrations. On the other hand, antioxidant interventions reduce ADMA overload and normalise NO synthesis.

It has therefore been hypothesised that a variety of cardiovascular risk factors and disease conditions that have been found to increase ADMA concentrations act via the increase of oxidative stress and that, consequently, ADMA might be an indirect indicator of oxidative burden since it is more stable, with a longer half-life, and can be measured in peripheral blood.

In prospective analyses, small and moderately-sized clinical studies have demonstrated relatively uniformly that there is an association between ADMA and adverse cardiovascular outcome. However, the risks appear to be inflated in smaller studies [41, 42], and further evidence is needed to evaluate the role of ADMA in cardiovascular disease. Furthermore, the value of all of the biomarkers mentioned above has been mostly assessed in cross-sectional or small, prospective studies. Clearly, information about their predictive ability has to be achieved across population-based cohorts and in different clinical settings. It has been demonstrated repeatedly that for risk indicators that performed well in initial studies, the overall gain of predictive information was rather moderate and did not merit inclusion in general risk prediction models [43]. In addition, the relevance of targeted intervention still remains unclear.

In summary, the assessment of oxidative stress by valid biomarkers may emerge as an attractive approach to assess an individual's response to oxidative challenges. However, the short-lived impact of acute oxidative stress and the rapid biological changes in oxidative status, in conjunction with the need for sophisticated measurement methods, unsolved pre-analytical issues and the lack of specificity are among the factors that have so far prevented the establishment of a well-accepted single marker (or distinct marker panel) to measure oxidative stress that fulfils stringent validity criteria [44].

MULTIPLE MARKER ASSESSMENT

After decades of single biomarker testing, another approach that has gained favour combines multiple circulating biomarkers representing different pathophysiological pathways (e.g. renal function, cardiac stress, haemostasis, inflammation and oxidative stress) to improve risk prediction beyond known risk factors. However, to date there are no convincing data to prove that the information on contemporary biomarkers substantially adds to standard risk factors [45], especially when cost-effectiveness is considered. A recent investigation suggested that a similar combination of blood markers of myocardial cell damage, left ventricular function, renal failure and inflammation may improve risk prediction compared to established risk factors in a selected cohort of lean elderly men [46]. The number of participants who changed risk categories, however, was only moderate, and additional costs for broad application of biomarker measurements were not calculated. More research is needed to establish whether or not current and future biomarkers can support risk assessment in primarily healthy individuals. Indeed, at present, the most promising progress in screening for atherosclerotic disease is being made with non-invasive or minimally invasive functional testing and imaging [47].

DIAGNOSIS OF DISEASE AND RISK STRATIFICATION IN SECONDARY PREVENTION

In contrast to primary prevention, a multimarker strategy has successfully been established to rule out acute myocardial infarction. The combination of necrosis markers with the early elevation of myoglobin, the MB isoenzyme of creatine kinase, and the later increase in troponins, which are highly specific for myocardial tissue injury, help the clinician to rule out acute myocardial damage within 6 hours after chest pain onset [48, 49]. Troponin elevation above the 99th percentile on any determination or creatine kinase concentration above the 99th percentile on two successive measurements are highly suspicious of myocardial ischaemia. As markers of diagnosis, severity and prognosis of acute coronary syndrome they have been a breakthrough for clinicians and patients faced with such a diagnosis.

TROPONINS

Cardiac troponins are highly sensitive for myocardial injury. While they also exhibit a high specificity for myocyte damage, they are not specific for ischaemic mechanisms and, importantly, are affected by renal function. Unstable angina with a high risk of recurrent ischaemic events yet no overt cardiac necrosis may be missed. The delayed elevation in troponin requires serial sampling. Therapeutic decisions are based on troponin concentrations and require early intervention and aggressive antithrombotic and antiplatelet treatment if the cut-off is met. There has been a demand for more sensitive assays, and novel tests are able to measure troponin concentrations in the picomolar range, which will significantly change reporting and interpretation of laboratory results [50]. Acute coronary syndromes may be detected at an earlier stage, but occurrence of more false positives with minor myocardial damage of questionable significance and non-invasive intervention will challenge clinician management. Further experience with the new generation of assays is needed and clinical trials will have to investigate age-and gender-specific cut-offs and provide data on optimal clinical care based on highly sensitive troponins.

More recent concepts of biomarkers in ACS comprise inflammation, oxidative stress and natriuretic peptides as markers of myocardial performance.

Plaque destabilisation and rupture is accompanied by increased inflammatory activity that can be measured systemically. ACS are characterised by higher CRP concentrations compared to stable coronary artery disease and are related to outcome [51]. However, neither the sensitivity nor the specificity of CRP are high enough to merit application of CRP to guidelines of ACS management or secondary prevention measures [18].

NATRIURETIC PEPTIDES

Natriuretic peptides as neurohumoral markers reflecting myocardial stress have been the focus of research since the 1950s when atrial natriuretic peptide (ANP) was isolated from atrial tissue. The almost ideal analytic characteristics and predominant myocardial origin of B-type natriuretic peptide (BNP) and the N-terminal fragment of the prohormone (NT-proBNP) have made them attractive biomarkers in cardiovascular disease. They have entered international guidelines for the differential diagnosis of heart failure in patients with dyspnoea and represent a valuable point-of-care clinical tool. BNP is also increased in ACS [52], especially in patients with large areas of myocardial ischaemia, pre-existing or concurrent heart failure, and multivessel or left main stem disease. For these reasons, the B-type natriuretic peptides are associated with mortality and incident heart failure independent of troponin concentrations [53, 54]. Other reasons for elevated BNP concentrations in ACS patients may be the delay between symptom onset and presentation to the emergency room, or renal impairment. The latter is more relevant for NT-proBNP, which has a predominant

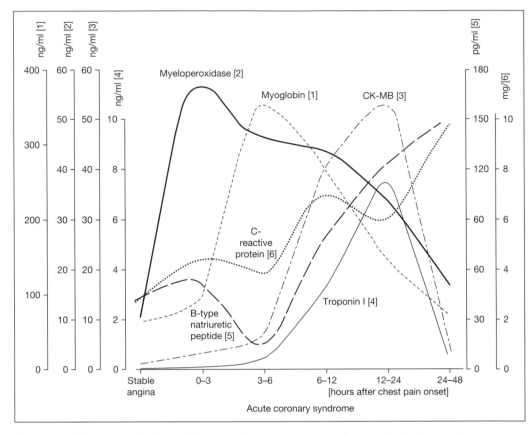

Figure 15.1 Time course of selected biomarkers in acute coronary syndrome patients after symptom onset in comparison with concentrations in patients with stable angina. CK-MB = creatine kinase MB isoenzyme.

renal excretion. BNP has been approved for prognosis assessment in ACS. Aggressive strategies have been recommended in patients with ACS and early elevation of BNP. However, to date, there is insufficient evidence from randomised trials to derive direct therapeutic implications. Similarly, NT-proBNP and BNP have consistently proven to be powerful predictors of cardiovascular outcome in patients at high risk for cardiovascular events [55, 56], but therapeutic implications in addition to closer monitoring and aggressive treatment of risk factors need to be established.

Furthermore, natriuretic peptides are good candidates for therapeutic monitoring in heart failure patients and those with ACS [57]. A decrease in BNP concentrations is correlated with clinical improvement and better prognosis.

Atrial natriuretic peptide is also related to cardiovascular outcome, but the short half-life and relative instability of the analyte have impaired large-scale investigations. More recently, stable fragments of the precursor of atrial natriuretic peptide have been identified. Their diagnostic and predictive capacity in comparison with BNP needs to be evaluated [58].

Whether screening of apparently healthy individuals helps the early identification of significant underlying cardiac structural and functional abnormalities and the propensity for future cardiovascular events is still under investigation [59].

OXIDATIVE STRESS

During ACS, free radicals are produced and oxidative stress is increased. Preceding the clinical event of plaque erosion and rupture, neutrophil granulocytes are recruited to the diseased vessel. Their major secretion product is the enzyme myeloperoxidase. In patients presenting with acute chest pain, the baseline myeloperoxidase measurement helps identify individuals who require revascularisation or have an adverse cardiac outcome during short-term and intermediate follow-up, even without elevated troponin concentrations [60, 61]. Of interest, myeloperoxidase is elevated within the first few hours after symptom onset in patients with initially negative troponin values. Several issues have to be addressed before myeloperoxidase can be evaluated for clinical application. The enzyme itself is not specific for cardiovascular diseases. Myeloperoxidase concentrations are elevated in various other conditions such as infections, and infiltrative and inflammatory disease processes. Furthermore, heparin appears to liberate enzyme normally bound to the vessel, resulting in a 1.6-fold increase in circulating plasma myeloperoxidase concentrations [62]. Recent studies have not adequately controlled for heparin, which is frequently administered in acute chest pain patients.

Efforts to identify early and specific biomarkers for the diagnosis of ACS that exceed a population-based threshold a short time period after symptom onset are ongoing (Figure 15.1). To date, only markers of necrosis in patients with suspected ACS have a clear indication and are routinely determined.

MULTIPLE MARKER STRATEGY

Whereas the bedside measurement of multiple necrosis markers is the standard of care for ACS, the combination of inflammatory markers and BNP for diagnosis and prognosis has not yet entered clinical practice. For markers like CRP, the incremental gain of information has remained inconsistent and for BNP, which is one of the strongest biomarkers in relation to cardiovascular disease outcomes, the lack of therapeutic consequences has hampered broad application [43, 46, 63].

DISCOVERY OF NEW BIOMARKERS

The identification of novel biomarkers is a rapidly evolving field of cardiovascular research.

Most of the above-mentioned biomarkers have a solid basis in prior pathophysiological research and their investigation is strongly hypothesis-driven. As a consequence, the results from studies of new biomarkers may show that they are highly correlated with known markers and thus provide redundant information. The emerging technology of mass array measurements, which generate enormous amounts of data, allows the systematic, unbiased characterisation of biological variations in genes, gene expression patterns, proteome and metabolome with almost hypothesis-free data generation (Figure 15.2). This approach has the potential to identify pathways and biomarkers that have not previously been related to cardiovascular disease and to provide orthogonal [64] and considerably less redundant information. Genomic microarrays will provide an unprecedented opportunity to dissect the genetic risk for complex cardiovascular diseases. A series of recent papers highlights associations of single nucleotide polymorphisms in relatively unknown areas of the genome with cardiovascular outcome [65–67].

Future investigations will unravel further genomic 'hot spots' in association with pre-clinical and manifest atherosclerotic disease. Approaches to collecting proteomic and metabolic biomarker information using different types of mass spectrometry have emerged as central tools. Whereas tissue samples might be the most informative and specific, blood or

assessment of large numbers of individuals. Their relevance at the population level is limited, but they provide valuable insights into disease pathways and may lead to the development of potent interventions.

When applying biomarkers in the setting of cardiovascular disease, one should keep in mind that the information they may provide should only be considered in the larger context of skilled clinical assessment. They can only provide supportive evidence to verify, or indeed rule out, a clinical diagnosis.

REFERENCES

1. Biomarkers Definitions Working Group. Biomarkers and surrogate endpoints: preferred definitions and conceptual framework. *Clin Pharmacol Ther* 2001; 69:89–95.
2. Yusuf S, Hawken S, Ounpuu S *et al*. Effect of potentially modifiable risk factors associated with myocardial infarction in 52 countries (the INTERHEART study): case-control study. *Lancet* 2004; 364:937–952.
3. Kannel WB, Dawber TR, Kagan A, Revotskie N, Stokes J 3rd. Factors of risk in the development of coronary heart disease – six year follow-up experience. The Framingham Study. *Ann Intern Med* 1961; 55:33–50.
4. D'Agostino RB Sr, Vasan RS, Pencina MJ *et al*. General cardiovascular risk profile for use in primary care: the Framingham Heart Study. *Circulation* 2008; 117:743–753.
5. Ross R, Harker L. Hyperlipidemia and atherosclerosis. *Science* 1976; 193:1094–1100.
6. Scandinavian Simvastatin Survival Group. Randomised trial of cholesterol lowering in 4444 patients with coronary heart disease: the Scandinavian Simvastatin Survival Study (4S). *Lancet* 1994; 344:1383–1389.
7. Shepherd J, Cobbe SM, Ford I *et al*. Prevention of coronary heart disease with pravastatin in men with hypercholesterolemia. West of Scotland Coronary Prevention Study Group. *N Engl J Med* 1995; 333:1301–1307.
8. Grundy SM, Cleeman JI, Merz CN *et al*. Implications of recent clinical trials for the National Cholesterol Education Program Adult Treatment Panel III guidelines. *Circulation* 2004; 110:227–239.
9. Kastelein JJ, van der Steeg WA, Holme I *et al*. Lipids, apolipoproteins, and their ratios in relation to cardiovascular events with statin treatment. *Circulation* 2008; 117:3002–3009.
10. Libby P. Inflammation in atherosclerosis. *Nature* 2002; 420:868–874.
11. Ernst E, Resch KL. Fibrinogen as a cardiovascular risk factor: a meta-analysis and review of the literature. *Ann Intern Med* 1993; 118:956–963.
12. Ridker PM, Rifai N, Rose L, Buring JE, Cook NR. Comparison of C-reactive protein and low-density lipoprotein cholesterol levels in the prediction of first cardiovascular events. *N Engl J Med* 2002; 347:1557–1565.
13. Koenig W, Lowel H, Baumert J, Meisinger C. C-reactive protein modulates risk prediction based on the Framingham Score: implications for future risk assessment: results from a large cohort study in southern Germany. *Circulation* 2004; 109:1349–1353.
14. Danesh J, Wheeler JG, Hirschfield GM *et al*. C-reactive protein and other circulating markers of inflammation in the prediction of coronary heart disease. *N Engl J Med* 2004; 350:1387–1397.
15. Wilson PW, Nam BH, Pencina M, D'Agostino RB Sr, Benjamin EJ, O'Donnell CJ. C-reactive protein and risk of cardiovascular disease in men and women from the Framingham Heart Study. *Arch Intern Med* 2005; 165:2473–2478.
16. Nissen SE, Tuzcu EM, Schoenhagen P *et al*. Statin therapy, LDL cholesterol, C-reactive protein, and coronary artery disease. *N Engl J Med* 2005; 352:29–38.
17. Ridker PM, Danielson E, Fonseca FAH *et al*, for the JUPITER Study Group. Rosuvastatin to prevent vascular events in men and women with elevated C-reactive protein. *N Engl J Med* 2008; 359:2195–2207.
18. Smith SC Jr, Anderson JL, Cannon RO *et al*. CDC/AHA Workshop on Markers of Inflammation and Cardiovascular Disease: Application to Clinical and Public Health Practice: report from the clinical practice discussion group. *Circulation* 2004; 110:e550–e553.
19. Harrison D, Griendling KK, Landmesser U, Hornig B, Drexler H. Role of oxidative stress in atherosclerosis. *Am J Cardiol* 2003; 91:7A–11A.
20. Hansson GK. Inflammation, atherosclerosis, and coronary artery disease. *N Engl J Med* 2005; 352:1685–1695.

21. Furchgott RF, Zawadzki JV. The obligatory role of endothelial cells in the relaxation of arterial smooth muscle by acetylcholine. *Nature* 1980; 288:373–376.

22. Zhang WZ, Venardos K, Finch S, Kaye DM. Detrimental effect of oxidized LDL on endothelial arginine metabolism and transportation. *Int J Biochem Cell Biol* 2008; 40:920–928.

23. Inoue T, Hayashi M, Takayanagi K, Morooka S. Lipid-lowering therapy with fluvastatin inhibits oxidative modification of low density lipoprotein and improves vascular endothelial function in hypercholesterolemic patients. *Atherosclerosis* 2002; 160:369–376.

24. Pierce GL, Beske SD, Lawson BR *et al.* Weight loss alone improves conduit and resistance artery endothelial function in young and older overweight/obese adults. *Hypertension* 2008; 52:72–79.

25. Cracowski JL, Durand T. Cardiovascular pharmacology and physiology of the isoprostanes. *Fundam Clin Pharmacol* 2006; 20:417–427.

26. Basarici I, Altekin RE, Demir I, Yilmaz H. Associations of isoprostanes-related oxidative stress with surrogate subclinical indices and angiographic measures of atherosclerosis. *Coron Artery Dis* 2007; 18:615–620.

27. Shishehbor MH, Aviles RJ, Brennan ML *et al.* Association of nitrotyrosine levels with cardiovascular disease and modulation by statin therapy. *JAMA* 2003; 289:1675–1680.

28. Shishehbor MH, Brennan ML, Aviles RJ *et al.* Statins promote potent systemic antioxidant effects through specific inflammatory pathways. *Circulation* 2003; 108:426–431.

29. Jones DP, Mody VC Jr, Carlson JL, Lynn MJ, Sternberg P Jr. Redox analysis of human plasma allows separation of pro-oxidant events of aging from decline in antioxidant defenses. *Free Radic Biol Med* 2002; 33:1290–1300.

30. Blankenberg S, Rupprecht HJ, Bickel C *et al.* Glutathione peroxidase 1 activity and cardiovascular events in patients with coronary artery disease. *N Engl J Med* 2003; 349:1605–1613.

31. Nygard O, Nordrehaug JE, Refsum H, Ueland PM, Farstad M, Vollset SE. Plasma homocysteine levels and mortality in patients with coronary artery disease. *N Engl J Med* 1997; 337:230–236.

32. Alfthan G, Aro A, Gey KF. Plasma homocysteine and cardiovascular disease mortality. *Lancet* 1997; 349:397.

33. Carson NA, Neill DW. Metabolic abnormalities detected in a survey of mentally backward individuals in Northern Ireland. *Arch Dis Child* 1962; 37:505–513.

34. Welch GN, Loscalzo J. Homocysteine and atherothrombosis. *N Engl J Med* 1998; 338:1042–1050.

35. Shirodaria C, Antoniades C, Lee J *et al.* Global improvement of vascular function and redox state with low-dose folic acid: implications for folate therapy in patients with coronary artery disease. *Circulation* 2007; 115:2262–2270.

36. Homocysteine Lowering Trialists' Collaboration. Dose-dependent effects of folic acid on blood concentrations of homocysteine: a meta-analysis of the randomized trials. *Am J Clin Nutr* 2005; 82:806–812.

37. Toole JF, Malinow MR, Chambless LE *et al.* Lowering homocysteine in patients with ischemic stroke to prevent recurrent stroke, myocardial infarction, and death: the Vitamin Intervention for Stroke Prevention (VISP) randomized controlled trial. *JAMA* 2004; 291:565–575.

38. Lonn E, Yusuf S, Arnold MJ *et al.* Homocysteine lowering with folic acid and B vitamins in vascular disease. *N Engl J Med* 2006; 354:1567–1577.

39. Albert CM, Cook NR, Gaziano JM *et al.* Effect of folic acid and B vitamins on risk of cardiovascular events and total mortality among women at high risk for cardiovascular disease: a randomized trial. *JAMA* 2008; 299:2027–2036.

40. Meuwese MC, Stroes ES, Hazen SL *et al.* Serum myeloperoxidase levels are associated with the future risk of coronary artery disease in apparently healthy individuals: the EPIC-Norfolk Prospective Population Study. *J Am Coll Cardiol* 2007; 50:159–165.

41. Valkonen VP, Paiva H, Salonen JT *et al.* Risk of acute coronary events and serum concentration of asymmetrical dimethylarginine. *Lancet* 2001; 358:2127–2128.

42. Schnabel R, Blankenberg S, Lubos E *et al.* Asymmetric dimethylarginine and the risk of cardiovascular events and death in patients with coronary artery disease: results from the AtheroGene Study. *Circ Res* 2005; 97:e53–e59.

43. Blankenberg S, McQueen MJ, Smieja M *et al.* Comparative impact of multiple biomarkers and N-Terminal pro-brain natriuretic peptide in the context of conventional risk factors for the prediction of recurrent cardiovascular events in the Heart Outcomes Prevention Evaluation (HOPE) Study. *Circulation* 2006; 114:201–208.

44. Manolio T. Novel risk markers and clinical practice. *N Engl J Med* 2003; 349:1587–1589.
45. Wang TJ, Gona P, Larson MG *et al*. Multiple biomarkers for the prediction of first major cardiovascular events and death. *N Engl J Med* 2006; 355:2631–2639.
46. Zethelius B, Berglund L, Sundstrom J *et al*. Use of multiple biomarkers to improve the prediction of death from cardiovascular causes. *N Engl J Med* 2008; 358:2107–2116.
47. Koenig W. Cardiovascular biomarkers: added value with an integrated approach? *Circulation* 2007; 116:3–5.
48. Thygesen K, Alpert JS, White HD *et al*. Universal definition of myocardial infarction. *Circulation* 2007;116: 2634–2653.
49. Anderson JL, Adams CD, Antman EM *et al*. ACC/AHA 2007 guidelines for the management of patients with unstable angina/non ST-elevation myocardial infarction: a report of the American College of Cardiology/American Heart Association Task Force on Practice Guidelines (Writing Committee to Revise the 2002 Guidelines for the Management of Patients With Unstable Angina/Non ST-Elevation Myocardial Infarction): developed in collaboration with the American College of Emergency Physicians, the Society for Cardiovascular Angiography and Interventions, and the Society of Thoracic Surgeons: endorsed by the American Association of Cardiovascular and Pulmonary Rehabilitation and the Society for Academic Emergency Medicine. *Circulation* 2007; 116:e148–e304.
50. Apple FS, Murakami MM. Serum and plasma cardiac troponin I 99th percentile reference values for 3 2nd-generation assays. *Clin Chem* 2007; 53:1558–1560.
51. Liuzzo G, Biasucci LM, Gallimore JR *et al*. The prognostic value of C-reactive protein and serum amyloid a protein in severe unstable angina. *N Engl J Med* 1994; 331:417–424.
52. de Lemos JA, Morrow DA, Bentley JH *et al*. The prognostic value of B-type natriuretic peptide in patients with acute coronary syndromes. *N Engl J Med* 2001; 345:1014–1021.
53. James SK, Lindahl B, Siegbahn A *et al*. N-terminal pro-brain natriuretic peptide and other risk markers for the separate prediction of mortality and subsequent myocardial infarction in patients with unstable coronary artery disease: a Global Utilization of Strategies To Open occluded arteries (GUSTO)-IV substudy. *Circulation* 2003; 108:275–281.
54. Morrow DA, de Lemos JA, Sabatine MS *et al*. Evaluation of B-type natriuretic peptide for risk assessment in unstable angina/non-ST-elevation myocardial infarction: B-type natriuretic peptide and prognosis in TACTICS-TIMI 18. *J Am Coll Cardiol* 2003; 41:1264–1272.
55. Schnabel R, Lubos E, Rupprecht HJ *et al*. B-type natriuretic peptide and the risk of cardiovascular events and death in patients with stable angina: results from the AtheroGene study. *J Am Coll Cardiol* 2006; 47:552–558.
56. Bibbins-Domingo K, Gupta R, Na B, Wu AH, Schiller NB, Whooley MA. N-terminal fragment of the prohormone brain-type natriuretic peptide (NT-proBNP), cardiovascular events, and mortality in patients with stable coronary heart disease. *JAMA* 2007; 297:169–176.
57. Kazanegra R, Cheng V, Garcia A *et al*. A rapid test for B-type natriuretic peptide correlates with falling wedge pressures in patients treated for decompensated heart failure: a pilot study. *J Card Fail* 2001; 7:21–29.
58. Jernberg T, Stridsberg M, Lindahl B. Usefulness of plasma N-terminal proatrial natriuretic peptide (proANP) as an early predictor of outcome in unstable angina pectoris or non-ST-elevation acute myocardial infarction. *Am J Cardiol* 2002; 89:64–66.
59. de Lemos JA, Hildebrandt P. Amino-terminal pro-B-type natriuretic peptides: testing in general populations. *Am J Cardiol* 2008; 101:16–20.
60. Brennan ML, Penn MS, Van Lente F *et al*. Prognostic value of myeloperoxidase in patients with chest pain. *N Engl J Med* 2003; 349:1595–1604.
61. Baldus S, Heeschen C, Meinertz T *et al*. Myeloperoxidase serum levels predict risk in patients with acute coronary syndromes. *Circulation* 2003; 108:1440–1445.
62. Baldus S, Rudolph V, Roiss M *et al*. Heparins increase endothelial nitric oxide bioavailability by liberating vessel-immobilized myeloperoxidase. *Circulation* 2006; 113:1871–1878.
63. Sabatine MS, Morrow DA, de Lemos JA *et al*. Multimarker approach to risk stratification in non-ST elevation acute coronary syndromes: simultaneous assessment of troponin I, C-reactive protein, and B-type natriuretic peptide. *Circulation* 2002; 105:1760–1763.
64. Gersa RE, Wang TJ. The search for new cardiovascular biomarkers. *Nature* 2008; 451:949–952.
65. Samani NJ, Erdmann J, Hall AS *et al*. Genomewide association analysis of coronary artery disease. *N Engl J Med* 2007; 357:443–453.

66. Schunkert H, Gotz A, Braund P et al. Repeated replication and a prospective meta-analysis of the association between chromosome 9p21.3 and coronary artery disease. *Circulation* 2008; 117:1675–1684.

67. Genome-wide association study of 14 000 cases of seven common diseases and 3000 shared controls. *Nature* 2007; 447:661–678.

68. Becker RC. The investigation of biomarkers in cardiovascular disease: time for a coordinated, international effort. *Eur Heart J* 2005; 26:421–422.

69. Loscalzo J. Association studies in an era of too much information: clinical analysis of new biomarker and genetic data. *Circulation* 2007; 116:1866–1870.

70. Bossuyt PM, Reitsma JB, Bruns DE et al. Towards complete and accurate reporting of studies of diagnostic accuracy: the STARD initiative. Standards for Reporting of Diagnostic Accuracy. *Clin Chem* 2003; 49:1–6.

71. McShane LM, Altman DG, Sauerbrei W, Taube SE, Gion M, Clark GM. Reporting recommendations for tumor marker prognostic studies. *J Clin Oncol* 2005; 23:9067–9072.

72. Cook NR. Use and misuse of the receiver operating characteristic curve in risk prediction. *Circulation* 2007; 115:928–935.

73. Lemeshow S, Hosmer DW Jr. A review of goodness of fit statistics for use in the development of logistic regression models. *Am J Epidemiol* 1982; 115:92–106.

16

Novel lipid-modifying agents

E. A. Stein, K. M. Kostner, D. R. Sullivan

INTRODUCTION

Despite the success of the statins, in the past 20 years, only one additional class of agents, specifically ezetimibe as a cholesterol absorption transport inhibitor (CAi), has been successfully developed and introduced for low-density lipoprotein cholesterol (LDL-C) lowering [1, 2].

New and additional LDL-C lowering agents are needed for the following reasons:

■ Clinical endpoint trials have confirmed that greater LDL-C reduction results in more cardiovasacular disease (CVD) risk reduction [3–5].

■ Clinical practice guidelines continue to propose lower LDL-C goals in high-and even lower-risk coronary heart disease (CHD) patients [6–8]. In addition, even with current therapies, many patients do not achieve these goals [9].

■ Special populations, such as those with familial and other forms of severe hypercholesterolaemia, often require significantly greater LDL-C reductions.

■ Particularly, there are a growing number of statin-adverse patients [10] in whom there are limited alternatives for achieving significant LDL-C reductions if even a low dose of a statin cannot be tolerated [11]. Although the focus for statin toxicity has been rare and potentially life-threatening rhabdomyolysis, occurrence of mild, non-specific muscle-related side-effects (in approximately 5–10% of those treated) has become a major impediment to instituting successful lipid-lowering therapy [10] (Table 16.1).

Despite achievement of very low LDL-C and use of other proven cardiovascular therapies, many patients still experience initial or recurrent CVD events. Because of the strong epidemiological inverse relationship between high-density lipoprotein cholesterol (HDL-C) and CVD risk, and tantalising evidence from clinical trials with drugs that raise HDL-C as well as lower LDL-C [12, 13], attention is now also focused on raising HDL-C as the next potential target for further reducing CVD events.

Evan A. Stein, MD, PhD, FRCP(C), FCAP, Voluntary Professor of Pathology and Laboratory Medicine, University of Cincinnati; Director, Metabolic and Atherosclerosis Research Center, Cincinnati, Ohio, USA

Karam M. Kostner, MD, FRACP, Consultant Cardiologist, Department of Cardiology, Mater Adult Hospital and University of Queensland, Brisbane, Queensland, Australia

David R. Sullivan, MBBS, FRACP, FRCPA, Senior Staff Specialist, Department of Clinical Biochemistry, Royal Prince Alfred Hospital, Camperdown, New South Wales, Australia

Table 16.1 PRIMO: risk of muscular symptoms with individual statins

Statin	Dosage	Patients with muscular symptoms*	Odds ratio[†] (95% CI)	P value[‡]
Pravastatin	40 mg/day	10.9%		
Atorvastatin	40–80 mg/day	14.9%	1.421 (1.171–1.723)	<0.001
Simvastatin	40–80 mg/day	18.2%	1.812 (1.463–2.245)	<0.001
Fluvastatin	80 mg/day	5.1%	0.437 (0.352–0.542)	<0.001

*Percentage values relative to the total number of patients with or without muscular symptoms.
[†]Odds ratios were calculated using pravastatin as the reference.
[‡]P values were determined by Pearson's Chi-squared test.

This chapter reviews a number of novel agents currently in various stages of clinical development or with potential for further development.

LDL-C LOWERING AGENTS

SQUALENE SYNTHASE INHIBITORS

For many years drugs inhibiting cholesterol synthesis were avoided as targets for lipid-lowering therapy because of a scandal involving a drug, triparanol, which inhibited the final step in cholesterol synthesis, conversion of demosterol to cholesterol [14, 15]. The compound led to baldness, cataracts and impotence, and was withdrawn in 1962 after it was found that pre-clinical data submitted to the Food and Drug Administration (FDA) had been falsified. It was nearly two decades before Brown and Goldstein discovered the major rate-limiting enzyme in cholesterol synthesis, 3-hydroxy-3-methylglutaryl coenzyme A (HMG-CoA) reductase, which in turn regulated hepatic LDL-receptor activity and uptake of circulating LDL-C [16]. Furthermore, it was required to show that inhibition of HMG-CoA reductase with statins and the resultant accumulation of 4-hydroxy-3-methoxy HMG-CoA was water soluble, recyclable and not toxic in either animals or humans.

There are other potential opportunities for inhibition of cholesterol synthesis but these must be prior to the cycliclisation and formation of squalene, a non-recyclable compound. One of these, squalene synthase, has been a desired target since 1970s. However only one, lapaquistat (TAK-475) has entered advanced development [17].

In addition to lowering plasma LDL-C by upregulation of the LDL receptor, as statins do (Figure 16.1), squalene synthase inhibitors (SSIs) may have the potential to reduce myalgias and other muscle-related side-effects with statins. This is because SSIs inhibit the synthetic pathway further downstream after formation of a number of key mevalonate-derived compounds involved in intracellular energy utilisation. Specifically, ubiquinone (coenzyme Q10) is a prenylated protein that is part of the electron chain which functions as an anti-oxidant in mitochondrial and other lipid membranes and is important in the normal functioning of skeletal muscle [18, 19]. Interestingly, athough a number of recent trials have assessed the potential effect of ubiquinone co-administration in patients with muscle-related side effects (MRSE) on statins, results have been variable but usually disappointing [20].

Inhibition of squalene synthase does result in accumulation of farnesyl pyrophosphate, the last water-soluble intermediate in the cholesterol synthetic pathway. While farnesyl pyrophosphate has known routes for metabolism, it is principally excreted in the urine as dicarboxylic acid [21]. Farnesyl-derived dicarboxylic acids (DCAs), have the potential to result in toxic acidosis and were increased sufficiently in animal studies with a number of

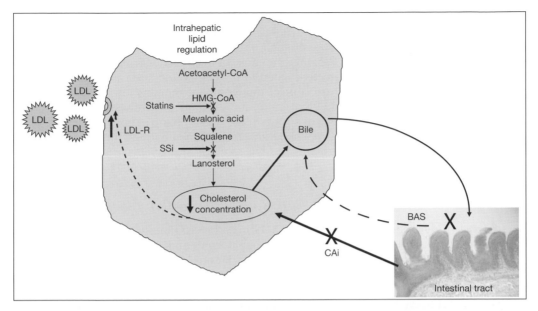

Figure 16.1 Mechanism for plasma LDL-C lowering by statins, squalene synthase inhibitors (SSi), cholesterol absorption inhibitors (CAi) and bile acid sequestrants (BAS).

SSIs, especially the zaragozic acids [22], causing them to be terminated prior to testing in humans. Preclinical studies with lapaquistat demonstrated no toxic acidosis although there was a mild increase in urinary levels of DCAs [17]. This was not sufficient to prevent the drug from entering human studies in which no significant acidosis was seen.

Lapaquistat undergoes rapid gastrointestinal absorption with a T_{max} ~3.5 hours and has high first pass clearance by the liver where it is converted to two active metabolites, MI and MII, which are excreted in the bile and subsequently the faeces, with minimal (0.2%), renal excretion [17]. While significantly metabolised via the cytochrome P450 3A4 system, lapaquistat does not appear to have significant interactions with statins, such as simvastatin and atorvastatin which are metabolised through the same CYP 3A4 system.

Lapaquistat has been extensively studied in a large, phase 3, global development programme involving well over 4000 patients exposed to the drug, mainly with a dose of 100 mg/day for up to 3 years. These have included a wide variety of hypercholesterolaemic patients including those with severe homozygous and heterozygous familial hypercholesterolaemia in whom lapaquistat 100 mg was added to maximal dose statin and in many patients also to ezetimibe and even bile acid sequestrants and niacin. A robust phase 2 dose-ranging trial evaluating the drug as monotherapy in approximately 60 patients per treatment arm (placebo, lapaquistat 25, 50 and 100 mg and atorvastatin 10 mg) has been presented [23]. Significant dose-related reductions in LDL-C of 16%, 18% and 26%, respectively, compared to placebo were seen. Similar reductions were seen in apolipoprotein B (apoB) lipoprotein, total cholesterol and triglycerides, with modest increases in HDL-C [23]. When assessed in a placebo-controlled trial in combination with stable doses of atorvastatin, an additional 20% decrease in LDL-C was found [24].

Initial safety and tolerability appeared good with the 100 mg dose, even in combination with the highest dose of the most efficacious statins. However one, and possibly two, patients developed both a sustained increase of >3 times the upper limit of normal range (ULN) for alanine transaminase/asparate transaminase (ALT/AST) and an increase in total bilirubin to 2 × ULN. This combination, given the term 'Hy's Law' [25], is viewed seriously by the FDA as an indirect indication of drug-associated hepatitis with the potential to lead to liver failure in approximately 10% of such patients. Subsequently, Takeda [26] terminated development in early 2008. Whether the cause of the liver abnormalities can be determined and whether these were directly related to the compound and can be overcome, or whether other SSIs will enter future clinical development remains uncertain. However, lapaquistat has clearly demonstrated that inhibition of squalene synthase can achieve significant additional LDL-C reductions of approximately 20% on top of both the highest dose of rosuvastatin and atorvastatin, even when they are combined with ezetimibe. This clearly indicates further capacity to upregulate the LDL receptor and achieve meaningful reductions in plasma LDL-C.

MICROSOMAL TRIGLYCERIDE TRANSFER PROTEIN INHIBITORS (MTPi)

Microsomal triglyceride transport protein (MTP) is a heterodimeric lipid transfer protein localised in the endoplasmic reticulum (ER) of hepatocytes and enterocytes, which plays a critical role in lipitation of apolipoprotein B (apoB) (Figure 16.2). It is vital to the formation of chylomicrons, very low-density lipoprotein (VLDL) and their downstream lipoproteins including remnants, intemediate-density lipoprotein (IDL) and LDL.

Since the discovery of MTP deficiency as the cause of a rare inherited disorder associated with very low levels of LDL-C, called abetalipoproteinaemia [27], this enzyme has been a therapeutic target. Abetalipoproteinaemia is also characterised by fat malabsorption, steatorrhoea and hepatic steatosis [28]. Prior to the development and treatment with water-soluble forms of vitamin E, the disorder was also associated with a number of serious neurological disorders due to both malabsorption of vitamin E as well as an inability to transport this lipid-soluble vitamin to the periphery and central nervous system (CNS), consequent on the very low levels of apoB-containing lipoproteins [29].

Systemic MTPi

Early animal and human studies confirmed that MTP inhibition reduces hepatic secretion of VLDL as well as intestinal secretion of chylomicrons [30–33]. Initial MTPi compounds were systemically active and inhibited the enzyme in both the liver and intestine. Although there may have been some modest differences between agents, all impacted on both apoB100 and apoB48 lipoprotein formation.

The first MTPi to be studied in humans, implitapide (BAY 13-9952) demonstrated significant effects on enzymes in the liver and intestine within 10 days [31]. Subsequently, BMS-201038 [34] and CP-346086 [35] also entered development. In 2001, Farnier and colleagues [36] reported a large, phase 2, dose-ranging, four-week, double-blind, placebo-controlled and parallel-group design study (MISTRAL), comparing the efficacy and the safety of 4 doses of implitapide (20, 40, 80 and 160 mg/day), placebo and cerivastatin (0.3 mg/day) in patients with primary hypercholesterolaemia. LDL-C reductions with implitapide ranged from 8.2% with 20 mg to 55.1% on 160 mg (P <0.001 compared to placebo), compared to a 33.3% reduction for 0.3 mg cerivastatin and 0.2% for placebo. In addition, dose-related reductions were seen in other apoB-related lipids, except lipoprotein (a) (Lp(a)). However, there were also dose-related reductions in HDL-C from 1.8–17.9% and in apoAI lipoprotein from 2–22.3%. Adverse events increased with the dose of implitapide with an unacceptably high incidence (mainly diarrhoea) in those receiving 80 and 160 mg/day. The percentages of patients with elevations in ALT >3 times the ULN were 8%, 8%, 27% and 25% in the groups receiving 20, 40, 80 and 160 mg of implitapide, respectively [36]. Further development of the compound was subsequently abandoned.

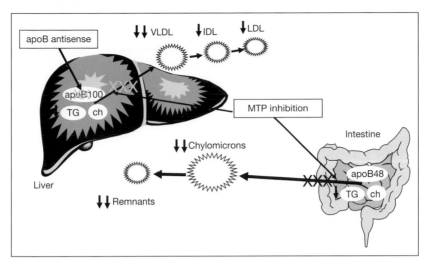

Figure 16.2 Reduction of plasma apoB containing lipoprotein entry into plasma by inhibiting apoB production or lipidation of apoB.

BMS-201038 was reported in a 7-day, ascending-dose, phase 1 study to produce large reductions in LDL-C ranging from 54–86% with doses of 25–100 mg [35]. However, there was a high rate of hepatosteatosis and adverse gastrointestinal effects, although the 25 mg dose was studied further in a longer phase 2 trial. Phase 2 data have not been reported for either the BMS or Pfizer compounds but both were apparently not carried into further development for similar reasons. An interesting observation from these trials was that, unlike statins, where after the starting dose additional LDL-C reduction when doubling the dose is approximately 6% [37], the dose–response with MTPi appeared quite steep.

After being abandoned by major pharmaceutical companies, both implitapide and BMS-201038 were provided to individual academic investigators, and small studies in homozygous familial hypercholesterolaemia (HoFH) and severe heterozygous familial hypercholesterolaemia (HeFH) were continued [38, 39]. In 2005, BMS-201038 was licensed to Aegerion, and renamed AEGR-733. In 2006, the same company obtained implitapide and renamed it AEGR-427. AEGR-733 entered new phase 2 trials at significantly lower doses (5, 7.5 and 10 mg/day) than the 25 mg/day dose originally investigated. It was administered for 4 weeks in a dose-escalating study with two other arms: ezetimibe only and a combination of ezetimibe and AEGR-733 [40]. Dose-related reductions in apoB and LDL-C were found; 30% for LDL-C with 10 mg dose. Triglyceride reductions were very modest, up to 10% with the 10 mg dose. In addition, there were significant reductions from 6.5–9.2% in HDL-C and 9–11% for apoAI with all doses. Thirty-two per cent of patients receiving AEGR-733 monotherapy discontinued treatment, mainly for frequent gastrointestinal side-effects. Elevated transaminases were also common.

Similar findings have also been reported with BMS-201038/AEGR-733 in HoFH patients [39]. Significant reductions in LDL-C up to approximately 50% were found with the 55–80 mg dose. Again, significant elevations of hepatic ALT were observed in more than 55% of subjects even at lower starting doses. Magnetic resonance imaging (MRI) showed hepatic fat accumulation in nearly all patients, even at lower doses.

The future of systemic MTPs appears uncertain because of their poor tolerability, transaminase elevations and probable hepatic steatosis, as well as the significant negative impact on apoAI lipoprotein and HDL-C.

Intestinal MTPi

Recently, Surface Logix Inc. described a MTPi, SLx-4090, that was minimally or not absorbed with effects only in the intestinal tract. SLx-4090 is a first-in-class inhibitor of enterocytic MTP, designed to overcome or reduce the inherent toxicity issues of systemic MTP inhibition. By inhibiting only MTPs in enterocytes, the drug reduces triglycerides and cholesterol transport into the lymphatic circulation and subsequent delivery to the liver.

Early results have promised that SLx-4090 might also achieve weight loss without hepatic and systemic effects [41].

APOLIPOPROTEIN B ANTISENSE

The other alternative approach to increasing LDL-C removal via the LDL receptor is inhibition of apoB lipoprotein production. apoB antisense inhibits only production of apoB100-containing lipoproteins which are found in the liver, whereas MTPi generally reduce both hepatic apoB100-containing lipoproteins as well as apoB48 lipoproteins, which are produced in the intestine and transport dietary fat via chylomicrons (Figure 16.2).

The principle for inhibiting apoB production is shown in Figure 16.3. The 'master blueprint' for apoB production is encoded in the two strands of deoxyribonucleic acid (DNA), one representing the 'sense' genetic code sequence and the other, containing complementary base pairs, the 'antisense' coding [42].

During transcription, the 'sense' and 'antisense' strands separate and the 'antisense' strand serves as a template for the production of a single-stranded messenger ribonucleic acid (mRNA). This mRNA has a base pairing matching the DNA antisense. On reaching the cytosol, ribosomes translate the mRNA to produce proteins, in this case apoB. It is possible to develop agents with RNase activity ('antisense'), which will degrade a specific mRNA, impairing its translation of the downstream protein (Figure 16.3). A potential advantage of antisense drugs is their increased specificity for proteins produced predominantly in the liver, such as apoB lipoprotein and other proteins important in lipid metabolism such as apoCIII, Lp(a) and proprotein convertase subtilisin/kexin 9 (PCSK9).

Initial investigation of antisense drugs showed they had predictable sites of accumulation, principally the liver, kidney, fat and reticular endothelium system [42]. All antisense drugs developed to date have been of single strand antisense nucleotide sequences that are complementary to mRNA, called antisense oligonucleotides (ASOs). Tissue levels are predictable from plasma concentrations, where they are 90% protein-bound, and correlate well with the pharmacology of ASOs. They disappear from the bloodstream rapidly but remain in tissue for prolonged periods, often months.

The only apoB antisense drug in clinical development is mipomersen [43]. It has a number of advantages over first-generation ASOs in that it has increased affinity for mRNA, is better tolerated, has increased resistance to nuclease activity and a prolonged half-life. Mipomersen is complementary to a 20-nucleotide segment of the coding region for the mRNA for apoB.

This selective hybridisation/binding of its cognate mRNA results in the RNase H-mediated degradation of the apoB message, thus inhibiting translation of the apoB protein [44].

There is also no cytochrome P450 (CYP450) metabolism and potential drug–drug interaction is anticipated to be minimal. Early studies have shown no interactions with simvastatin or ezetimibe [45].

Side-effects are apparently related mainly to the ASOs, rather than the target mRNA sequence to apoB, and predominantly relate to injection site reactions (ISR) and liver enzyme elevation [45].

Current ASOs are poorly absorbed [42] and need to be given parenterally. Initial administration in humans was intravenous to achieve faster hepatic concentrations and proof of efficacy in the limited time-frame associated with phase 1 trials. However, as the drug has

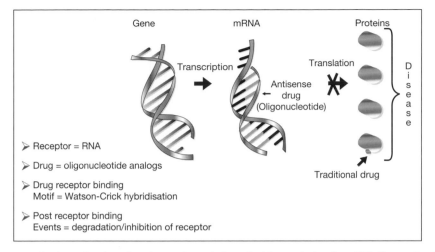

Figure 16.3 Mechanism of action of antisense drugs (adapted with permission from ISIS Pharma Inc.).

advanced in longer-term studies, it has been given subcutaneously, approximately weekly. Mipomersen has been assessed in a number of phase 2 trials, initially as monotherapy, followed by combinations with lower-dose statins and then high-dose statins and other lipid-lowering agents [45–47].

It is estimated that up to 6 months may be required for mipomersen to achieve a steady state. Thus it is likely the initial phase 2 trials, of 6–12 weeks, underestimated the final achievable reductions in LDL-C and other apoB-related lipoproteins. The initial dose-ranging study was carried out in 50 patients with moderately elevated LDL-C on diet alone [45]. Mipomersen 50, 100, 200, 300 and 400 mg was administered weekly for 12 weeks and patients then monitored for a further 90 days. A progressive dose-related reduction in LDL-C and apoB was found, reaching nearly 70% at the 400 mg per week dose after 12 weeks. Indeed, in many of the patients treated with 400 mg dose, LDL-C and apoB reached barely detectable levels. The sustained reduction in LDL-C and apoB was noteworthy and even 90 days after cessation of treatment, levels had not yet returned to pre-treatment values.

Additional studies have been performed in patients with heterozygous [46] and homozygous FH [47]. In both trials, mipomersen was added to maximal therapy which included the highest doses of simvastatin, atorvastatin or rosuvastatin, usually combined with ezetimibe, and in some patients, resins and niacin. Weekly doses of 50–300 mg were assessed. Robust dose-and time-related reductions in LDL-C (36% and 4.6% after 6 and 13 weeks, respectively, of the 300 mg dose), apoB, triglycerides, non-HDL-C and Lp(a) were also noted, with no significant change in HDL-C or apoAI lipoprotein.

As for all effective lipid-lowering agents, long-term viability often hinges on safety and tolerability. For mipomersen, the most common side-effect observed to date has been ISR, in more than 90% of subjects. These are usually mild, painless and associated with transient slight erythema. Histologically, ISRs consist of activated polymorphonuclear leucocytes and macrophages. There is no anamnestic response.

The major long-term safety concerns relate to potential liver toxicity because of prior data concerning drugs that inhibit assembly and release of apoB-containing lipoproteins such as the MTP inhibitors. However, only at the very highest dose of mipomersen tested (400 mg) were there significant numbers of patients with sustained increases in ALT of >3 times ULN, many of these having undetectable LDL-C levels. The dose selected for further development, 200 mg, was associated with minimal sustained ALT abnormalities. No cases of concomitant increases in bilirubin have been reported in these early trials.

CHOLESTEROL ABSORPTION INHIBITORS (CAi)

Inhibition of cholesterol absorption with ezetimibe has been shown to reduce LDL-C levels by approximately 18%, whether as monotherapy or in combination with agents such as statins [1] or fibrates.

Ezetimibe, the first of the cholesterol absorption inhibitors, has a mechanism of action that is consistent with binding to and blockade of a sterol transporter on the brush border membrane of intestinal epithelial cells, a Niemann–Pick C1-like 1 protein/transporter (NPC1L1) [48].

Through inhibition of intestinal cholesterol absorption, ezetimibe effectively increases net cholesterol excretion as two-thirds of cholesterol absorbed via the gut is recycled cholesterol and not just dietary. In addition, by reducing delivery of cholesterol to the liver via apoB48 lipoproteins, chylomicrons and remnants, there is a resultant increase in LDL receptor expression and this increases removal of LDL-C.

A number of other CAis are, or have been, in early phase 2 development, including compounds from AstraZeneca (AZD-4121) [49], Microbia (MCP 201) [50] and Sanofi (AVE 5530) [51], with only the latter now entering further phase 3 clinical development as monotherapy and in combination with statins [52].

PROPROTEIN CONVERTASE SUBTILISIN/KEXIN TYPE 9 (PCSK9) INHIBITORS

In 2003, Abifadel and colleagues [53] described a new form of autosomal dominant hypercholesterolaemia (ADH), which was not associated with mutations in the genes coding for the receptor or its ligand, apoB. They reported two mutations in the gene encoding PCSK9 that were responsible for hypercholesterolaemia. PCSK9 is a member of the nuclear protease family involved in degradation of the LDL/apoB receptor (Figure 16.4). The mechanism by which PCSK9 increases proteolysis of the LDL receptor was originally thought to be via enzymatic degradation. The mechanism has recently been elucidated more clearly, with recognition that the interaction between the LDL receptor and PCSK9 is important [54]. If the LDL cholesterol receptor is depleted from reduced endogenous synthesis or reduced delivery from the gut, key transcription factors termed sterol receptor element binding proteins, (SREBPs) are activated, leading to increased levels of mRNA and increased synthesis of the LDL receptor. There appears to be concomitant increased synthesis of PCSK9 [54]. As PCSK9 results in degradation of LDL receptors, this action is mostly likely a counter-regulatory mechanism to prevent excessive cellular uptake of cholesterol.

While mutations leading to increased PCSK9 activity have been associated with increased LDL-C as found in ADH, mutations which lead to loss of function result in lower levels of LDL-C [55]. These mutations and reduced LDL-C levels are also associated with reduced cardiovascular risk [56] (Figure 16.5).

These exciting findings have generated considerable interest because reduction in PCSK9 has no apparent negative clinical associations and thus appears an ideal therapeutic target. Furthermore, in addition to maintaining increased LDLR longevity, recycling and activity with downregulation of PCSK9, there may be added benefit with combination with statins and other drugs which upregulate LDLR activity. This is because statins have been shown to increase plasma PCSK9 levels [57].

Development of a therapeutic agent that targets PCSK9 may prove difficult. It has been shown that even mutations or changes in PCSK9 that alter its functional ability or even its binding domain to the LDLR, do not reduce its ability to redirect the receptor toward a path of increased catabolism.

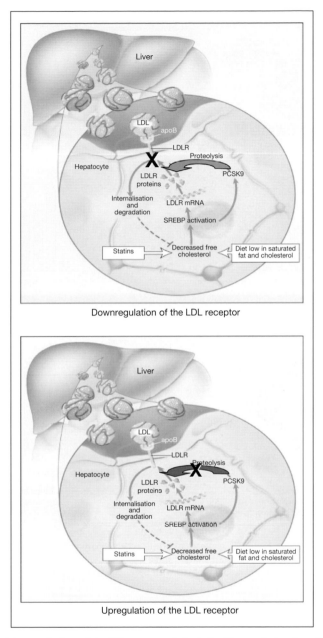

Figure 16.4 PCSK9 and its regulation of the LDL receptor (adapted with permission from Tall A. Protease variants, LDL, and coronary disease. *N Engl J Med* 2006; 354:1310–1312). LDL = low-density lipoprotein; LDLR = low-density lipoprotein receptor; mRNA = messenger ribonucleic acid; PCSK9 = proprotein convertase subtilisin/kexin 9; SREBP = sterol receptor element binding protein.

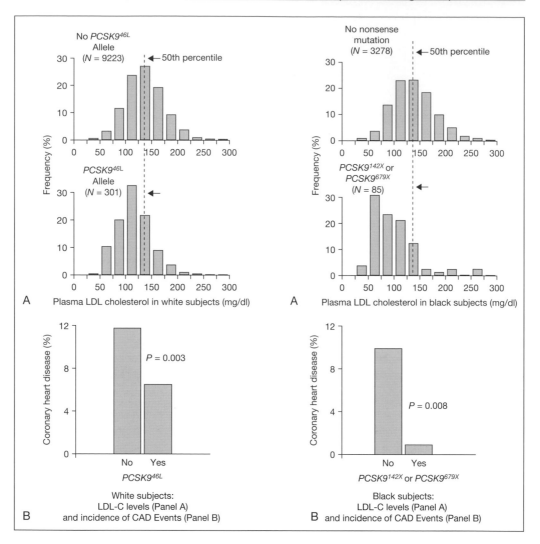

Figure 16.5 Distribution of plasma LDL cholesterol levels and coronary events among white subjects, according to the presence or absence of a PCSK9[46L] allele and black subjects, according to the presence or absence of a PCSK9[142X] or PCSK9[679X] allele (adapted with permission from [56]).

Small molecules that target PCSK9 could:

■ Prevent the autocatalytic process that results in the formation of mature PCSK9; this would have to be very specific to PCSK9 and not result in possible toxicity from formation of alternative forms of PCSK9; or
■ Block the ability of PCSK9 to bind to the LDLR.

However, an alternative approach using the same antisense technology described previously for apoB has already been successfully demonstrated in an animal model, in which a second-generation antisense ASO directed at murine PCKS9 reduced PCSK9 expression and decreased LDL-C by 38% in 6 weeks [58]. This study also showed that inhibition of PCSK9 expression was associated with a 2-fold increase in hepatic LDLR protein levels. Based on the promise shown in these animal experiments combined with the human experience with the apoB ASO, mipomersen, in May 2007 ISIS Pharmaceuticals and Bristol-Myers Squibb announced a collaboration to '*discover, develop and commercialise novel antisense drugs targeting proprotein convertase subtilisin kexin 9 (PCSK9) for the prevention and treatment of cardiovascular disease*' [59]. The first of these is anticipated to enter human studies in 2009.

HDL-INCREASING AGENTS

NIACIN FORMULATIONS

Niacin or nicotinic acid is a vitamin (vitamin B_3), a low dose of which is essential for human health. As a pharmacological agent, it was initially used to treat schizophrenia, but that use has since been abandoned. Niacin favourably affects all major lipid fractions and it is the most potent HDL-raising drug currently available in clinical practice. It also significantly lowers apoB-containing lipoproteins including VLDL and LDL, thereby reducing triglycerides and LDL-C. It is also the only currently available lipid-lowering drug that reduces Lp(a), one of the most atherogenic lipoproteins [60].

The use of niacin has been shown to lead to regression of coronary atherosclerosis and intima-media thickness in several studies, especially in combination with statins [60] and it was the first lipid-altering agent to significantly reduce cardiovascular events in the Coronary Drug Project (CDP). This clinical trial, which randomised 8341 men, demonstrated that 6 years of niacin therapy reduced the risk for non-fatal myocardial infarction [61]. An 11% reduction in all-cause mortality compared with placebo was seen in a 15-year follow-up study [61].

Although niacin is often used in the management of dyslipidaemia, especially in the United States, adherence to therapy is significantly affected by flushing, which is the major reason for discontinuation. Different niacin formulations vary in their flushing adverse experience (AE) rate as well as their effect on lipids. Immediate-release (IR) niacin, which is the oldest form of niacin, causes more flushing (25–40%) than extended-release niacin (niacin-ER), which is the most widely used form [61]. Nicotinic acid-induced flushing involves binding of nicotinic acid to its receptor and the production of prostaglandin D_2 (PGD_2) in epidermal Langerhans cells. PGD_2 binds to the prostaglandin receptor DP1 to induce vasodilation of dermal blood vessels. Recently, niacin-ER has been combined with laropiprant, a DP1 inhibitor, which has been shown to reduce flushing further [62].

Niacin has several modes of action:

■ Reduced free fatty acid mobilisation from adipose tissue via the G protein-coupled 109A niacin receptor has been one of the suggested mechanisms by which niacin decreases triglycerides (TG) (Figure 16.6).
■ New findings indicate that niacin also works via other important pathways and inhibits hepatocyte diacylglycerol acyltransferase–2, a key enzyme for TG synthesis [63].
■ The inhibition of TG synthesis by niacin results in accelerated intracellular hepatic apoB degradation and the decreased secretion of VLDL and LDL particles [63].
■ Decreased HDL–apoAI catabolism by niacin partially explains the increases in HDL half-life, which augments reverse cholesterol transport [63]. Unlike some other HDL-raising drugs such as fenofibrate, niacin does not inhibit scavenger receptor-B1 (SR-B1) [64].

Niacin can be used alone or in combination with statins, which augments reductions of apoB-containing lipoproteins and triglycerides as well as increases in HDL. It is not surprising therefore, that a combination of extended-release niacin and simvastatin has been recently approved by the FDA in the USA.

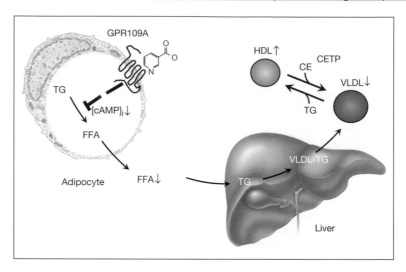

Figure 16.6 Niacin: mechanisms of action. Niacin decreases the mobilisation of free fatty acids (FFA) from adipose tissues, resulting in decreased hepatic triglyceride (TG) levels which reduce hepatic synthesis and triglyceride content of VLDL and lower LDL levels. Niacin also increases the degradation of apoB100 which is required for the assembly of VLDL particles. Niacin reduces the clearance of HDL particles from the plasma. This increases HDL-C concentration by reducing HDL turnover. Niacin also has effects on PPAR-γ and inhibits CETP (adapted from Soudijn W, van Wijngaarden I, Ijzerman AP. Nicotinic acid receptor subtypes and their ligands. *Med Res Rev* 2007; 27:417–433).

Two large mortality trials are currently underway looking at clinical endpoint reduction with niacin and statin compared to statin alone [60]. The Atherothrombosis Intervention in Metabolic Syndrome With Low HDL/High Triglycerides and Impact on Global Health Outcomes (AIM-HIGH) is comparing simvastatin plus extended-release niacin (Niaspan; Abbott Laboratories, Abbott Park, IL) with simvastatin monotherapy in 3300 patients at high risk, with cardiovascular disease, low HDL-C and high triglycerides. The Heart Protection Study 2: Treatment of HDL to Reduce the Incidence of Vascular Events (HPS2-THRIVE) is testing simvastatin plus extended-release niacin plus a D prostanoid 1 receptor antagonist, MK 0524, to inhibit the flushing side-effect in comparison with simvastatin monotherapy in 20 000 patients with coronary disease. These trials, which are due to be completed between 2010 and 2012, will provide important clinical outcome data.

CHOLESTERYL ESTER TRANSFER PROTEIN (CETP) INHIBITORS

CETP mediates exchange of esterified cholesterol and triglyceride between apoB-containing particles and HDL. Torcetrapib was the first of a new class of drugs that inhibit CETP [65], one of the effects of which is to elevate plasma HDL-C levels. In humans, torcetrapib, has been shown to increase plasma HDL by up to 100% and apoAI by 35% [66]. This increase in apoAI is due to decreased fractional catabolism of apoAI [66]. In subjects with low HDL-C levels, CETP inhibition with torcetrapib markedly increased HDL-C levels and also decreased LDL-C levels, both when administered as monotherapy and in combination with a statin [67].

On 2nd December 2006, development of torcetrapib was ceased due to an excess rate of mortality in a large clinical events trial, ILLUMINATE (Investigation of Lipid Level Management to Understand its Impact in Atherosclerotic Events) [68]. This has shown that systolic blood pressure in the cohort of the ILLUMINATE study increased significantly in patients receiving torcetrapib, the increase being apparent after about 12 weeks of therapy and being in part due to particularly large increases in a relatively small proportion of patients [69]. Furthermore, *post hoc* analyses showed that torcetrapib use was associated with an increase in aldosterone level accompanied by changes in electrolytes that were consistent with mineralocorticoid excess [70].

The lack of clinical benefit in ILLUMINATE [68] was supported by observations in other studies that torcetrapib did not slow progression of carotid intima-medial thickness [71] and coronary atherosclerosis [72] in atorvastatin-treated patients. The mechanism underlying the lack of clinical benefit of torcetrapib remains to be fully elucidated. It is not clear to date, however, whether the large, cholesterol-and apoE-rich particles formed by CETP inhibition are truly functional in reverse cholesterol transport and have anti-atherogenic properties [73]. However, the fact that the overall efflux capacity of HDL and faecal sterol excretion is not impaired following administration of torcetrapib suggests that HDLs created by CETP-inhibition are functional [74]. A recent publication by Nicholls and colleagues showed that raising HDL-C with torcetrapib was associated with a beneficial impact on progression of coronary atherosclerosis, and plaque regression was observed in those subjects who achieved the highest levels of HDL-C [75].

JTT-705 is another drug being developed to inhibit CETP [76]. This compound has been shown to increase HDL in animals and humans [77]. A single published study of JTT-705 in combination with a statin using a fixed dose of pravastatin 40 mg stated that '*no dose-related changes of vital signs, blood pressure and body weight were observed*' [78]. Phase 2 and 3 trials currently being conducted with JTT-705 will determine whether this drug provides additional benefits to statin therapy and whether this approach is safe.

Anacetrapib (MK0859) is another CETP inhibitor that is currently undergoing phase 2 and 3 studies. Anacetrapib has been shown to increase HDL without affecting blood pressure in healthy individuals [79].

PLASMA DELIPIDATION (PD)

Extracorporeal delipidation with organic solvents has been developed to remove lipids from circulating lipoproteins such as HDL and then return the delipidated lipoprotein particles to the bloodstream where they may promote reverse cholesterol transport [80]. This has been shown to lead to regression of atherosclerosis and mobilisation of adipose tissue in animal studies [81]. The benefits of infusing lipid-deplete forms of HDL have prompted the development of technologies that enable delipidation of an individual's own HDL, which can then be reinfused as acute therapy [82]. The effect of delipidation therapy is currently being tested in humans.

DIRECT HDL-THERAPY: ApoAI /SYNTHETIC PEPTIDES/ApoAI$_{MILANO}$ PHOSPHOLIPID COMPLEXES

Currently, the most direct approach to increasing HDL is the infusion of HDL, recombinant apoAI or apoAI-phospholipid complexes. Several apoAI analogues: AI, pro apoAI, recombinant apoAI$_{Milano}$, as well as mimetic peptides and small molecules such as ETC-462, ETC-216, 5F and D-4F, are currently under investigation. In one early study, apoAI/phosphatidyl choline discs were infused over 4 hours into 7 healthy men [83]. The authors concluded that the infusion of apoAI phosphatidyl complexes resulted in an increased intravascular production of small pre-beta-HDL *in vivo* and that this was associated with an increase in the efflux of unesterified cholesterol from fixed tissues.

In another study, Ericksson and colleagues [86] explored the effect of pro apoAI/phospholipid complexes on faecal sterol excretion as the final step in the reverse cholesterol transport pathway. There was a 30% increase in faecal bile salt excretion and a 39% increase in neutral sterol excretion, corresponding to the removal of approximately 500 mg of excess cholesterol after infusion. Lathosterol, a marker for the rate of cholesterol synthesis *in vivo*, was unchanged, suggesting that the net increase in cholesterol excretion reflected enhanced reverse cholesterol transport.

In a landmark study by Nissen and co-workers, five weekly infusions of a complex consisting of apoAI$_{Milano}$ and phospholipids resulted in significant regression of atherosclerosis in patients with acute coronary syndromes. The total atheroma volume decreased by 4.2% on intravascular ultrasound [85]. However, the study group was small and there is currently no evidence that infusion of apoAI$_{Milano}$ is more beneficial than wild-type apoAI or phospholipid complexes. In a similar study of patients following an acute coronary syndrome, serial coronary intravascular ultrasound imaging was performed to monitor the effects of four weekly infusions of either saline or apoAI/phospholipid complexes (CSL-111). Patients receiving infusions of CSL-111 demonstrated a trend toward regression and an increase in echogenicity, which is an intravascular ultrasound surrogate marker of plaque composition [86].

ApoAI mimetic peptides consisting of amino acid D-isomers remain active after oral administration and have been shown to inhibit the formation of atherosclerotic plaques in a hyperlipidaemic mouse model [87].

The clinical impact and safety of these direct HDL therapies has yet to be established in large clinical trials.

ENDOTHELIAL LIPASE INHIBITORS

Endothelial lipase (EL) is a 482-amino-acid protein from the triglyceride lipase gene family that uses a Ser-His-Asp triad for catalysis. Its expression in endothelial cells and preference for phospholipids rather than triglycerides are unique. Animal models in which it is overexpressed or knocked out indicate EL levels are inversely correlated with HDL-C. Endothelial lipase promotes hydrolysis of HDL phospholipid, increasing apoAI catabolism and decreasing HDL-C levels [88]. The findings that inhibition of EL reduces formation of lesions in animal models [89], and of a relationship between EL activity and coronary calcification in humans, suggest that inhibitors of EL may be beneficial [90].

NUCLEAR RECEPTORS AND TRANSCRIPTION FACTORS

Other targets for anti-atherosclerotic therapy affecting HDL are the transcription factors peroxisome proliferator-activated receptor (PPAR) α, γ, δ, LXRα, RXRα and other members of the orphan nuclear receptor gene family.

Greater insight into the impact of PPAR agonists on HDL levels and functionality have led to considerable efforts to develop more potent PPAR-α agonists than currently available fibrates, as well as agents that interact with multiple PPAR receptors (α, γ and δ).

Natural agonists of LXRα (oxysterols) and RXRα (retinoids), which improve cholesterol efflux from macrophages, and have a beneficial impact on reverse cholesterol transport [91], reduce lesion formation in animal models of atherosclerosis [92]. However, increased fatty acid and triglyceride synthesis as a result of an upregulation of hepatic expression of SREBP has limited development of potentially efficacious LXR agonists [93]. Only synthetic agonists that specifically exert non-hepatic effects are currently under investigation [94].

OTHER TARGETS FOR HDL THERAPIES

The use of endocannabinoid receptor (CB1) antagonists such as rimonabant to achieve weight loss has been associated with substantial improvement in HDL-C, particularly when combined with fenofibrate [95]. Unfortunately, the development of CB1 antagonists has been curtailed due to adverse effects on mood. Three other targets for potential anti-atherogenic treatments involving HDL metabolism are being actively pursued. Stimulation of apoAI synthesis and secretion, stimulation of ABCA1 expression and upregulation of SR-BI are all currently being tested [96].

REFERENCES

1. Davidson MH, Ballantyne CM, Kerzner B *et al*; Ezetimibe Study Group. Efficacy and safety of ezetimibe coadministered with statins: randomised, placebo-controlled, blinded experience in 2382 patients with primary hypercholesterolemia. *Int J Clin Pract* 2004; 58:746–755.
2. Stein EA, Ose L, Retterstol K *et al*. Further reductions in low-density lipoprotein cholesterol and C-reactive protein with the addition of ezetimibe to maximum dose rosuvastatin in patients with severe hypercholesterolemia. *J Clin Lipidol* 2007; 1:280–286.
3. LaRosa JC, Grundy SM, Waters DD *et al*. Treating to New Targets (TNT) Investigators. Intensive lipid lowering with atorvastatin in patients with stable coronary disease. *N Engl J Med* 2005; 352:1425–1435.
4. Pedersen TR, Faergeman O, Kastelein JJ *et al*. Incremental Decrease on End Points Through Aggressive Lipid Lowering (IDEAL) Study Group. *JAMA* 2005; 294:2437–2445.
5. Cannon CP, Braunwald E, McCabe CH *et al*. Pravastatin or Atorvastatin Evaluation and Infection Therapy – Thrombolysis In Myocardial Infarction 22 Investigators. Intensive versus moderate lipid lowering with statins after acute coronary syndromes. *N Engl J Med* 2004; 350:1495–1504.
6. Grundy SM, Cleeman JI, Merz CN *et al*.; National Heart, Lung, and Blood Institute; American College of Cardiology Foundation; American Heart Association. Implications of recent clinical trials for the National Cholesterol Education Program Adult Treatment Panel III guidelines. *Circulation* 2004; 110:227–239.
7. Smith SC Jr, Allen J, Blair SN *et al*.; AHA/ACC; National Heart, Lung, and Blood Institute. AHA/ACC guidelines for secondary prevention for patients with coronary and other atherosclerotic vascular disease: 2006 update: endorsed by the National Heart, Lung, and Blood Institute. *Circulation* 2006; 113:2363–2372.
8. Graham I, Atar D, Borch-Johnsen K *et al*.; for the Task Force European guidelines on cardiovascular disease prevention in clinical practice: Executive Summary. *Atherosclerosis* 2007; 194:1–45.
9. Davidson MH, Maki KC, Pearson TA *et al*. Results of the National Cholesterol Education (NCEP) Program Evaluation ProjecT Utilizing Novel E-Technology (NEPTUNE) II survey and implications for treatment under the recent NCEP Writing Group recommendations. *Am J Cardiol* 2005; 96:556–563.
10. Bruckert E, Hayem G, Dejager S, Yau C, Begaud B. Mild to moderate muscular symptoms with high-dosage statin therapy in hyperlipidemic patients – the PRIMO study. *Cardiovasc Drugs Ther* 2005; 19:403–414.
11. Stein EA, Ballantyne CM, Windler E *et al*. Efficacy and tolerability of fluvastatin XL 80 mg alone, ezetimibe alone, and the combination of fluvastatin XL 80 mg with ezetimibe in patients with a history of muscle-related side effects with other statins: A randomized, double-blind, double-dummy trial. *Am J Cardiol* 2008; 101:490–496.
12. Gordon DJ, Rifkind BM. High density lipoprotein – the clinical implications of recent studies. *N Engl J Med* 1989; 321:1311–1316.
13. Chapman MJ, Assmann G, Fruchart JC, Shepherd J, Sirtori C. Raising high-density lipoprotein cholesterol with reduction of cardiovascular risk: the role of nicotinic acid – a position paper developed by the European Consensus Panel on HDL-C. *Curr Med Res Opin* 2004; 20:1253–1268.
14. Steinberg D, Avigan J, Feigelson EB. Effects of triparanol (MER-29) on cholesterol biosynthesis and on blood sterol levels in man. *J Clin Invest* 1961; 40:884–893.
15. Triparanol Side Effects. Time Magazine, 3 April, 1964.
16. Brown MS, Goldstein JL. A receptor-mediated pathway for cholesterol homeostasis. *Science* 1986; 232:34–47.
17. Amano Y, Nishimoto T, Tozawa R *et al*. Lipid-lowering effects of TAK-475, a squalene synthase inhibitor, in animal models of familial hypercholesterolemia. *Eur J Pharmacol* 2003; 466:155–161.
18. Folkers K, Langsjoen P, Willis R *et al*. Lovastatin decreases coenzyme Q levels in humans. *Proc Natl Acad Sci USA* 1990; 87:8931–8934.
19. Ghirlanda G, Oradei A, Manto A *et al*. Evidence of plasma CoQ10-lowering effect by HMG-CoA reductase inhibitors: a double-blind, placebo-controlled study. *J Clin Pharmacol* 1993; 33:226–229.
20. Marcoff L, Thompson PD. The role of coenzyme Q10 in statin-associated myopathy. *J Am Coll Cardiol* 2007; 49:2231–2237.
21. Bostedor RG, Karkas JD, Arison BH *et al*. Farnesol-derived dicarboxylic acids in the urine of animals treated with zaragozic acid A or with farnesol. *J Biol Chem* 1997; 272:9197–9203.
22. Vaidya S, Bostedor R, Kurtz MM, Bergstrom JD, Bansal VS. Massive production of farnesol-derived dicarboxylic acids in mice treated with the squalene synthase inhibitor zaragozic acid A. *Arch Biochem Biophys* 1998; 355:84–92.

23. Piper E, Price G, Chen Y. TAK-475, a squalene synthase inhibitor improves lipid profile in hyperlipidemic subjects. *Circulation* 2006; 114(18 suppl II):II-288, Abstract 1493.

24. Piper E, Price G, Munsaka M, Karim a. TAK-475, a squalene synthase inhibitor, coadministered with atorvastatin: a pharmacokinetic study. American Society for Clinical Pharmacology and Therapeutics Annual Meeting 21–24 March, 2007 Anaheim, CA (PI-75). *Clin Pharmacol Ther* 2007; 91(suppl 1):S37.

25. CDER-PHRMA-AASLD CONFERENCE 2000. Clinical White Paper. November 2000 http://www.fda.gov/Cder/livertox/clinical.pdf

26. Discontinuation of Development of TAK-475, A Compound for Treatment of Hypercholesterolemia http://www.takeda.com/press/article_29153.html (accessed 28 March, 2008).

27. Wetterau JR, Aggerbeck LP, Bouma ME *et al*. Absence of microsomal triglyceride transfer protein in individuals with abetalipoproteinemia. *Science* 1992; 258:999–1001.

28. Scriver CR, Sly WS, Childs B, Beaudet AL, Valle D, Kinzler KW (eds). *The Metabolic and Molecular Bases of Inherited Disease*, 8th edition. McGraw-Hill Professional, 2000.

29. Rader DJ, Brewer HB Jr. Abetalipoproteinemia: new insights into lipoprotein assembly and vitamin E metabolism from a rare genetic disease. *JAMA* 1993; 270:865–869.

30. Stein EA, Isaacsohn JL, Mazzu A, Ziegler R. Effect of BAY 13-9952, a microsomal triglyceride transfer protein inhibitor on lipids and lipoproteins in dyslipoproteinemic patients. *Circulation* 1999; 100(18 suppl 1):Abstract 1342.

31. Stein EA, Ames SA, Moore LJ, Isaacsohn JL, Laskarzewski PM. Inhibition of post-prandial fat absorption with the MTP inhibitor BAY 13-9952. *Circulation* 2000; 102(18 suppl II):II-601, Abstract 2193 [presented at AHA national meeting, New Orleans LA, Nov 12–15, 2000].

32. Zaiss S, Gruetzmann R, Ulrich M. BAY 13-9952, an inhibitor of the microsomal triglyceride transfer protein (MTP), dose-dependently blocks the formation of atherosclerotic plaques and renders them more stable in apoE knockout mice. *Circulation* 1999; 100(18 suppl 1):Abstract 1343.

33. Bischoff H, Denzer D, Gruetzmann R, Muller U. BAY 13-9952 (implitapide): pharmacodynamic effects of a new and highly active inhibitor of the microsomal-triglyceride-transfer-protein (MTP). *Eur Heart J* 2000; 21(suppl):Abstract TuP9:W16.

34. Wetterau JR, Gregg RE, Harrity TW *et al*. An MTP inhibitor that normalizes atherogenic lipoprotein levels in WHHL rabbits. *Science* 1999; 282:751–754.

35. Chandler CE *et al*. CP-346086: an MTP inhibitor that lowers plasma total, VLDL, and LDL cholesterol and triglycerides by up to 70% in experimental animals and in humans. *J Lipid Res* 2003; 44:1887–1901.

36. Farnier M, Stein E, Megnien S *et al*. Efficacy and safety of implitapide, a microsomal triglyceride transfer protein inhibitor in patients with primary hypercholesterolemia. Abstract Book of the XIV International Symposium on Drugs Affecting Lipid Metabolism in New York, 9–12 September 2001, p 46.

37. Roberts WC. The rule of 5 and the rule of 7 in lipid-lowering by statin drugs. *Am J Cardiol* 1997; 80:106–107.

38. http://www.clinicaltrials.gov/ct/show/NCT00079859

39. Cuchel M, Bloedon LT, Szapary PO *et al*. Inhibition of microsomal triglyceride transfer protein in familial hypercholesterolemia. *N Engl J Med* 2007; 356:148–156.

40. Samaha FF, McKenney J, Bloedon LT, Sasiela WJ, Rader DJ. Inhibition of microsomal triglyceride transfer protein alone or with ezetimibe in patients with moderate hypercholesterolemia. *Nat Clin Pract Cardiovasc Med* 2008; 5:497–505.

41. Surface logix achieves big objectives with SLx-4090 in Phase 2a clinical trial: http://www.surfacelogix.com/news/news_080129.htm (accessed 29 January 2008).

42. Crooke ST (ed). *Antisense Drug Technology. Principles, Strategies and Applications*, 2nd edition. Marcel Dekker, Inc., New York, USA, 2008.

43. Crooke RM, Graham MJ, Lemonidis KM, Whipple CP, Koo S, Perera RJ. An apolipoprotein B antisense oligonucleotide lowers LDL cholesterol in hyperlipidemic mice without causing hepatic steatosis. *J Lipid Res* 2005; 46:872–884.

44. Monia BP, Lesnik EA, Gonzalez C *et al*. Evaluation of 2′-modified oligonucleotides containing 2′-deoxy gaps as antisense inhibitors of gene expression. *J Biol Chem* 1993; 268:14514–14522.

45. Kastelein JJ, Wedel MK, Baker BF *et al*. Potent reduction of apolipoprotein B and low-density lipoprotein cholesterol by short-term administration of an antisense inhibitor of apolipoprotein B. *Circulation* 2006; 114:1729–1735.

46. Kastelein JJ *et al*. Presented at Drugs Affecting Lipid Metabolism, New York, 4–7 October 2007.

47. Stein EA. High LDL-C on Three Drugs (abstract). Presented to the American College of Cardiology, New Orleans, March 2007.

48. Altmann SW, Davis HR Jr, Zhu LJ *et al*. Niemann-Pick C1 Like 1 protein is critical for intestinal cholesterol absorption. *Science* 2004; 303:1201–1204.

49. http://www.myfatdog.com/phase_ii_pipeline

50. Microbia MD-0727/MCP 201: http://www.microbia.com/pdfs/MicrobiaFinancing030107.pdf

51. Kramer W, Girbig F, Corsiero D *et al*. Aminopeptidase N (CD13) is a molecular target of the cholesterol absorption inhibitor ezetimibe in the enterocyte brush border membrane. *J Biol Chem* 2005; 280:1306–1320.

52. A Study Evaluating the Safety and Efficacy of AVE 5530 (4 Weeks) in Patients With Mild to Moderate Hypercholesterolemia. ClinicalTrials.gov identifier: NCT00440154. http://clinicaltrials.gov/ct2/show/NCT00440154

53. Abifadel M, Varret M, Rabès JP *et al*. Mutations in PCSK9 cause autosomal dominant hypercholesterolemia. *Nature Genetics* 2003; 34:154–156.

54. McNutt MC, Lagace TA, Horton JD. Catalytic activity is not required for secreted PCSK9 to reduce low density lipoprotein receptors in HepG2 cells. *J Biol Chem* 2007; 282:20799–20803.

55. Alborn WE, Cao G, Careskey HE *et al*. Serum proprotein convertase subtilisin kexin type 9 is correlated directly with serum LDL cholesterol. *Clin Chem* 2007; 53:1814–1819.

56. Cohen JC, Boerwinkle E, Mosley TH Jr, Hobbs HH. Sequence variations in PCSK9, low LDL, and protection against coronary heart disease. *N Engl J Med* 2006; 354:1264–1272.

57. Dubuc G, Chamberland A, Wassef H *et al*. Statins upregulate PCSK9, the gene encoding the proprotein convertase neural apoptosis regulated convertase-1 implicated in familial hypercholesterolemia. *Arterioscler Thromb Vasc Biol* 2004; 24:1454–1459.

58. Graham MJ, Lemonidis KM, Whipple CP *et al*. Antisense inhibition of proprotein convertase subtilisin/kexin type 9 reduces serum LDL in hyperlipidemic mice. *J Lipid Res* 2007; 48:763–767.

59. Bristol-Myers Squibb selects ISIS drug targeting PCSK9 as development candidate for prevention and treatment of cardiovascular disease. Carlsbad, Calif., 8 April 2008. /PRNewswire-FirstCall

60. Kostner KM, Gupta S. Niacin: a lipid polypill? *Expert Opin Pharmacother* 2008; 9:2911–2920.

61. Canner PL, Berge KG, Wenger NK *et al*. Fifteen year mortality in coronary drug project patients: long-term benefit with niacin. *J Am Coll Cardiol* 1986; 8:1245–1255.

62. Cheng K, Wu TJ, Wu KK *et al*. Antagonism of the prostaglandin D2 receptor 1 suppresses nicotinic acid-induced vasodilation in mice and humans. *Proc Natl Acad Sci USA* 2006; 103:6682–6687.

63. Kamanna VS, Moti LK. Mechanism of action of niacin. *Am J Cardiol* 2008; 101(8 suppl 1):20B–26B.

64. Nieland TJ, Shaw JT, Jaipuri FA *et al*. Influence of HDL-cholesterol-elevating drugs on the in vitro activity of the HDL receptor SR-B1. *J Lipid Res* 2007; 48:1832–1845.

65. Davidson MH, McKenney JM, Shear CL, Revkin JH. Efficacy and safety of torcetrapib, a novel cholesteryl ester transfer protein inhibitor, in individuals with below-average high-density lipoprotein cholesterol levels. *J Am Coll Cardiol* 2006; 48:1774–1781.

66. Brousseau ME, Diffenderfer MR, Millar JS *et al*. Effects of cholesteryl ester transfer protein inhibition on high-density lipoprotein subspecies, apolipoprotein A-I metabolism, and fecal sterol excretion. *Arterioscler Thromb Vasc Biol* 2005; 25:1057–1064.

67. Brousseau ME, Schaefer EJ, Wolfe ML *et al*. Effects of an inhibitor of CETP on HDL cholesterol. *N Engl J Med* 2004; 350:1505–1515.

68. Barter PJ, Caulfield M, Eriksson M *et al*. Effects of torcetrapib in patients at high risk for coronary events. *N Engl J Med* 2007; 357:2109–2122.

69. Howes LG, Kostner K. The withdrawal of torcetrapib from drug development: implications for the future of drugs that alter HDL metabolism. *Expert Opin Investig Drugs* 2007; 16:1509–1516.

70. Kontush A, Guerin M, Chapman MJ. Spotlight on HDL-raising therapies: insights from torcetrapib trials. *Nat Clin Pract Cardiovasc Med* 2008; 5:329–336.

71. Bots ML, Visseren FL, Evans GW *et al*. Torcetrapib and carotid intima-media thickness in mixed dyslipidaemia (RADIANCE 2 study): a randomised, double-blind trial. *Lancet* 2007; 370:153–160.

72. Nissen SE, Tardif JC, Nicholls SJ *et al*. Effect of torcetrapib on the progression of coronary atherosclerosis. *N Engl J Med* 2007; 356:1304–1316.

73. Kostner KM, Cauza E. HDL therapy: the next big step in the treatment of atherosclerosis? *Future Cardiology* 2005; 1:767–773.

74. Tall AR, Yvan-Charvet L, Wang N. The failure of torcetrapib: was it the molecule or the mechanism? *Arterioscler Thromb Vasc Biol* 2007; 27:257–260.

75. Nicholls SJ, Brennan DM, Wolski K *et al*. Changes in levels of high-density lipoprotein cholesterol predict the impact of torcetrapib on progression of coronary atherosclerosis: insights from ILLUSTRATE. *Circulation* 2007; 116:II_127.

76. Kobayashi J, Okamoto H, Otabe M, Bujo H, Saito Y. Effect of HDL, from Japanese white rabbit administered a new cholesteryl ester transfer protein inhibitor JTT-705, on cholesteryl ester accumulation induced by acetylated low density lipoprotein in J774 macrophage. *Atherosclerosis* 2002; 162:131–135.

77. de Grooth GJ, Kuivenhoven JA, Stalenhoef AF *et al*. Efficacy and safety of a novel cholesteryl ester transfer protein inhibitor, JTT-705, in humans: a randomized phase II dose-response study. *Circulation* 2002; 105:2159–2165.

78. Kuivenhoven JA, de Grooth GJ, Kawamura H *et al*. Effectiveness of inhibition of cholesteryl ester transfer protein by JTT-705 in combination with pravastatin in type II dyslipidemia. *Am J Cardiol* 2005; 95:1085–1088.

79. Krishna R, Anderson MS, Bergman AJ *et al*. Effect of the cholesteryl ester transfer protein inhibitor, anacetrapib, on lipoproteins in patients with dyslipidemia and on 24-h ambulatory blood pressure in healthy individuals: two double-blind, randomised placebo-controlled phase I studies. *Lancet* 2007; 370:1907–1914.

80. Kostner K, Smith J, Dwivedy A. Lecithin-cholesterol acyltransferase activity in normocholesterolaemic and hypercholesterolaemic roosters: modulation by lipid apheresis. *Eur J Clin Invest* 1997; 27:212–218.

81. Cham BE, Kostner KM, Shafey TM, Smith JL, Colquhoun DM. Plasma delipidation process induces rapid regression of atherosclerosis and mobilisation of adipose tissue. *J Clin Apher* 2005; 20:143–153.

82. Brewer HB Jr. Focus on high-density lipoproteins in reducing cardiovascular risk. *Am Heart J* 2004; 148:S14–S18.

83. Nanjee MN, Cooke CJ, Garvin R *et al*. Intravenous apoA-I/lecithin discs increase pre-beta HDL concentration in tissue fluid and stimulate reverse cholesterol transport in humans. *J Lipid Res* 2001; 42:1586–1593.

84. Ericksson M, Carlson LA, Miettinen T, Angeliu B. Stimulation of fecal steroid excretion after infusion of recombinant proapolipoprotein A-I. *Circulation* 1999; 100:594–598.

85. Nissen SE, Tsunoda T, Tuzcu EM *et al*. Effect of recombinant Apo AI Milano on coronary atherosclerosis in patients with acute coronary syndromes: a randomized controlled trial. *JAMA* 2003; 290:2292–2300.

86. Tardif JC, Grégoire J, L'Allier PL *et al*. Effects of reconstituted high-density lipoprotein infusions on coronary atherosclerosis: a randomized controlled trial. *JAMA* 2007; 297:1675–1682.

87. Navab M, Anantharamaiah GM, Hama S *et al*. Oral administration of an oral Apo A-1 mimetic peptide dramatically reduces atherosclerosis in mice independent of plasma cholesterol. *Circulation* 2002; 105:290–292.

88. Maugeais C, Tietge UJ, Broedl UC *et al*. Dose-dependent acceleration of high-density lipoprotein catabolism by endothelial lipase. *Circulation* 2003; 108:2121–2126.

89. Jin W, Millar JS, Broedl U, Glick JM, Rader DJ. Inhibition of endothelial lipase causes increased HDL cholesterol levels in vivo. *J Clin Invest* 2003; 111:357–362.

90. Badellino KO, Wolfe ML, Reilly MP, Rader DJ. Endothelial lipase concentrations are increased in metabolic syndrome and associated with coronary atherosclerosis. *PLoS Med* 2006; 3:e22.

91. Naik SU, Wang X, Da Silva JS *et al*. Pharmacological activation of liver X receptors promotes reverse cholesterol transport in vivo. *Circulation* 2006; 113:90–97.

92. Joseph SB, McKilligin E, Pei L *et al*. Synthetic LXR ligand inhibits the development of atherosclerosis in mice. *Proc Natl Acad Sci USA* 2002; 99:7604–7609.

93. Li AC, Glass CK. PPAR-and LXR-dependent pathways controlling lipid metabolism and the development of atherosclerosis. *J Lipid Res* 2004; 45:2161–2173.

94. Von Eckardstein A. Therapeutic approaches for the modification of HDL. *Drug Discovery Today* 2004; 1:177–187.

95. Florentin M, Liberopoulos EN, Filippatos TD *et al*. Effect of rimonabant, micronized fenofibrate and their combination on cardiometabolic risk in overweight/obese patients: a pilot study. *Expert Opin Pharmacother* 2008; 9:2741–2750.

96. Hersberger M, Von Echardstein A. Modulation of HDL cholesterol metabolism and reverse cholesterol transport. *Handbook of Experimental Pharmacology* 2005; 170:529–554.

17

The enhanced evidence base and translation into improved outcomes

A. M. Tonkin

INTRODUCTION

The evidence base supporting the value of lowering cholesterol is arguably as robust as any in cardiovascular medicine. Many landmark clinical trials have clearly established benefit of the 3-hydroxy 3-methylglutaryl coenzyme A (HMG-CoA) reductase inhibitors (statins), in particular, in various patient groups [1]. There is also evidence from large-scale trials, although less extensive, to support use of fibrates [2], niacin [3] and dietary interventions [4, 5]. Furthermore, mortality and other outcomes, at least for secondary prevention in coronary heart disease (CHD) patients, are related to whether or not statins and other guideline (evidence-based) therapies such as aspirin and β-blockers are used. For example, propensity analysis of a multicentre registry of patients following myocardial infarction showed that the adjusted hazard ratio for 12-month all-cause mortality was 2.86 (95% confidence interval [CI] 1.47–5.55) in those who discontinued a statin at one month [6] (Figure 17.1). Similar findings have been found in another recent Canadian study [7]. In the Global Registry of Acute Coronary Events (GRACE) [8], medical variables including a history of hypertension or heart failure, presentation with myocardial infarction rather than unstable angina, and specialist care were found to be important determinants of medication use. Other studies [6, 7] found that demographic and socioeconomic rather than simply clinical variables were most important. It has been suggested that these might operate through factors other than simply an absence of clinical benefit, and possibly reflect self-care behaviours.

Despite the strength of the evidence base, studies in many different regions of the world have consistently documented the failure of appropriate implementation of proven therapies such as statins in usual clinical practice.

The recent Reduction of Atherosclerosis for Continued Health (REACH) Registry collected data in 2003 and 2004 concerning cardiovascular disease (CVD) risk factors and treatment in 44 countries [9]. The registry included 67 888 patients, with mean age of 68.5 years, and 36.3% women, who had either established CHD, cerebrovascular disease (n = 18 843), peripheral arterial disease (n = 12 389), or three or more risk factors for atherosclerosis (Table 17.1). A total of 44% of patients were recruited from family practice and the remainder from office-based specialists. Patients in different regions of the world had similar risk factor profiles but were generally under-treated (Figure 17.2). In all, 72.4% had elevated cholesterol levels (arbitrarily >200 mg/dl, 5.18 mmol/l). Statins were being administered to 69.4% of all

Andrew M. Tonkin, MBBS, MD, FRACP, FCSANZ, Professor of Medicine; Consultant Cardiologist; Head, Cardiovascular Research Unit, Department of Epidemiology and Preventive Medicine, School of Public Health and Preventive Medicine, Monash University, Melbourne, Australia

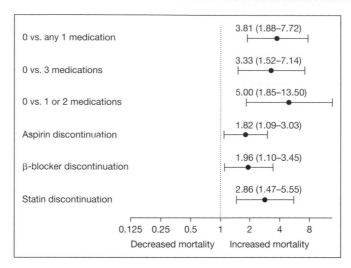

Figure 17.1 Adjusted hazard ratios for 12-month mortality following myocardial infarction in a multicentre registry according to whether or not drug therapies were discontinued by one month after the event (with permission from [6]).

individuals; to 76.2% of those with CHD, 56.4% with cerebrovascular disease and 64.2% with peripheral arterial disease. Other lipid-lowering agents were being given to 12.0% of all patients. There were regional variations in statin usage; North America 76.9%; Latin America 64.2%; Western Europe 69.9%; Eastern Europe 57.6%; Middle East 82.4%; Asia 60.5%; Australia 78.8%; Japan 44.6%. Cardiologists (79.1%) prescribed statins more frequently than other specialists such as neurologists who ranked lowest (45.2%) or family practitioners (69.4%). Highlighting that poor control and under-treatment are general, rates of current tobacco use (14.4% in those with established vascular disease) and inadequate treatment of blood pressure (50%) were also high.

Similar observations have been found in many other important surveys conducted in Europe [10, 11], North America [12] and elsewhere [13].

Inadequate treatment impacts not only on individual outcomes but also at population level and can increase healthcare costs [14].

Non-adherence is a particular problem in primary prevention. One cohort study of statin use showed that over a 2-year period, adherence was approximately 40% in patients following acute coronary syndromes, 36% in those with chronic CHD and 25% in primary prevention [15].

The importance of delivery of the most appropriate care, including the use of cholesterol-lowering agents, will be accentuated by the increasing epidemic of overweight and progressive ageing of many populations. For example, it has been projected that in the US, on the basis of adolescent overweight in 2000 and historical trends regarding overweight adolescents who become obese adults, there will be an increase in the prevalence of CHD by 5–16% by 2035 and 100 000 excess cases of CHD attributable to increased obesity [16]. Similarly, it has been estimated that ageing of the 'baby boomer' segment of the US population born between 1946 and 1964 will increase CHD prevalence by more than 50% from 2000 to 2030 [17].

THE ENHANCED EVIDENCE BASE: THE JUPITER STUDY

Recently, a further landmark study, the Justification for the Use of Statins in Primary prevention: an Intervention Trial Evaluating Rosuvastatin (JUPITER) has been published [18]. The

Table 17.1 Baseline demographics of population in the REACH registry

	Percentage of Population*					
	Total (N= 67 888)	Symptomatic (n=55 499)	CAD (n = 40 258)	CVD (n = 18 843)	PAD (n = 8273)	≥3 Risk factors (n =12 389)
Age, mean (SD), y	68.5 (10.1)	68.4 (10.1)	68.3 (10.1)	69.4 (10.0)	69.2 (9.8)	69.0 (9.8)
Men	63.7	66.9	69.8	59.5	70.7	49.5
Diabetes	44.3	37.5	38.3	37.4	44.2	74.9
Hypertension*	81.8	80.0	80.3	83.3	81.0	90.3
Hypercholesterolaemia **	72.4	70.2	77.0	58.2	66.7	82.2
Obesity+	46.6	44.0	45.4	42.6	44.1	58.4
Overweight (BMI, 25–<30)	39.8	40.9	41.7	39.4	40.3	35.0
Obesity Class I BMI, 30–<35)	19.9	18.8	20.3	16.5	17.2	24.8
Class II BMI, 35–<40)	6.7	5.8	6.4	4.9	4.6	10.6
Class III BMI, ≥40)	3.6	2.8	3.2	2.3	2.0	7.0
Smoker Former	41.6	44.6	47.1	38.6	50.9	28.4
Current	15.3	14.4	13.0	14.3	24.5	19.2

* Patients currently treated with medication
** Total cholesterol >200mg/dl (5.18 mmol/l)
+ Men: waist circumference 102 cm. Women: waist circumference >88 cm

results will almost certainly lead to a paradigm shift in thinking about high sensitivity C-reactive protein (hs-CRP) as a marker of increased vascular risk associated with inflammation [19], and, pending further analyses including cost-effectiveness, probable modification of guidelines concerning primary prevention.

The JUPITER study was undertaken in 17 802 apparently healthy subjects from 26 countries who were enrolled if they had neither previous cardiovascular disease nor diabetes, were aged 50 years or over if male and 60 years or over if female, and had a low-density lipoprotein cholesterol (LDL-C) level <130 mg/dl (3.4 mmol/l) and hs-CRP of 2 mg/l or higher. They were randomised to receive rosuvastatin 20 mg daily or placebo.

At 12 months, LDL-C was reduced from a baseline average of 108 mg/dl to a median of 55 mg/dl (1.4 mmol/l; interquartile range 44; 72 mg/dl), and hs-CRP from 4.2 to 2.2 mg/l (interquartile range 1.2; 4.4 mg/l). The trial was terminated early after a median of 1.9 years follow-up (planned 3.5 years) because of a highly significant reduction in the primary endpoint of the study, a composite of myocardial infarction, stroke, arterial revascularisation, hospitalisation for unstable angina, or death from cardiovascular causes (hazard ratio [HR] 0.56; 95% CI 0.46–0.69; P <0.00001). In absolute terms, events were reduced from 1.36 to 0.77 per 100 person-years of follow-up (number needed to treat [NNT] extrapolated to 5 years = 25). There was also a significant reduction in all-cause mortality (HR 0.80; 95% CI 0.67–0.97; P = 0.02). The primary endpoint was significantly reduced in all published subgroups, including women (38% of the cohort), minorities, those with body mass index (BMI) at baseline <25 kg/m^2, non-smokers and with low Framingham risk score (<10% CHD risk over 10

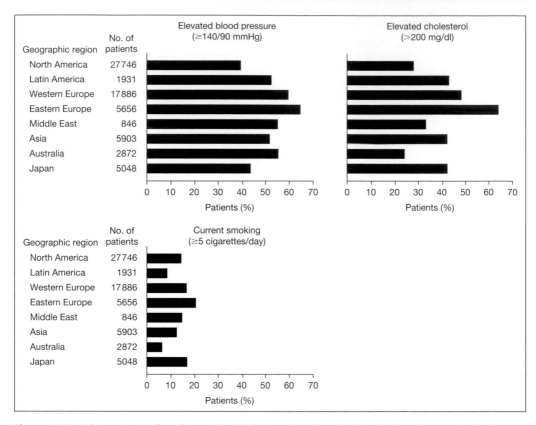

Figure 17.2 Undertreatment of cardiovascular risk factors, including cholesterol, in various regions in the REACH registry of 67 888 patients (with permission from [9]).

years). Apart from an increase in self-reported diabetes, there was no increase in adverse effects in those assigned rosuvastatin despite the low LDL-C levels achieved.

In previous studies, the levels of LDL-C and hs-CRP achieved following statins have been largely unrelated [20]. The relative importance of these effects of rosuvastatin in the JUPITER study is unclear from the present results. However, the observation that the observed treatment effect was not only greater than expected but also greater than predicted from the proportional 20–25% reduction in vascular events per 1 mmol/l lower LDL-C in the Cholesterol Treatment Trialists' (CCT) Collaboration [1], is consistent with the important pleiotropic effects of rosuvastatin on inflammation (Figure 17.3). Also, no insights are provided as to whether hs-CRP is only a risk marker or a causal mediator. The genetic epidemiology is uncertain, although the balance of evidence shows no association between alleles which are associated with high CRP levels and incident cardiovascular events [21]. However, a recent genome-wide association study in 6345 apparently healthy women found that loci associated with high CRP levels were closely related to loci associated with potential putative factors for CVD including insulin resistance, weight homeostasis and the metabolic syndrome, inflammation and premature atherothrombosis [22]. Whether CRP is directly involved in atherothrombotic processes may be further elucidated by studies of direct CRP inhibitors [23] or other anti-inflammatory therapies such as low-dose methotrexate [24].

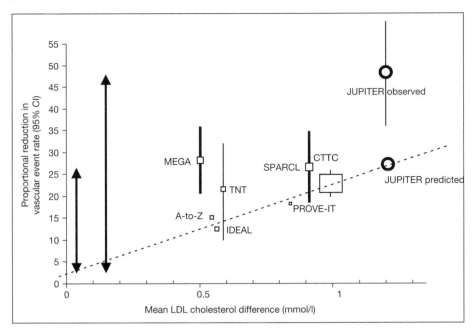

Figure 17.3 The relationship between the reduction in LDL-C and proportional reduction in major vascular events in the Cholesterol Treatment Trialists' Collaboration and subsequent major statin trials. The observed treatment effect in the JUPITER study was much greater than expected, consistent with pleiotropic effects of rosuvastatin on inflammation in subjects identified to be at higher risk because of baseline elevation in hs-CRP >2mg/l (adapted with permission from SEARCH Study Collaborative Group, Bowman L, Armitage J, Bulbulia R, Parish S, Collins R. Study of the effectiveness of additional reductions in cholesterol and homocysteine (SEARCH): characteristics of a randomized trial among 12 064 myocardial infarction survivors. *Am Heart J* 2007; 154:815–823).

Pending further analyses of absolute effects in subgroups (and cost-effectiveness which should include the initial costs associated with screening) and bearing in mind the age of the JUPITER cohort, elevated hs-CRP >2 mg/l may identify a new group for aggressive primary prevention, but sensibly after an initial period of lifestyle therapy if this is appropriate. In addition, guidelines concerning low hs-CRP are incorporated into risk assessment in those who are apparently healthy without CVD or diabetes could be reviewed [25].

FACTORS CONTRIBUTING TO THE EVIDENCE–TREATMENT GAP

Many factors contribute to the lack of implementation of guidelines and failure of persistence with therapy. They can be broadly categorised as related to patient characteristics, the therapy itself, providers and the healthcare system [26].

SOCIETAL FACTORS

Access to effective treatments can be a major problem, particularly in those countries which do not have local manufacturing facilities. In many countries, the cost of pharmaceuticals is seen as prohibitive. However, incremental cost-effectiveness is the critical issue. There is a direct relationship between the risk for future vascular events of the cohort enrolled in clinical trials or the individual(s) treated and the absolute reduction in event rate with treatment. It follows that lipid-lowering therapy is most cost-effective and should be targeted for support if resources are limited, especially when preferentially directed to those at highest risk.

PROVIDER FACTORS

Health professionals may not implement proven therapies for diverse reasons. These include lack of acceptance of guidelines, particularly if they are regarded as being out-of-date or do not have local 'champions', lack of resources and time pressures. Despite the universal nature of the evidence, international guidelines for lipid lowering differ. Such inconsistencies can also lead to inertia.

The complexity of clinical practice guidelines may also be a source of tension for busy professionals. However, for lipid-lowering therapy, the broad indications are relatively simple. Those who have clinical events associated with CHD [27] or with a previous stroke [27, 28] should be treated without a need to focus on cholesterol levels. An overview of 23 studies showed that the annual death rate in such patients in the absence of preventative treatments is at least 5% [29]. Statins should at least be considered in all people with diabetes, including those with type 1 as well as type 2 diabetes [30]. Finally, the estimation of absolute risk rather than cholesterol levels alone should be used to guide indications for treatment of those adults who are apparently healthy. Without preventative treatments, the annual death rate in men without CVD and aged about 60 years with cholesterol level >80th percentile has been estimated to be only about 0.6% [29].

CHARACTERISTICS OF THE PATIENTS AND THERAPY

Primary non-adherence – patients not filling the first prescription they are given – may be a greater problem than secondary non-adherence (after therapy is started, either failing to follow instructions for use, or failing to refill prescriptions) [7]. However, both are important.

A number of different factors contribute to primary and secondary non-adherence. These include the costs, complexity and inconvenience of treatment, concerns about safety, preference for non-drug therapies, inadequate understanding of the potential gains with treatment, and a poor relationship between the clinician and patient. Advanced age, cognitive impairment and depression may also be major contributing factors [26, 31].

MEASURES TO SUPPORT USE OF PROVEN THERAPIES

Because of the disparate nature of the factors outlined, efforts to improve outcomes must also be multifaceted.

UNDERSTANDING THE COMPLEMENTARY NATURE OF SOCIETAL AND INDIVIDUAL APPROACHES TO THE PREVENTION OF CVD EVENTS

Modelling of the decrease in age-standardised CHD mortality in various populations in recent decades has shown that this relates particularly to the decreased prevalence of risk factors and, to a lesser extent, to improved treatments and decrease in case-fatality rates [32].

Population-based and high-risk individualised strategies for CVD prevention are complementary. The Global Burden of Disease Study group has analysed the costs and gain in disability-adjusted life years with both 'non-personal' interventions such as the use of media for health education and 'personal' interventions such as cholesterol-or blood pressure-lowering drugs [33]. Their analyses again highlighted the much greater cost-effectiveness of drugs such as statins and antihypertensive agents when their use is based on absolute risk assessment rather than threshold levels of individual risk factors (Figure 17.4).

An important recent study used a Markov cost-effectiveness model to estimate the incremental cost-effectiveness of providing Medicare beneficiaries in the US with full coverage of secondary prevention therapies after myocardial infarction [34]. It was estimated that this would result in both greater functional life expectancy (an average of 0.35 quality-adjusted life years) and save money (an average of US$ 2500) from a societal perspective. Such stud-

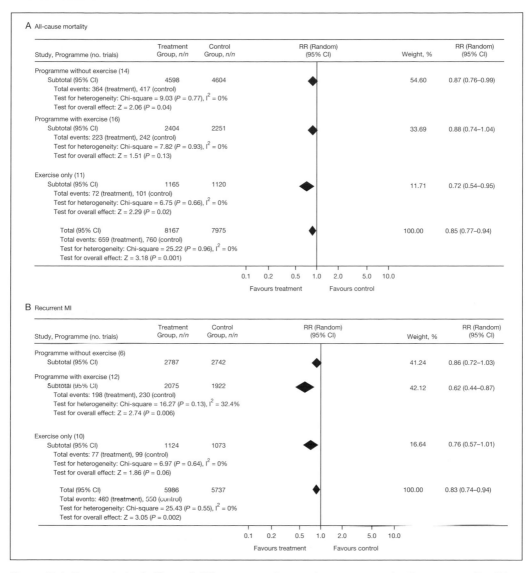

Figure 17.4 Meta-analysis of effects of different types of prevention programmes in all-cause mortality (A) and recurrent myocardial infarction (B) (with permission from [38]).

ies are most relevant when undertaken in the context of the local health system but may inform more effective use of 'health dollars'.

THE NEED TO TREAT 'NEGLECTED' GROUPS

For some years, there was uncertainty concerning the benefit of statin therapy in women. The initial landmark trials of statins were not sufficiently powered to detect significant benefits in females. However, there was no evidence of statistical heterogeneity in treatment effect. Similarly, under-treatment of the elderly has also been documented [35]. The Heart Protection Study [27] has now conclusively demonstrated benefits in both women and the elderly.

Often, treatment may be withheld in the elderly because of their shorter life expectancy. However, an analysis of the Long-Term Intervention with Provastatin in Ischemic Disease (LIPID) study of 9014 CHD patients aged 65–74 years at baseline has shown that the incremental cost-effectiveness of pravastatin was greater among those aged 65 years and over compared to younger patients [36]. Despite the shorter life expectancy of older patients, the lesser impact of treatment on this was more than offset by their greater risk of events and longer duration of hospital stay.

ESTABLISHMENT OF 'FORMAL' SECONDARY PREVENTION PROGRAMMES

Cardiac rehabilitation programmes were originally conceived to support the return of patients to the workplace following myocardial infarction. Subsequently, it was shown that exercise-based rehabilitation has a beneficial effect on outcomes in CHD patients [37].

These original concepts have been expanded with the recognition that formal programmes can provide the platform for ongoing effective secondary prevention in those who have had CHD events. The importance of this is highlighted by the fact that linkage of administrative datasets has shown that about half of all CHD deaths and non-fatal myocardial infarctions occur in the small percentage (around 5%) of the population who have already been diagnosed with CHD [Michael Hobbs, Western Australia, personal communication].

A meta-analysis of 63 randomised trials evaluating secondary prevention programmes in 21 295 patients following myocardial infarction demonstrated a reduction in both all-cause mortality and recurrent myocardial infarction [38] (Figure 17.5). The risk ratio (RR) avoid splittuy numles 21 295 for all-cause mortality was 0.85 (95% CI 0.77–0.94), but varied with time (RR 0.97; 95% CI 0.82–1.14 at 12 months and RR 0.53; 95% CI 0.35–0.81 after this). The risk ratio for recurrent myocardial infarction was 0.83 (95% CI 0.74–0.94) over a median follow-up of 12 months. These benefits were similar for programmes that included coronary risk factor education or counselling with a supervised and structured exercise component, and for programmes with only one of these two elements. The beneficial effects on all-cause mortality were also similar in more recent trials to those observed in trials performed some decades ago before the widespread use of statins and other therapies.

Flexibility of such programmes is important. Depending on the societal context, cultural diversity and use of information technology which supports programme delivery to more remote regions may be important.

EARLY FOLLOW-UP AND SHARED CARE OF PATIENTS AFTER DISCHARGE

Most quality improvement initiatives for management of CHD patients have concentrated on the hospital setting. However, the interplay between hospital specialists and primary care practitioners is an important factor in guideline implementation. Primary care physicians are less likely to initiate a therapy but will usually continue treatment which is initiated in hospital.

Current guidelines recommend that patients are followed up within a few weeks of hospital discharge after acute myocardial infarction [39]. Although this recommendation had been largely based on expert opinion, a recent analysis of the Prospective Registry Evaluating Myocardial Infarction: Events and Recovery (PREMIER) registry in the United States supports this [40].

Of 1516 patients hospitalised with acute myocardial infarction between January 2003 and June 2004 and who completed follow-up interviews at one-and six months, 34% had no follow-up visit within one month, 52% had follow-up within one month by either a primary care physician or cardiologist, and 14% had follow-up within one month by both. Discharge medication rates were similar among these groups. Adjusting for relevant patient and clinical characteristics, patients followed up within one month were more likely to be still receiving a statin at 6 months (75.9% vs. 68.6%; $P = 0.005$). Similar results were found

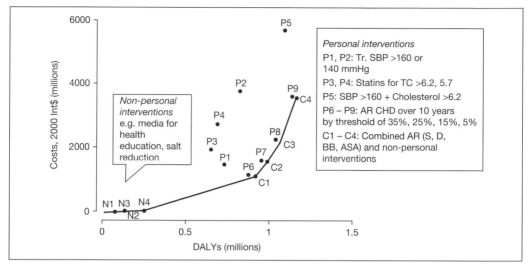

Figure 17.5 Modelling by the Global Burden of Disease Study Group showing the complementary nature of population and high-risk approaches to prevention of cardiovascular disease, and the importance of basing the high-risk approach on absolute risk rather than systolic blood pressure or cholesterol alone (adapted with permission from [33]). AR = absolute risk; ASA = aspirin; BB = beta blocker; C = combined personal and non-personal interventions; D = drugs for blood pressure; N = non-personal interventions; P = personal interventions; S = statin; Tr. = treatment.

with persistence of use of β-blockers (80.1% vs. 71.3%; $P = 0.001$) and aspirin (82.9% vs. 77.1%; $P = 0.01$). A further analysis showed that statin use at six months was significantly higher in patients seen within one month after discharge by both a primary care physician and a cardiologist [40].

THE IMPORTANT ROLE OF PRIMARY CARE PRACTITIONERS

Health systems in developed countries often focus particularly on specialists for the delivery of evidence-based care. This probably reflects the fact that in many societies, the major proportion of direct costs associated with CVD relates to hospital care.

However primary healthcare if adequately resourced, may be more accessible, equitable and, indeed, cost-effective for delivery of preventive therapies. Primary care initiatives which have been shown to be effective in implementing guidelines include maintenance of registers of CHD patients (which can be linked to electronic prescribing), support for risk factor assessment, care plans which might help employer-, patient- and nurse-led secondary prevention services.

Incentive funding can be important. One such programme is the Quality and Outcomes Framework in the United Kingdom National Health Service which was directed towards improving primary care practice. A key aspect was additional funding if quality of clinical care could be demonstrated. Coronary heart disease and diabetes were among conditions for which quality indicators were introduced. For CHD these included not only a process indicator related to the creation of a disease register of CHD patients, but an outcome measure, the proportion of patients in whom cholesterol levels were recorded and with their last cholesterol level ≤5mmol/l. Not only have standards of care risen in primary care in the UK, but there appears to have been a narrowing of the gap between measures in those from the least-and most-deprived areas.

It has also been shown that non-physician healthcare workers can competently assess and manage cardiovascular risk in primary care [41]. This is particularly relevant in settings in which physicians are not available.

APPROPRIATE PROGRAMMES

Coronary heart disease and cardiovascular risk factors tend to segregate in families. The cultural and social environment of family members is often similar in addition to their 'shared' lifestyle.

An important study compared outcomes in 30–59-year-old American siblings of patients who had had a CHD event before the age of 60 years [42]. The 364 subjects studied had blood pressure ≥149/90 mmHg, LDL-C ≥3.37 mmol/l (130 mg/dl) or were current smokers. They were randomised to receive 'enhanced' primary care or community-based care from a nurse practitioner and a community health worker and followed for one year. The community-based care programme was designed by a community advisory panel. 'Enhanced' primary care included patient materials, free medications, exercise opportunities and comprehensive screening with dissemination of guidelines. Despite this enhancement, after adjustment for age, sex, education and baseline use of medications, LDL-C goals were more likely to be achieved in those receiving community-based care (relative odds 2.2; 95% CI 1.11–4.20). Community-based care was also associated with lower LDL-C levels (3.59 ± 1.0 mmol/l at baseline decreasing to 3.06 ± 1.0 mmol/l at one year compared with 3.51 ± 1.0 mmol/l decreasing to 3.33 ± 1.0 mmol/l; P <0.0001) and also lower levels of blood pressure, blood glucose, Framingham risk score and greater usage of both lipid-lowering and anti-hypertensive agents (all P <0.0001).

It seems logical that, as an extension, the effect of family-based community interventions should be investigated, particularly among patients with CHD and their children. In this context, both primary and secondary prevention might be enhanced because of mutual family support.

DETECTING AND IMPROVING NON-ADHERENCE

Markers for non-adherence include missed appointments, lack of anticipated response (e.g. in LDL-C) and missed refills [26].

Adherence is often not explored in the patient encounter. Non-judgemental questions which the patient should be asked and which have been validated include: *'Do you ever forget to take your medication?'*; *'Are you irregular or inconsistent at times about taking your medicines?'*; *'When you feel better, do you sometimes stop taking your medication?'*; *'Sometimes, if you feel worse when you are taking your medicine, do you stop taking it?'* [43].

Strategies to improve adherence to medication include simplification of the treatment regimen, provision of simple, clear instructions, encouraging use of a medication-taking system, telephone calls and other prompts, obtaining support from family and others in the community, and reinforcement of the benefits of treatment [26].

THE NEED FOR POLICY-MAKERS TO IMPLEMENT STRATEGIES TO IMPACT SPECIFICALLY ON HEALTH INEQUALITIES

Socioeconomic inequalities in health are a major problem worldwide [44]. Furthermore, in many countries, cardiovascular disease is the major cause of such inequalities. Although absolute differences in health outcomes between the vulnerable, disadvantaged and the advantaged in some societies may have decreased, relative inequalities have often widened.

Some countries have suggested specific strategies to reduce health inequalities [45, 46] and it has also been suggested that all strategies should be monitored for the extent to which they impact on inequalities [45]. As one specific example, patients less likely to attend and to complete secondary prevention programmes include those among the groups at highest risk: women, the elderly, low-income groups and ethnic minorities [47].

IMPROVING RISK COMMUNICATION

The term 'concordance' encompasses the concept of a consensual agreement between the patient and his or her practitioner. It establishes the appropriate basis for improving outcomes through effective use of therapies.

Risk communication is one important aspect of this interaction between the provider and patient. This is because the patients' understanding of their risk of future events and of the benefits of both lifestyle and pharmacological therapies, influences behaviour and can improve compliance. However, in clinical practice, little attention is paid to the process of communication.

Communication can occur in a number of ways, including verbally, as written statements, or in graphical or other visual formats [48]. Materials can also allow presentation of the positive effect of change. Flexibility is important, not only to allow for variable degrees of health literacy and user preferences but also to permit subsequent discussion with family members and others. Communication is enhanced when information is framed in a positive way, e.g. in terms of benefit or survival rather than the chance of death [48].

Atherosclerosis develops over many decades. This would suggest the particular value of presenting risk over a very long time-frame, even as lifelong risk. However, our own focus group testing has shown that depiction of risk over a shorter time-frame, e.g. 5 rather than 10 years is more meaningful to those who are apparently healthy [S Hill et al., submitted]. Risk within 10 years was seen as too remote, leading individuals to perhaps defer lifestyle change. Another strategy that has been proposed is to present a cardiovascular risk-adjusted age as a contrast to the true age of an individual [49].

It is likely that active involvement of consumers in the development of health information materials which should supplement guidelines and be a focus of communication between the health professional and consumer would also enhance the implementation of guidelines. Although these concepts may appear simple, e.g. couching risk in terms of betting odds (6 or 7 to 1) rather than percentages (16%), there are large potential gains from further research and education related to methods of communication.

ADDRESSING COSTS AND INCONVENIENCE

The concept of a 'polypill', the cheap co-formulation of generic cardiovascular agents was based on an analysis of the independent beneficial effects of statins, blood pressure lowering, aspirin and folic acid in clinical trials [50]. The case for folic acid was subsequently challenged because lowering of homocysteine levels has not translated to a reduction in CHD events [51]. Polypills (excluding folic acid) are about to enter clinical trials in a number of countries. The primary endpoint of these randomised studies comparing the polypill with usual management with the individual agents will often be compliance or measures related to this such as cholesterol and blood pressure levels. A prospective meta-analysis of these trials could examine the effects of the polypill on 'hard' clinical endpoints.

It was initially proposed that population groups who should be given the polypill were those with known CVD, people with diabetes and others aged ≥55 years [49]. It was argued that these broad categories should be treated without reference to risk factor levels because of the absence of a threshold in the association with clinical events and the fact that most myocardial infarctions and strokes occur in people with near-average cholesterol and blood pressure levels. Antagonists of the polypill argue that the approach mitigates against dosing flexibility and may therefore increase side-effects. They have also expressed concerns about 'medicalisation' of what is largely a disease of lifestyle and behaviour. Indeed, similar methodology to the seminal polypill paper [50] has been applied to dietary factors [52]. Modelling suggested a similar reduction in risk of CVD events with a 'polymeal' – an evidence-based recipe of wine, fish, dark chocolate, fruit and vegetables, garlic and almonds!

ALLAYING CONCERNS ABOUT THE SAFETY OF TREATMENT

The popular media has caused substantial harm by sensational over-reporting of the possible danger of low cholesterol levels. Such reporting has encompassed conditions such as cancer, suicide and memory loss.

Observational studies have shown that low cholesterol levels are associated with increased mortality from diseases such as cancers, chronic respiratory disease, chronic kidney disease and haemorrhagic stroke [53, 54]. These observations may often reflect reverse causality. The significance of these observational data was magnified in the eyes of some by other isolated reports, such as the increase in breast cancer among women in the CARE (Cholesterol And Recurrent Events) study [55] or in gastrointestinal cancer in the PROSPER (Prospective Study of Pravastatin in the Elderly at Risk) study [56]. However, the first cycle of analyses of individual data from 90 056 participants in 14 trials in the CCT Collaboration [1] showed no difference in non-vascular deaths (either total deaths or for a specific cause of death) among those assigned statin (3.8%) or control treatment (4.0%; $P = 0.1$). There was also no association between statin treatment and cancer. The five-year follow-up in this analysis was probably too short to exclude without reasonable doubt any possible association with non-vascular death, particularly from cancer. Further reassurance has come from published extended follow-up to 10 and 12 years in 4S (Scandinavian Simvastatin Survival Study [57]) and LIPID [58]) respectively.

A significant number of patients complain of muscle pains while taking a statin. However, meta-analyses have found no difference in myopathy – muscle pain or weakness with creatinine kinase >10 times upper limit of normal between those assigned placebo or a statin [1, 59, 60]. Rhabdomyolysis is a potentially fatal but rare adverse event, occurring much less frequently than potentially fatal haemorrhage in patients taking low-dose aspirin. The incidence of myopathy does not appear to be significantly increased with higher doses of statins.

Although statins may be associated with asymptomatic elevation in serum transaminase levels, typically within the first few months of starting treatment, transaminase levels nearly always normalise on stopping treatment or reducing the dose. There is also no evidence that an increase in serum transaminase levels is associated with development of chronic liver disease.

Studies involving formal neurophysiological testing [61] and controlled trial data should also allay anxiety concerning early reports related to depression [62] and memory loss [63].

Papers discussing safety (rather than harm) do not receive the attention they warrant. There has been an excellent discussion of this elsewhere [64].

FACILITATING PATIENT ASSESSMENT: NON-FASTING SAMPLES IN FUTURE PRACTICE?

It is currently recommended that lipid parameters are assessed from blood samples taken after 8–12 hours fasting. This is because of the increase in plasma triglyceride levels after food is taken and the fact that the Friedewald equation used to calculate indirect LDL-C concentration (the cornerstone for conventional assessment) includes a correction for fasting triglyceride levels.

In addition, the importance of fasting triglyceride levels as an independent risk factor for CVD has been debated. This partly reflects the inverse correlation between triglyceride and high-density lipoprotein cholesterol (HDL-C) levels and studies which have shown that correction for HDL-C attenuates the risk associated with triglyceride levels.

In many societies, humans spend much of their time in the non-fasting state. Early research showed that postprandial plasma triglyceride levels were higher in CHD patients than in controls [65]. Recent studies have shown a significant association between non-fasting (but not fasting) triglyceride levels and adjusted risk of future cardiovascular events. The association was stronger for levels taken 2–4 hours after a meal, corresponding to the time course of postprandial triglyceride metabolism [66].

Therefore, future wider availability of direct assays for LDL-C, coupled with the importance of non-fasting triglyceride levels hold promise for simplifying the point-of-contact assessment of lipid profiles. More importantly, increasing data, including from the landmark INTERHEART study [67] support the proposition that non-fasting apoB/apoA1 ratio (or perhaps HDL and non-HDL levels) could replace LDL-C and HDL-C and triglycerides as the lipid parameters which should be assessed.

RECOGNITION THAT LIFESTYLE APPROACHES ARE FUNDAMENTAL IN ALL APPROACHES TO PREVENTION

Atherosclerosis is largely a disease of lifestyle and behaviour. It is essential that all therapeutic approaches are underpinned by attention to lifestyle [68]. It was estimated from the Nurses' Health Study that in women maintaining an appropriate weight, eating a healthy diet, having regular physical activity, not smoking and with moderate alcohol intake, risk might be reduced by about 85% [69]. The Nurses' Health Study demonstrated the beneficial effects of a dietary pattern low in trans fatty acids and glycaemic load, high in cereal fibre and omega-3 fatty acids, and with a high polyunsaturated:saturated fat ratio on risk of both coronary heart disease [69] and diabetes [70]. Randomised trials have also shown the benefit of maintenance of healthy diets in patients following myocardial infarction [4, 5].

The benefits of physical activity in reducing CHD events have also been shown, both in men [71] and women [72]. Beneficial effects on stroke are less consistent but still exist [73, 74]. Protective mechanisms include reducing adiposity, blood pressure, dyslipidaemia, diabetes and decreasing inflammation and improving endothelial function [75]. Concerning dyslipidaemia, one controlled study suggested that improvements in lipid profiles were related particularly to the amount and not the intensity of physical activity [76].

It is important that the sustained benefits of healthy lifestyle have been demonstrated whether or not individuals are taking lipid- and blood pressure-lowering agents [77].

Lifestyle approaches are not only the domain of the individual and health professional. Governments have a critical role to play through measures such as the provision of supportive environments through urban planning and, potentially, policies that encourage the provision of nutritious rather than energy-dense, nutrient-poor products.

CONCLUSIONS

Irrefutable evidence from very large randomised trials supports the benefit of lipid-lowering agents, particularly statins in many population groups, including those people with known CHD, previous stroke, diabetes and subgroups of the general population who are apparently healthy. The case for a more aggressive approach to LDL-C lowering is also proven. Despite this evidence, studies throughout the world have repeatedly documented under-utilisation of treatment with statins as well as other therapies, such as aspirin and β-blockers. As might be expected, suboptimal treatment leads to worsening of patient outcomes.

There are many and varied reasons underlying failure to implement proven therapies. Accordingly, strategies to overcome barriers must be multifaceted and directed towards policy and healthcare systems, clinical practice and individual patients.

REFERENCES

1. Cholesterol Treatment Trialists' (CTT) Collaborators. Efficacy and safety of cholesterol-lowering treatment: prospective meta-analysis of data from 90 056 participants in 14 randomised trials of statins. *Lancet* 2005; 366:1276–1278.

2. Rubins HB, Robins SJ, Collins D *et al*. For the Veterans Affairs High-Density Lipoprotein Cholesterol Intervention Trial Study Group. Gemfibrozil for the secondary prevention of coronary heart disease in men with low levels of high-density lipoprotein cholesterol. *N Engl J Med* 1999; 341:410–418.

3. Canner PL, Berge KG, Wenger NK *et al*. Fifteen year mortality in Coronary Drug Project patients: long-term benefit with niacin. *J Am Coll Cardiol* 1986; 8:1245–1255.

4. de Lorgeril M, Salen P, Martin JL *et al*. Mediterranean diet, traditional risk factors and the rate of cardiovascular complications after myocardial infarction: final report of the LYON Diet Heart Study. *Circulation* 1999; 99:779–785.

5. GISSI – Prevenzione Investigators. Dietary supplementation with n-3 polyunsaturated fatty acids and vitamin E after myocardial infarction: results of the GISSI-Prevenzione trial. Gruppo Italiano per lo Studio della Sopravvivenza nell'Infarto miocardico. *Lancet* 1999; 354:447–455.

6. Ho PM, Spertus JA, Masoudi FA *et al*. Impact of medication therapy discontinuation on mortality after myocardial infarction. *Arch Intern Med* 2006; 166:1842–1847.

7. Jackevicius CA, Li P, Tu JV. Prevalence, predictors and outcomes of primary nonadherence after acute myocardial infarction. *Circulation* 2008; 117:1028–1036.

8. Eagle KA, Kline-Rogers E, Goodman SG *et al*. Adherence to evidence-based therapies after discharge for acute coronary syndromes: an ongoing prospective observational study. *Am J Med* 2004; 117:73–81.

9. Bhatt DL, Steg PG, Ohman EM *et al*. International prevalence, recognition and treatment of cardiovascular risk factors in outpatients with atherothrombosis. *JAMA* 2006; 295:180–189.

10. Bowker TJ, Clayton TC, Ingham JE *et al*. A British Cardiac Society survey of the potential for secondary prevention of coronary disease: ASPIRE (Action on Secondary Prevention through Intervention to Reduce Events). *Heart* 1996; 75:334–342.

11. EUROASPIRE II Steering Group. Clinical reality of coronary prevention guidelines: a comparison of EUROASPIRE I and II in nine countries. *Lancet* 2001; 357:995–1001.

12. Pearson TA, Laurora I, Chu H *et al*. The Lipid Treatment Assessment Project (L-TAP). A multicentre survey to evaluate the percentages of dyslipidemic patients receiving lipid-lowering therapy and achieving low-density lipoprotein cholesterol goals. *Arch Intern Med* 2000; 160:459–467.

13. Vale MJ, Jelinek MV, Best JD *et al*. How many patients with coronary heart disease are not achieving their risk-factor targets? Experience in Victoria 1996–1998 versus 1999–2000. *Med J Aust* 2002; 176:211–215.

14. Connor J, Rafter N, Rodgers A. Do fixed-dose combination pills or unit-of-use packaging improve adherence? A systematic review. *Bull World Health Organ* 2004; 82:935–939.

15. Jackevicius CA, Mamdani M, Tu JV. Adherence with statin therapy in elderly patients with and without acute coronary syndromes. *JAMA* 2002; 288:462–467.

16. Bibbins-Domingo K, Coxson P, Pletcher MJ *et al*. Adolescent overweight and future adult coronary heart disease. *N Engl J Med* 2007; 357:2371–2379.

17. Foot DK, Lewis RP, Pearson TA *et al*. Demographics and cardiology, 1950–2050. *J Am Coll Cardiol* 2000; 35:1067–1081.

18. Ridker PM, Danielson E, Fonseca FAH *et al*. Rosuvastatin to prevent vascular events in men and women with elevated C-reactive protein. *N Engl J Med* 2008; 359:2195–2207.

19. Danesh J, Wheeler JG, Hirschfield GM *et al*. C-reactive protein and other circulatory markers of inflammation in the prediction of coronary heart disease. *N Engl J Med* 2004; 350:1387–1397.

20. Ridker PM, Cannon CP, Morrow D. C-reactive protein levels and outcomes after statin therapy. *N Engl J Med* 2005; 352:20–28.

21. Zacho J, Tybjaerg-Hansen A, Jensen JS *et al*. Genetically elevated C-reactive protein and ischaemic vascular disease. *N Engl J Med* 2008; 359:1897–1908.

22. Ridker PM, Pare G, Parker A *et al*. Loci related to metabolic syndrome pathways including LEPR, HNFIA, IL6R, and GCKR associate with plasma C-reactive protein. The Women's Genome Health Study. *Am J Hum Genet* 2008; 82:1185–1192.

23. Pepys MB, Hirschfield GM, Tennent GA *et al*. Targeting C-reactive protein for the treatment of cardiovascular disease. *Nature* 2006; 440:1217–1221.

24. Ridker PM. The time for cardiovascular inflammation reduction trials has arrived. How low to go for hsCRP? *Arterioscler Thromb Vasc Biol* 2008; 28:1222–1224.

25. Pearson T, Mensah GA, Alexander W *et al*. Markers of inflammation and cardiovascular disease: application to clinical and public health practice: a statement for healthcare professionals from the Centers for Disease Control and Prevention and the American Heart Association. *Circulation* 2003; 107:499–511.

26. Osterberg L, Blashke T. Adherence to Medication. *N Engl J Med* 2005; 353:487–497.

27. Heart Protection Study Collaborative Group. MRC/BHF Heart Protection Study of cholesterol lowering with simvastatin in 20,536 high-risk individuals: a randomised placebo-controlled trial. *Lancet* 2002; 360:7–22.

28. The Stroke Prevention by Aggressive Reduction in Cholesterol Levels (SPARCL) Investigators. High-dose atorvastatin after stroke or transient ischemic attack. *N Engl J Med* 2006; 355:549–559.

29. Law MR, Watt HC, Wald NJ. The underlying risk of death after myocardial infarction in the absence of treatment. *Arch Intern Med* 2002; 162:2405–2410.

30. Cholesterol Treatment Trialists' (CTT) Collaborators. Efficacy of cholesterol-lowering therapy in 18,686 people with diabetes in 14 randomised trials of statins: a meta-analysis. *Lancet* 2008; 371:117–125.

31. Ziegelstein RC, Bush DE, Fauerback JA. Depression, adherence behaviour and coronary disease outcomes. *Arch Intern Med* 1998; 58:808–809.

32. Ford ES, Capewell S. Coronary heart disease mortality among young adults in the U.S. from 1980 through 2002. *J Am Coll Cardiol* 2007; 50:2128–2132.

33. Murray CJ, Lauer JA, Hutubessy RC *et al*. Effectiveness and costs of interventions to lower systolic blood pressure and cholesterol: a global and regional analysis on reduction of cardiovascular disease risk. *Lancet* 2003; 361:717–725.

34. Choudhry NK, Patrick AR, Elliot MS *et al*. Cost-effectiveness of providing full drug coverage to increase medication adherence in post-myocardial infarction Medicare beneficiaries. *Circulation* 2008; 117:1261–1268.

35. Ko DT, Mamdani M, Alter DA. Lipid-lowering therapy with statins in high-risk elderly patients: the treatment-risk paradox. *JAMA* 2004; 291:1864–1870.

36. Tonkin AM, Eckermann S, White H *et al*.; on behalf of the LIPID Study Group. Cost-effectiveness of cholesterol-lowering therapy with pravastatin in patients with previous acute coronary syndromes aged 65–74 years compared with younger patients: results from the LIPID study. *Am Heart J* 2006; 151:1305–1312.

37. Taylor RS, Brown A, Ebrahim S *et al*. Exercise-based rehabilitation for patients with coronary heart disease: systematic review and meta-analysis of randomised controlled trials. *Am J Med* 2004; 116:682–692.

38. Clark AM, Hartling L, Vandermeer B *et al*. Meta-analysis: secondary prevention programs for patients with coronary artery disease. *Ann Intern Med* 2005; 143:659–672.

39. Anderson JL, Adams CD, Antman EM *et al*. Writing committee to revise the 2002 Guidelines for the Management of Patients with Unstable Angina/Non-ST Elevation Myocardial Infarction. ACC/AHA Guideline revision: ACC/AHA 2007 Guidelines for the Management of Patients with Unstable Angina/Non-ST-Elevation Myocardial Infarction. *Circulation* 2007; 116:e148–e304.

40. Daugherty SL, Ho M, Spertus J *et al*. Association of early follow-up after acute myocardial infarction with higher rates of medication use. *Arch Intern Med* 2008; 168:485–491.

41. Abegunde DO, Bakuti S, Luyten A *et al*. Can non-physical healthcare workers assess and manage cardiovascular risk in primary care? *Bull World Health Organ* 2007; 85:432–440.

42. Becker DM, Yanek LR, Johnson WR *et al*. Impact of a community-based multiple risk factor intervention on cardiovascular risk in black families with a history of premature coronary disease. *Circulation* 2005; 111:1298–1304.

43. Morisky DE, Green LW, Levine DM. Concurrent and predictive validity of a self-reported measure of medication adherence. *Med Care* 1986; 24:67–74.

44. WHO Health. *The health for all policy framework for the WHO region*. World Health Organization, Copenhagen, 1999.

45. Acheson D, Barker D, Chambers J *et al*. *Independent inquiry into inequalities in health*. The Stationery Office, London, 1998.

46. Ostlin P, Diderichsen F. *Equality-orientated national strategy for public health in Sweden. A case study. Policy Learning Curve Series 1*. European Centre for Health Policy, Brussels, 2000.

47. Cooper AF, Jackson G, Weinman J, Horne R *et al*. Factors associated with cardiac rehabilitation attendance: a systematic review of the literature. *Clin Rehabil* 2002; 16:541–552.

48. Edwards A, Elwyn G, Mulley AI. Explaining risks: turning numerical data into meaningful pictures. *Br Med J* 2002; 324:827–830.

49. Goldman RE, Parker DR, Eaton CB *et al*. Patients' perception of cholesterol, cardiovascular disease risk, and risk communication strategies. *Ann Fam Med* 2006; 4:205–212.

50. Wald N, Law M. A strategy to reduce cardiovascular disease by more than 80%. *Br Med J* 2003; 326:1419–1424.

51. Heart Outcomes Prevention Evaluation (HOPE) 2 Investigators. Homocysteine lowering with folic acid and B vitamins in vascular disease. *N Engl J Med* 2006; 354:1567–1577.

52. Franco OH, Bonneux L, de Laet C *et al*. The polymeal: a more natural, safer, and probably tastier (than the Polypill) strategy to reduce cardiovascular disease by more than 75%. *Br Med J* 2004; 329:1447–1450.

53. Neaton, JD, Blackburn H, Jacobs D *et al*. for the Multiple Risk Factor Intervention Trial Research Group. Serum cholesterol level and mortality findings for men screened in the Multiple Risk Factor Intervention Trial. *Arch Intern Med* 1992; 152:1490–1500.

54. Muldoon MF, Manuck SB. Ischemic heart disease and cholesterol. Safety of cholesterol reduction remains in doubt. *Br Med J* 1994; 308:1104–1105.

55. Sacks FM, Pfeffer MA, Moye LA *et al*. for the Cholesterol and Recurrent Events Trial Investigators: The effect of pravastatin on coronary events after myocardial infarction in patients with average cholesterol levels. *N Engl J Med* 1996; 335:1001–1009.

56. Shepherd I, Blauw GJ, Murphy MB *et al*.; on behalf of the PROSPER Study Group: Pravastatin in elderly individuals at risk of vascular disease (PROSPER): A randomised controlled trial. *Lancet* 2002; 360:1623–1630.

57. Strandberg TE, Pyörälä PK, Cook TJ *et al*. Morality and incidence of cancer during 10-year follow-up of the Scandinavian Simvastatin Survival Study (4S). *Lancet* 2002; 359:1379–1387.

58. Long-term effectiveness and safety of pravastatin in 9014 patients with coronary heart disease and average cholesterol concentrations: the LIPID trial follow-up. *Lancet* 2002; 359:1379–1387.

59. Pfeffer MA, Keech A, Sacks FM *et al*. Safety and tolerability of pravastatin in long-term clinical trials: Prospective Pravastatin Pooling (PPP) Project. *Circulation* 2002; 105:2341–2346.

60. Newman CB, Palmer G, Silbershatz H *et al*. Safety of atorvastatin derived from analysis of 44 completed trials in 9416 patients. *Am J Cardiol* 2003; 92:670–676.

61. Stewart R, Sharples K, North F *et al*. Long-term assessment of psychological well-being in a randomised placebo-controlled trial of cholesterol reduction with pravastatin. *Arch Intern Med* 2000; 160:3144–3152.

62. Morgan RE, Palinkas LA, Barrett-Connor EL *et al*. Plasma cholesterol and depressive symptoms in older men. *Lancet* 1993; 341:75–79.

63. Wagstaff LR, Mitton MW, Arvik BM *et al*. Statin-associated memory loss: analysis of 60 case reports and review of the literature. *Pharmacotherapy* 2003; 23:871–880.

64. Armitage J. The safety of statins in clinical practice. *Lancet* 2007; 370:1781–1790.

65. Brown D, Heslin A, Doyle J. Postprandial lipemia in health and in ischaemic heart disease. *N Engl J Med* 1961; 264:733–737.

66. Bansal S, Buring JE, Rifai N *et al*. Fasting compared with nonfasting triglycerides and risk of cardiovascular events in women. *JAMA* 2007; 298:309–316.

67. McQueen MJ, Howken S, Wang X *et al*., for the INTERHEART study investigators. Lipids, lipoproteins and apolipoproteins as risk markers of myocardial infarction in 52 countries (the INTERHEART study): a case-control study. *Lancet* 2008; 372:324–333.

68. Pearson TA, Blair SN, Daniels SR *et al*. AHA guidelines for primary prevention of cardiovascular disease and stroke: 2002 update. *Circulation* 2002; 106:388–391.

69. Stampfer MJ, Hu FB, Manson JE *et al*. Primary prevention of coronary heart disease in women through diet and lifestyle. *N Engl J Med* 2000; 343:16–22.

70. Hu FB, Manson JE, Stampfer MJ *et al*. Diet, lifestyle and the risk of type 2 diabetes mellitus in women. *N Engl J Med* 2001; 345:790–797.

71. Berlin JA, Colditz GA. A meta-analysis of physical activity in the prevention of coronary heart disease. *Am J Epidemiol* 1990; 132:612–628.

72. Manson JE, Greenland P, LaCroix AZ *et al*. Walking compared with vigorous exercise for the prevention of cardiovascular events in women. *N Engl J Med* 2002; 347:716–725.

73. Hu FB, Stampfer MJ, Colditz GA *et al*. Physical activity and risk of stroke in women. *JAMA* 2000; 283:2961–2967.

74. Lee IM, Hennekens CH, Berger K *et al*. Exercise and risk of stroke in male physicians. *Stroke* 1999; 30:1–6.

75. Bassuk SS, Manson JE. Physical activity and the prevention of cardiovascular disease. *Curr Atheroscler Rep* 2003; 5:299–307.

76. Kraus WE, Houmard JA, Duscha BD *et al*. Effects of the amount and intensity of exercise on plasma lipoproteins. *N Engl J Med* 2002; 347:1483–1492.

77. Chiuve SE, McCullough ML, Sacks FM *et al*. Healthy lifestyle factors in the primary prevention of coronary heart disease among men: benefits among users and nonusers of lipid-lowering and antihypertensive medications. *Circulation* 2006; 114:160–167.

Abbreviations

4D	Deutsche Diabetes Dialyse Study
4S	Scandinavian Simvastatin Survival Study
ABCA1	ATP binding cassette transporter A1
ABCG1	ATP binding cassette transporter G1
ACAPS	Asymptomatic Carotid Artery Progression Study
ACAT	acyl-coenzyme A:cholesterol acyltransferase
ACC	American College of Cardiology
ACCORD	Action to Control Cardiovascular Risk in Diabetes
ACE	angiotensin converting enzyme/angiotensin controlling enzyme (*check context*)
ACHIEVE	Assessment of Coronary Health Using an Intima-Media Thickness Endpoint for Vascular Effects
ACS	acute coronary syndrome(s)
ACTIVATE	ACAT Intravascular Atherosclerosis Treatment Evaluation
ADA	American Diabetes Association
ADH	autosomal dominant hypercholesterolaemia
ADMA	asymmetric dimethylarginine
AE	adverse experience(s)
AFCAPS/TexCAPS	Air Force Texas Coronary Atherosclerosis Prevention Study
AHA	American Heart Association
AIDS	acquired immune deficiency syndrome
AIM-HIGH	Atherothrombosis Intervention in Metabolic Syndrome With Low HDL/High Triglycerides and Impact on Global Health Outcomes
ALERT	Assessment of Lescol in Renal Transplantation
ALLHAT	Antihypertensive and Lipid-Lowering Treatment to Prevent Heart Attack Trial
ALLIANCE	Aggressive Lipid Lowering Initiation Abates New Cardiac Events
ALT	alanine transaminase
ANP	atrial natriuretic peptide
APCSC	Asia Pacific Cohort Studies Collaboration
A-PLUS	Avasimibe and Progression of coronary Lesions assessed by intravascular Ultrasound
apoAI	apolipoprotein AI
apoAII	apolipoprotein AII
apoB	apolipoprotein B
apoE	apolipoprotein E
AngII	angiotensin II
ARB	angiotensin receptor blocker(s)

ARBITER	Arterial Biology for the Investigation of Treatment Effects of Reducing Cholesterol
ARR	absolute risk reduction(s)
ASAP	Atorvastatin versus Simvastatin Atherosclerosis Progression
ASBT	(ileal) apical sodium-dependent bile acid transporter
ASCOT	Anglo-Scandinavian Cardiac Outcomes Trial
ASCT	autologous stem cell transplantation
ASO	antisense oligonucleotide
ASPEN	Atorvastatin Study for Prevention of Coronary Heart Disease Endpoints in Non-Insulin-Dependent Diabetes Mellitus
ASSIGN	cardiovascular risk score chosen for use by SIGN (Scottish Intercollegiate Guidelines Network)
ASSIST	Asymptomatic aortic Sclerosis/Stenosis: Influence of Statins
AST	aspartate transaminase
ASTEROID	A Study to Evaluate the Effect of Rosuvastatin on Intravascular Ultrasound-Derived Coronary Atheroma Burden
ASTRONOMER	Aortic Stenosis Progression Observation: Measuring the Effect of Rosuvastatin
AT-1R	angiotensin-1 receptor
ATP	adenosine triphosphate
ATPIII	Adult Treatment Panel III
A to Z	Aggrastat to Zocor trial
AUC	area under the curve
aVIC	activated valve interstitial cells
AVS	aortic valve stenosis
BAS	bile acid sequestrants
BECAIT	Bezafibrate Coronary Atherosclerosis Intervention Trial
BHAT	β-Blocker Heart Attack Trial
BIP	Bezafibrate Infarction Prevention
BMI	body mass index
BMP	bone morphogenetic protein
BNP	B-type/brain natriuretic peptide
BP	blood pressure
BPLA	Blood-Pressure Lowering Arm
CABG	coronary artery bypass graft
CAD	coronary artery disease
CAi	cholesterol absorption inhibitor
CARDS	Collaborative Atorvastatin Diabetes Study
CARE	Cholesterol And Recurrent Events
CDP	Coronary Drug Project
CE	cholesteryl ester
CETP	cholesteryl ester transfer protein
CHD	coronary heart disease
CHICAGO	Carotid Intima-Media Thickness in Atherosclerosis Using Pioglitazone
CHIPS	Control of Hypertension In Pregnancy Study
CI	confidence interval
cIMT	carotid artery intima-media thickness

CK	creatine kinase
CKD	chronic kidney disease
CK-MB	creatine kinase, muscle and brain (subunits)
CLP	caecal ligation and perforation
CNS	central nervous system
CORONA	Controlled Rosuvastatin Multinational Study in Heart Failure
COX	cyclooxygenase
CRP	C-reactive protein
CTT	Cholesterol Treatment Trialists
CV	cardiovascular
CVD	cardiovascular disease
CYP7A1	cholesterol 7 alpha hydroxylase (cytochrome P450, family 7, subfamily A, polypeptide 1)
DAIS	Diabetes Atherosclerosis Intervention Study
DALY	disability-adjusted life year
DAS28	28-joint Disease Activity Score
DBP	diastolic blood pressure
DC	dendritic cells
DCA	dicarboxylic acid
DMARD	disease-modifying antirheumatic drugs
DNA	deoxyribonucleic acid
DP1	prostaglandin D_2 receptor 1
DPP	Diabetes Prevention Program
DPS	Diabetes Prevention Study
EBCT	electron-beam computed tomography
ECG	electrocardiogram
ECG-LVH	electrocardiographically-determined left ventricular hypertrophy
EEM	external elastic membrane
EL	endothelial lipase
ENHANCE	Ezetimibe and Simvastatin in Hypercholesterolemia Enhances Atherosclerosis Regression
eNOS	endothelial nitric oxide synthase
ER	endoplasmic reticulum / extended release (*check context*)
ESC	European Society of Cardiology
ESKD	end-stage kidney disease
ESR	eosinophil sedimentation rate
ESTABLISH	Early Statin Treatment in Patients With Acute Coronary Syndrome. Demonstration of the Beneficial Effect on Atherosclerotic Lesions by Serial Volumetric Intravascular Ultrasound Analysis During Half a Year After Coronary Event
ET-1	endothelin-1
EULAR	European League Against Rheumatism
FC	free cholesterol
FDA	United States Food and Drug Administration
FDB	familial defective apolipoprotein B
FH	familial hypercholesterolaemia
FIELD	Fenofibrate Intervention and Event Lowering in Diabetes
FMD	flow-mediated dilatation
FPP	farnesyl-pyrophosphate

GAIN	German Atorvastatin Investigation
GFR	glomerular filtration rate
GISSI-HF	Gruppo Italiano per lo Studio della Sopravvivenza nell'Infarto Miocardico - Heart Failure
GPP	geranylgeranyl-pyrophosphate
GPx-1	glutathione-peroxidase-1
GRACE	Global Registry of Acute Coronary Events
GTPase	guanosine triphosphatase
GWAS	genome-wide association studies
HATS	HDL-Atherosclerosis Treatment Study
HbA_{1c}	glycosylated haemoglobin A_{1c}
HCTZ	hydrochlorothiazide
HDL	high-density lipoprotein(s)
HDL-C	high-density lipoprotein cholesterol
HeFH	heterozygous familial hypercholesterolaemia
HF	heart failure
HL	hepatic lipase
HMG-CoA	3-hydroxy 3-methylglutaryl coenzyme A
HoFH	homozygous familial hypercholesterolaemia
HPS	Heart Protection Study
HPS-THRIVE	Heart Protection Study – Treatment of HDL to Reduce the Incidence of Vascular Events
HR	hazard ratio
hs-CRP	high-sensitivity C-reactive protein
ICAM-1	intercellular adhesion molecule-1
IDF	International Diabetes Federation
IDEAL	Incremental Decrease in End Points Through Aggressive Lipid-Lowering
IDL	intermediate-density lipoprotein
IFNγ	interferon-gamma
IGF	insulin-like growth factor
IL	interleukin
ILLUMINATE	Investigation of Lipid Level Management to Understand its Impact in Atherosclerotic Events
ILLUSTRATE	Investigation of Lipid Level Management Using Coronary Ultrasound To Assess Reduction of Atherosclerosis by CETP Inhibition and HDL Elevation
IMPROVE IT	Reduction of Outcomes: Vytorin Efficacy International Trial
IMT	intima-media thickness
iNOS	indicible nitric oxide synthase
INR	International Normalized Ratio
IORRA	Institute of Rheumatology and Rheumatoid Arthritis
IR	immediate-release
ISA	intrinsic sympathomimetic activity
ISR	injection site reaction
IVUS	intravascular ultrasound
JBS	Joint British Societies
JUPITER	Justification for the Use of Statins in Primary Prevention: an Intervention Trial Evaluating Rosuvastatin

LAARS	LDL-Apheresis Atherosclerosis Regression Study
LACMART	Low Density Lipoprotein Apheresis Coronary Morphology and Reserve Trial
LCAT	lecithin:cholesterol acyltransferase
LDL	low-density lipoprotein
LDL-C	low-density lipoprotein cholesterol
LDL P	low-density lipoprotein particle number
LDLR	low-density lipoprotein receptor
LIPID	Long-Term Intervention with Pravastatin in Ischaemic Disease
LLA	Lipid Lowering Arm
Lp(a)	lipoprotein (a)
LPS	lipopolysaccharides
MAAS	Multicentre Anti-Atherosclerosis Study
MAP-kinase	mitogen-activated protein kinase
MARS	Monitored Atherosclerosis Regression Study
MCP	monocyte chemoattractant protein
MCVE	major cardiovascular event
MEGA	Management of Elevated Cholesterol in the Primary Prevention Group of Adult Japanese
METEOR	Measuring Effects on Intima-Media Thickness: an Evaluation of Rosuvastatin
MI	myocardial infarction
MIRACL	Myocardial Ischemia Reduction with Aggressive Cholesterol Lowering
MISTRAL	Safety and Efficacy Study of Implitapide Compared With Placebo in Patients With Heterozygous Familial Hypercholesterolemia (HeFH) on Maximal Concurrent Lipid-Lowering Therapy
MLD	minimum lumen diameter
MMP	matrix metalloproteinase
MRC	Medical Research Council
MRFIT	Multiple Risk Factor Intervention Trial
MRI	magnetic resonance imaging
mRNA	messenger ribonucleic acid
MRSE	muscle-related side-effects
MTP	microsomal triglyceride transfer protein
MTPi	microsomal triglyceride transfer protein inhibitor
n3-PUFA	n3-polyunsaturated fatty acids
NADPH	nicotinamide adenine dinucleotide phosphate
NCEP	National Cholesterol Education Program
NHFA/CSANZ	National Heart Foundation of Australia and Cardiac Society of Australia and New Zealand
NNT	number needed to treat
NO	nitric oxide
NPC1L1	Niemann–Pick C 1-like 1 protein/transporter
NSAID	non-steroidal anti-inflammatory drug
NT-proBNP	N-terminal prohormone brain natriuretic peptide
NYHA	New York Heart Association
obVIC	osteoblastic valve interstitial cells
OCT	optical coherence tomography

OECD	Organisation for Economic Cooperation and Development
OR	odds ratio
ORION	Outcome of Rosuvastatin Treatment on Carotid Artery Atheroma: a Magnetic Resonance Imaging Observation
oxLDL	oxidized low-density lipoprotein
PACT	Pravastatin in Acute Coronary Treatment
PAF	platelet activation factor
PAI-1	plasminogen activator inhibitor-1
PAR	population attributable risk
PCI	percutaneous coronary intervention
PCSK9	proprotein convertase subtilisin/kexin 9
PD	plasma delipidation
PGD$_2$	prostaglandin D$_2$
PLA$_2$	phospholipase A$_2$
PLAC-1	Pravastatin Limitation of Atherosclerosis in the Coronary Arteries
POSCH	Program on the Surgical Control of the Hyperlipidemias
PPAR	peroxisome proliferator-activated receptor
PPP	Prospective Pravastatin Pooling
PREMIER	Prospective Registry Evaluating Myocardial Infarction: Events and Recovery
PRINTO	Paediatric Rheumatology International Trial Organization
PROBE	Prospective Randomised Open Blinded Endpoint
PROGRESS	Perindopril Protection against Recurrent Stroke Study
PROSPER	Prospective Study of Pravastatin in the Elderly at Risk
PROVE IT-TIMI 22	Pravastatin or Atorvastatin Evaluation and Infection Therapy
PSC	Prospective Studies Collaboration
PVD	peripheral vascular disease
pVIC	progenitor valve interstitial cells
QALY	quality-adjusted life year
QRISK	cardiovascular disease risk calculator
qVIC	quiescent valve interstitial cells
RA	rheumatoid arthritis
RAAVE	Rosuvastatin Affecting Aortic Valve Endothelium
RADIANCE	Rating Atherosclerotic Disease change by Imaging with A New CETP Inhibitor
RANTES	regulated upon activation T cells expressed and secreted
REACH	Reduction of Atherosclerosis for Continued Health
REGRESS	Regression Growth Evaluation Statin Substudy
REVERSAL	Reversal of Atherosclerosis with Aggressive Lipid Lowering
rHDL	reconstituted HDL
ROS	reactive oxygen species
RR	relative risk/risk ratio (*check context*)
RRR	relative risk reduction
SALTIRE	Scottish Aortic Stenosis Lipid Lowering Trial, Impact on Regression
SCORE	Systematic Coronary Risk Evaluation
SEARCH	Study of the Effectiveness of Additional Reductions in Cholesterol and Homocysteine
SEAS	Simvastatin and Ezetimibe in Aortic Stenosis
SBP	systolic blood pressure

SHARP	Study of Heart and Renal Protection
SI	special intervention
sICAM-1	soluble intercellular adhesion molecule-1
SIEC	Italian Society of Cardiovascular Echography
sJIA	systemic juvenile idiopathic arthritis
SLE	systemic lupus erythematosus
SPARCL	Stroke Prevention by Aggressive Reduction in Cholesterol Levels
SR-B1	scavenger receptor-B1
SREBP	sterol receptor element binding protein
SSi	squalene synthase inhibitor
STARS	St Thomas' Atherosclerosis Regression Study
TARA	Trial of Atorvastatin in Rheumatoid Arthritis
TC	total cholesterol
TF	tissue factor
TG	triglycerides
TGF-β	transforming growth factor-beta
Th1	T helper cells
TIA	transient ischaemic attack
TLC	therapeutic lifestyle change
TNF-α	tumour necrosis factor-alpha
TNT	Treatment to New Targets
TOMHS	Treatment of Mild Hypertension Study
tPA	tissue plasminogen activator
tRNA	transfer ribonucleic acid
UC	usual care
UKPDS	United Kingdom Prospective Diabetes Study
ULN	upper limit of normal
USRDS	United States Renal Data System
VA-HIT	Veterans Affairs High-Density Lipoprotein Intervention Trial
VAS	visual analogue scale
VCAM-1	vascular cell adhesion molecule-1
VEGF	vascular endothelial growth factor
VIC	valve interstitial cells
VLDL	very low-density lipoprotein(s)
VLDL-C	very low-density lipoprotein cholesterol
WHO Monica	World Health Organization Monitoring of Trends and Determinants in Cardiovascular Disease
WMD	weighted mean difference
WOSCOPS	West of Scotland Coronary Prevention Study

Index

2nd Joint British Societies, guidelines for statin therapy 168–9

4D (Die Deutsche Diabetes Dialyse) study 136

4S (Scandinavian Simvastatin Survival Study) 35, 48, 98, 143, 150, 158, 256

4th European Joint Task Force, guidelines for statin therapy 168–9, 170

A to Z (Aggrastat to Zocor) trial 62, 65, 66, 67, 68

A-PLUS (Avasimibe and Progression of coronary Lesions assessed by intravascular Ultrasound) study 202

A1 HDLs 34

ABCs (ATP binding cassettes) 30–1

abetalipoproteinaemia 127, 230

absolute risk 157

absolute risk assessment
   Framingham risk equations, validity in other populations 159–60
   future developments 170–1
   as guideline to therapy 167, 170
   inclusion of new markers 166–7
   in people with diabetes 165, 166
   population-specific tools 162–5
   tools derived from Framingham Heart Study 159
   tools from populations other than FHS participants 160–1
   in women 161, 166
   in younger adults 161

absolute risk reduction 158

ACAPS (Asymptomatic Carotid Artery Progression Study) 198

ACAT (acyl-coenzyme A: cholesterol acyltransferase) inhibitors 126–7
   site of action 124

ACE (angiotensin-converting enzyme) inhibitors, lipid and lipoprotein effects 112

acebutolol, effect on lipids and lipoproteins 113

ACHIEVE (Assessment of Coronary Health Using an Intima–Media Thickness Endpoint for Vascular Effects) 122, 125

acipimox 24

ACTIVATE (ACAT Intravascular Atherosclerosis Treatment Evaluation) study 202

acute coronary syndromes (ACS)
   biomarkers 217–19
   early risk of recurrent events 64
   follow-up and shared care 252–3
   secondary prevention programmes 252
   trials of statin therapy 63–4
      meta-analyses 66–9

adhesion molecule expression, effect of statins 188

AEGR-427 231

AEGR-733 231

AFCAPS/TexCAPS 35, 48, 50, 98, 158

age-related prevalence, CVD 3

ageing population 246

AIM-HIGH trial 24–5, 72, 238

alanine transaminase (ALT)
   effect of lapaquistat 229
   effect of mipomersen 233–4
   effect of statins 21, 256

ALERT (Assessment of Lescol in Renal Transplantation) study 137–8

ALLHAT (Antihypertensive and Lipid-Lowering Treatment to Prevent Heart Attack Trials) 98, 109, 158

ALLIANCE (Aggressive Lipid Lowering Initiation Abates New Cardiac Events) study 80–1

alpha-HDLs 34

alpha-I antagonists, lipid and lipoprotein effects 112

amiodarone, interaction with statins 21

amlodipine, synergy with atorvastatin 111

AMORIS study 48, 50
anacetrapib (MK0859) 126, 130, 239
angiogenesis promotion, HDLs 33
anti-inflammatory activity, HDLs 31–3
anti-oxidant activity, HDLs 31
anticoagulant control, effect of statins 21
antifungals, interaction with statins 21
antihypertensive drugs
    development 111
    effects on lipids and lipoproteins 112–13
antisense drugs
    mipomersen 232–4
    PCSK9 inhibition 236–7
aortic valve stenosis
    pathways 181
    value of statins 180–3
apical sodium-dependent bile acid
    transporter (ASBT) inhibition 124, 127
apoAI analogue therapy 239–40
apolipoprotein B (apoB) 43, 55
    APOB mutations 117–18
    apoB48 44
    apoB100 44, 93
    apoB antisense drugs 127, 130, 232–4
    apoB/apoA ratio 8, 257
    correlation with non-HDL-C 50–2
    as determinant of atherosclerosis 50
    heterogeneity 45
    as marker of adequacy of LDL-lowering
        therapy 52
    as measure of cardiovascular risk
        comparison with LDL-C 47–8
        comparison with non-HDL-C 48–50
apolipoprotein composition, HDLs 34
ARBITER (Arterial Biology for the
    Investigation of Treatment Effects of
    Reducing Cholesterol) study 198–9
ARBs (angiotensin receptor blockers), lipid
    and lipoprotein effects 112
arrhythmias, effect of statins 145
arthritis, value of statins 183–6
ASAP (Atorvastatin versus Simvastatin
    Atherosclerosis Progression) trial 119,
    198
ASCOT (Anglo–Scandinavian Cardiac
    Outcomes Trial) 78, 98, 109–11, 158, 178
Asia Pacific Cohort Studies Collaboration
    (APCSC) 5–6, 7, 161
Asian countries, risk prediction tools 161
aspartate transaminase (AST)
    effect of lapaquistat 229
    effect of statins 21, 256

ASPEN (Atorvastatin Study for Prevention of
    Coronary Heart Disease Endpoints in
    Non-Insulin-Dependent Diabetes
    Mellitus) 98, 158
ASSIGN score 162, 167
ASSIST (Asymptomatic aortic
    Sclerosis/Stenosis: Influence of Statins)
    study 183
ASTEROID (A Study to Evaluate the Effect of
    Rosuvastatin on Intravascular Ultrasound-
    Derived Coronary Atheroma Burden) 145,
    200
ASTRONOMER (Aortic Stenosis Progression
    Observation: Measuring the Effect of
    Rosuvastatin) 183
asymmetric dimethylarginine (ADMA) 216
atenolol, effect on lipids and lipoproteins 114
atherogenesis
    apoB concentration as determinant 50
    role of LDL cholesterol
        epidemiology 17–18
        pathophysiology 16–17
atherosclerotic plaques
    compliance and strain assessment 204
    stabilisation, statins 82
    structure 17
    see also plaque regression
atorvastatin
    4D study 136–7
    comparison with simvastatin in FH 119,
        121
    effect in aortic valve stenosis 180–2
    effect on cIMT 198
    effect in rheumatoid arthritis 185
    effect in systemic juvenile idiopathic
        arthritis 184, 185
    efficacy and safety 20
    risk of muscular symptoms 228
    serial IVUS study 199–200
    SPARCL study 78–80
    synergy with amlodipine 111
    use in hypertension (ASCOT) 109–11
    see also statins
ATPIII, definition of metabolic syndrome 90
atrial natriuretic peptide 218
autoimmune disease, effects of statins
    183–4
autonomic system, effect of statins 145
avasimibe 126
    IVUS study 202
AVE 5530 234
AZD-4121 234

B-type (brain) natriuretic peptide (BNP)
   217–18
BAY 13-9952 (implitapide) 230, 231
BECAIT (Bezafibrate Coronary
   Atherosclerosis Intervention Trial) 197
bendroflumethiazide 111
   lipid and lipoprotein effects 112
beta-blockers
   interaction with statins 146
   lipid and lipoprotein effects 112, 113, 114
bezafibrate, angiographic studies 197
   BIP study 35, 97, 99
BHAT (Beta-Blocker Heart Attack Trial)
   114
bile acid sequestrants (resins) 24, 72–3, 97
   mechanism of action 121, 124, 229
   use in FH 124
bile acids
   intestinal uptake 124
   synthesis 120
biomarkers 211
   future in cardiovascular disease 221–2
   general characteristics 212
   of inflammation 213–14
   multiple marker assessment
      in ACS 219
      in primary prevention 216
   natriuretic peptides 217–18
   novel markers, discovery and assessment
      219–21
   of oxidative stress 214–16
   troponins 217
bioprosthetic valve protection, statins
   179–80
BIP (Bezafibrate Infarction Prevention) study
   35, 97, 99
blood pressure 107
   in definition of metabolic syndrome 90
   relationship to cardiovascular disease
      107–8
   relationship to CHD risk 5, 6, 8
   stroke risk 77
   trends 3, 4
   see also hypertension
Blood Pressure Lowering Arm (BPLA),
   ASCOT 110–11
BMS-201038 127, 230–1
body mass index (BMI), trends 3
bone formation, effect of statins 180
brain (B-type) natriuretic peptide (BNP)
   217–18
Brazil, obesity rates 4

C-index 47
C-reactive protein (CRP)
   as biomarker 213–14, 217, 218, 247, 248–9
   effect of statins 179, 200
   inclusion in risk prediction tools 166–7
   relationship to outcomes in rosuvastatin
      therapy 148, 149, 150
calcification, inhibition by statins 180
calcium blockers, lipid and lipoprotein effects
   112
Canadian Cardiovascular Society, guidelines
   for statin therapy 168–9
CAPTIVATE trial 123
cardiac rehabilitation programmes 252
cardiovascular diseases
   association with risk factors, global
      differences 5–6, 9–10
   global impact 1–2, 155
   rationale for absolute risk assessment
      156–7
cardiovascular health strategies 156
Cardiovascular Health Study 48
cardiovascular risk, relationship to blood
   pressure 107–8
CARDS (Collaborative Atorvastatin Diabetes
   Study) 78, 98, 158, 178
CARE (Cholesterol and Recurrent Events)
   study 35, 63, 98, 139, 158, 256
Carotid IMT 50
carotid intima–media thickness (cIMT),
   measurement in clinical trials 197–9
Casale Monferrato Study 48, 50
Cdc42, effect of statins 178
central adiposity 89
cerivastatin 20
   effect on coronary calcification 203
   effect in sepsis 187
   see also statins
CHICAGO (Carotid Intima–Media Thickness
   in Atherosclerosis Using Pioglitazone)
   study 199
children, management of FH 128–9
China
   atherothrombotic conditions 2
   total cholesterol levels, trends 4
Chinese Heart Study 48, 50
chlorthalidone 111
   lipid and lipoprotein effects 112, 113
chlorthiazide 111
cholesterol
   intestinal uptake 124
   safety of low levels 256

cholesterol (continued)
  see also high-density lipoprotein
    cholesterol (HDL-C); low-density
    lipoprotein cholesterol (LDL-C); non-
    HDL-C; total cholesterol
cholesterol absorption inhibitors (CAi) 234
  mechanism of action 229
  see also ezetimibe
cholesterol efflux, role of HDLs 30–1, 32
cholesterol synthesis 120, 178, 229
Cholesterol Treatment Trialists (CTT)
  collaboration 60, 78, 96, 100, 256
cholesteryl ester transfer protein (CETP) 37,
  46–7, 238
cholesteryl ester transfer protein inhibitors
  238–9
  animal studies 34
  clinical trials 36–7
    effect on cIMT 199
    IVUS studies 201–2
  use in FH 125–6, 130
chronic kidney disease (CKD) 135–6, 140–1
  4D study 136–7
  ALERT (Assessment of Lescol in Renal
    Transplantation) study 137–8
  effects of lipid-lowering 141
  lipid-lowering in early disease 138–40
  relationship between lipids and CVD 136
chylomicron remnants 44
chylomicrons 44
ciclosporin
  interaction with ezetimibe 23
  interaction with statins 21
clarithromycin, interaction with statins 21
clinical trials, imaging endpoints 195, 204–5
  carotid intima–media thickness 197–9
  computed tomography 203
  coronary angiography 195–7
  intravascular ultrasound 199–203
  magnetic resonance imaging 204
clusterin (apolipoprotein J) 177
clustering of risk factors 108, 156
coenzyme Q10 228
  effect of statins 146
colesevelam 24
  use in FH patients 122, 124
    children 128
  see also bile acid sequestrants
colestipol 24
  see also bile acid sequestrants
colestyramine 24
  angiographic study 196

Lipid Research Clinics Primary Prevention
  Trial 35
  use in FH patients 124
  see also bile acid sequestrants
communication with patients 255
community-based interventions 254
computed tomography, use in clinical trials
  203
concordance 255
Copenhagen City Heart Study 48
Copenhagen Risk Score 162
core lipid exchange, lipoprotein particles
  46–7
CORONA (Controlled Rosuvastatin
  Multinational Study in Heart Failure)
  68–9, 146–9, 150–1
coronary angiography, use in clinical trials
  195–7
coronary atheroma, effect of rosuvastatin
  145
coronary calcification quantification 203
Coronary Drug Project 24, 96, 237
coronary heart disease (CHD)
  mortality, decline in developed countries
    157
  see also acute coronary syndromes (ACS)
coronary heart disease patients
  absolute risk 59–60
  cholesterol levels 59, 60
  stable
    benefits of LDL-C reduction 60–1
    intensive statin therapy 61–3
  statin therapy 63–6
  triglyceride and HDL-C levels 70–2
coronary heart disease risk
  relationship to HDL-C 29, 30
  relationship to total cholesterol levels 5, 6,
    7, 17–18
cost-effectiveness of CVD prevention 250–1,
  252
CP-346086 230
creatine kinase (CK) levels
  statin therapy 20, 21
  CK-MB, in ACS 218
CUORE risk equation 162

Da Qing IGT and Diabetes Study 100
DAIS (Diabetes Atherosclerosis Intervention
  Study) 99, 197
dalcetrapib 126, 130
DECODE risk scores 162
delipidation therapy 239

developing countries
    age-related prevalence of CVD 3
    cardiovascular risk factors 4
    epidemiological transition 1–2
diabetes
    association with metabolic syndrome 91
    cardiovascular disease risk 88
    dyslipidaemia 93–4, 101
        treatment 94–100
    increasing incidence 3, 4
    prevalence 87–8
    risk assessment 165, 166
Diabetes Prevention Programme (DPP) 100
Diabetes Prevention Study (DPS) 100
dialysis, effect on cholesterol levels 135–6
Die Deutsche Diabetes Dialyse (4D) study
    136
diet, relationship to blood pressure 107
dietary intervention 245, 257
    LDL reduction 19
    value in diabetes and metabolic syndrome
        100
discoidal HDLs 30–1, 32, 34
drug interactions
    bile acid sequestrants 24
    statins 20, 21, 70
Dubbo risk equation 162

E-selectin expression, effect of HDLs 32
EGIR (European Group for the study of
    Insulin Resistance), definition of metabolic
    syndrome 90
elderly people, statin therapy 20, 251–2
end-stage kidney disease (ESKD) 135
    4D study 136–7
endocannabinoid receptor (CB1) antagonists
    240
endothelial function, effect of statins 145,
    179, 188
endothelial lipase inhibitors 240
endothelial repair, effect of HDLs 33
endothelium relaxant factor 214
ENHANCE (Ezetimibe and Simvastatin in
    Hypercholesterolaemia Enhances
    Atherosclerosis Regression) trial 73, 121,
    123, 125, 198
epidemiological transition 1–2, 9
erythrocyte glutathione-peroxidase-1 (GPx-1)
    215
erythromycin, interaction with statins 21
ESTABLISH study 200
evidence base 245–6

JUPITER study 246–9
evidence-treatment gap 245, 246, 248
    contributing factors 249–50
exercise 257
    effect on lipid profile in diabetes 100
    lack of 9
    relationship to blood pressure 107
    secondary prevention programmes 252
ezetimibe 22–4, 73, 97, 234
    combination with simvastatin 73, 198
    mechanism of action 119, 124
    use in FH 119, 121, 122, 123, 130
        children 128

F_2-isoprostanes 215
factor analysis, metabolic syndrome 91
familial defective apolipoprotein B 118
familial dysbetalipoproteinaemia (type III
    hyperlipoproteinaemia) 49–50, 52
familial hypercholesterolaemia (FH) 45,
    117–18, 130
    children 128–9
    clinical trials 23–4, 122–3
        ENHANCE study 198
    homozygous disease 130
    pre-clinical phase treatments
        apical sodium-dependent bile acid
            transporter (ASBT) inhibition 127
        gene therapy 128
        PCSK9 inhibition 127
    pregnancy 129–30
    treatment options 118–19
        bile acid sequestrants 24, 121, 124
        ezetimibe 119, 121
        LDL apheresis 124–5
        plant sterols and stanols 125
        statins 119
    treatment in development
        ACAT inhibitors 126–7
        apoB antisense drugs 127, 232–4
        CETP inhibitors 125–6
        MTP inhibitors 127, 230–2
        niacin (nicotinic acid) 125
        squalene synthase inhibitors 126,
            229–30
    treatment goals 118
Familial Hypercholesterolaemia Regression
    Study 196
family-based interventions 254
farnesyl-pyrophosphate (FPP) 177, 178, 228
fasting blood samples, rationale 256–7
fatty streaks 16

fenofibrate
   angiographic study 197
   clinical trials FIELD study 35, 97, 99
fibrates 73, 97, 100
   angiographic studies 197
   clinical trials 35
   evidence base 245
   interaction with statins 21
   use in diabetes 99
FIELD (Fenofibrate Intervention and Event
   Lowering in Diabetes) study 35, 97, 99
FINRISK equation 162
flushing, niacin-induced 237
fluvastatin
   ALERT study 137–8
   effect on synoviocytes 186
   efficacy and safety 20
   risk of muscular symptoms 228
   see also statins
foam cells 16–17
follow-up after myocardial infarction 252–3
Framingham Heart Study, risk prediction
   tools 159
Framingham Offspring Study 47–8, 49, 50,
   54, 55, 108
Framingham risk equations 162–3
   validity in other populations 159–60
Friedwald equation 15–16, 213, 256

GAIN (German Atorvastatin Investigation)
   study 199–200
gamma-HDLs 34
gel electrophoresis, HDLs 34
gemfibrozil
   clinical trials 35, 99
   see also fibrates
gene therapy, FH 128
geranylgeranyl-pyrophosphate (GPP) 177,
   178
GISSI-HF trial 149, 150–1
Global Burden of Disease Study group 250,
   253
global impact, cardiovascular diseases 1–2
global trends, cardiovascular risk factors 3–5
glomerular flow rate (GFR), effect of statin
   therapy 140
glucose levels, in definition of metabolic
   syndrome 90
glutathione 215
GRACE (Global Registry of Acute Coronary
   Events) 245
guidelines 250

haemodialysis, cholesterol levels 135–6
haemorrhagic stroke risk
   relationship to cardiovascular risk factors
     5, 6
   SPARCL study 80
HATS (HDL-Atherosclerosis Treatment
   Study) 197
health inequalities 254–5
Health Professionals' Follow-up Study 48, 50
heart failure
   causes of death 144
   cholesterol levels 144
   mortality according to stain treatment 147
   statin therapy 143, 151–2
     clinical trials 146–51
     possible harmful effects 145–6
     potential beneficial effects 144
heart failure risk, effect of intensive statin
   therapy 68–9
Heart Protection Study (HPS) 60, 94, 96, 98,
   108, 139, 158
   HPS-THRIVE 72, 238
   myopathy risk 21
   stroke prevention 78
Heart and Soul Study 183
Helsinki Heart Study 35, 97, 99
heparin, effect on myeloperoxidase
   concentrations 219
hepatic steatosis, as side effect of MTPis 231
high baseline risk strategy 167
high-density lipoprotein cholesterol (HDL-C)
   29, 37
   in chronic kidney disease 135
   in definition of metabolic syndrome 90
   effect of antihypertensive drugs 112
   effect of niacin 97
   effect of statins 19, 186
   effect of torcetrapib 36–7
   HDL infusion therapy 36, 239–40
   as measure of cardiovascular risk 5, 48
   raising levels
     effect on cIMT 198–9
     niacin formulations 237–8
     serial IVUS studies 200–1
   and risk of recurrent CHD 71–2
   role in heart failure 145
   as therapeutic target in FH 125
high-density lipoproteins (HDLs)
   evidence for protective effect
     animal studies 34–5
     clinical trials 35–6
   protective functions 29–30, 31

anti-inflammatory activity 31–3
anti-oxidant activity 31
cholesterol efflux promotion 30–1, 32
endothelial repair 33
thrombosis inhibition 33
subpopulations 34
3-HMG-CoA 119, 120, 178
homocysteine 215
HPS2-THRIVE trial 25
hydralazine, lipid and lipoprotein effects
112
hydrochlorothiazide 111
hypertension 107
antihypertensives, effects on lipids and
lipoproteins 112–13
in definition of metabolic syndrome 90
historical background 111–12
relationship to cardiovascular risk 107–8
stroke risk 77
trends 3, 4
value of cholesterol lowering 108–11
see also blood pressure
hypertriglyceridaemia 49
correlation between non-HDL-C and apoB
51
see also triglycerides
Hy's Law 229–30

IDEAL (Incremental Decrease in End Points
Through Aggressive Lipid-Lowering) trial
61, 62, 63, 68, 80
recent MI subset 65
IDF (International Diabetes Federation),
definition of metabolic syndrome 90
ileal bypass 73
ILLUMINATE (Investigation of Lipid Level
Management to Understand its Impact in
Atherosclerotic Events) 36, 238–9
ILLUSTRATE (Investigation of Lipid Level
Management Using Coronary Ultrasound
To Assess Reduction of Atherosclerosis by
CETP Inhibition and HDL Elevation) 36,
37, 201–2, 203
imaging endpoints, clinical trials 204–5
carotid intima–media thickness 197–9
computed tomography 203
coronary angiography 195–7
intravascular ultrasound 199–203
magnetic resonance imaging 204
implitapide (BAY 13-9952) 230, 231
IMPROVE IT 73, 121
incentive funding, primary care 253

indapamide, lipid and lipoprotein effects
112, 113
India cardiovascular risk factors 5
Indonesia, dietary changes 4
inequalities in healthcare 254–5
inflammation
biomarkers 213–14
effects of statins 145, 179, 180, 183–4
in arthritis 184–6
in sepsis 186–9
inhibition by HDLs 31–3
reduction after ACS 66
role in metabolic syndrome 92
insulin resistance 88–9, 90
intensive statin therapy
in ACS 65–6
costs 70
meta-analyses 66–9
safety and efficacy 69–70
stable CHD patients 61–3
stroke prevention 80–1, 83
intercellular adhesion molecule-1 (1CAM-1)
expression, effect of HDLs 32
INTERHEART study 7–8, 93, 157, 212–13,
257
interleukin 8 expression, effect of statins 188
intermediate-density lipoproteins (IDLs) 44
effect of statins 19
intestinal MTPi 232
intravascular ultrasound (IVUS), use in
clinical trials 199–203
ischaemic stroke, relationship to
cardiovascular risk factors 5, 6
ISIS 301012 127
isoprene synthesis 177, 178
isoprostanes 215
itraconazole, interaction with statins 21

JTT-130 127
JTT-705 239
JUPITER (Justification for the Use of statins
in Prevention: an Intervention Trial
Evaluating Rosuvastatin) 158, 214, 246–9

ketoconazole, interaction with statins 21
kidney disease see chronic kidney disease
(CKD); end-stage kidney disease (ESKD)
kidney function, effect of statin therapy 140
kidney transplant recipients, ALERT study
137–8
Kuopio Atherosclerosis Prevention Study
198

LAARS (LDL-Apheresis Atherosclerosis Regression Study) 196
LACMART (Low density Lipoprotein-Apheresis Coronary Morphology and Reserve Trial) 199
lapaquistat 228–30
    trial in FH 123
laropiprant (MK0524) 25, 122, 125, 130, 237
lathosterol 239–40
lecithin:cholesterol acyltransferase (LCAT) 32
left ventricular remodelling, effect of statins 145
Leiden Heart Study 50
life expectancy, global increases 1
lifestyle changes, developing countries 4
lifestyle modification 157, 257
    in FH 118
    value in diabetes and metabolic syndrome 100
LIPID (Long-Term Intervention with Pravastatin in Ischaemic Disease) trial 35, 48, 50, 63, 98, 111, 139, 158, 252, 256
    conenzyme Q10 concentrations 146
lipid exchange, lipoprotein particles 46–7
Lipid Lowering Arm (LLA), ASCOT 110
Lipid Research Clinics Primary Prevention Trial 35
lipoprotein (a) (Lp(a)) 44
lipoproteins 15
    core lipid exchange 46–7
    structure 16
    see also high-density lipoproteins (HDLs); intermediate-density lipoproteins (IDLs); low-density lipoproteins (LDLs); very low-density lipoproteins (VLDLs)
liver enzymes
    effect of ezetimibe 23
    effect of lapaquistat 229–30
    effect of mipomersen 233–4
    effect of statins 21, 69, 256
lovastatin
    AFCAPS/TexCAPS 35
    effect on cIMT 198
    efficacy and safety 20
    see also statins
low cholesterol levels, safety 256
low-density lipoprotein, oxidised 215
low-density lipoprotein cholesterol (LDL-C) 25
    in chronic kidney disease 135
    correlation and concordance with aopB 51

effect of antihypertensive drugs 112, 113
LDL apheresis 124–5, 130
    clinical trials 196, 199
LDL-lowering therapy, apoB as marker of adequacy 52
    as measure of cardiovascular risk 47–8
    measurement 15–16, 257
    reduction 18–19
        dietary intervention 19
        ezetimibe 22–4
        niacin (nicotinic acid) 24–5
        relationship to reduction in CHD 63
        relationship to stroke risk 79
        resins 24
        statins 19–22
    relationship to LDL particle size and composition 54–5
    relationship to LDL particles 45
    role in atherogenesis 16–18
    role in heart failure 145
    stable CHD patients, benefits of reduction 60–1
    therapeutic targets 52, 53
        in FH 118
        in stroke prevention 80–2
low-density lipoprotein cholesterol receptor (LDLR) 117–18, 120
    regulation by PCSK9 234, 235
low-density lipoprotein particles 15, 44
    core lipid exchange 46–7
    in diabetes and metabolic syndrome 93–4
    as measure of cardiovascular risk 47–8
    size and composition, relationship to LDL-C and triglycerides 54–5
    subclasses 45, 93
low-risk patients, benefits of statins 198
LXRα agonists 240

MAAS (Multicentre Anti-Atherosclerosis Study) 196
magnetic resonance imaging, use in clinical trials 204
MARS (Monitored Atherosclerosis Regression Study) 196, 198
MCP 201 234
MCP-1, effect of statins 188
meaningful re-classification, new biomarkers 220–1
MEGA (Management of Elevated Cholesterol in the Primary Prevention Group of Adult Japanese) study 158
metabolic syndrome 88–9

aetiology 91–2
clinical utility 89, 91
definitions 89
dyslipidaemia 93–4, 101
    treatment 94–100
METEOR (Measuring Effects on
    Intima–Media Thickness: an Evaluation of
    Rosuvastatin) study 198
methyl dopa, lipid and lipoprotein effects
    112
mevalonate pathway, effect of statins 145–6
microalbuminuria, in definition of metabolic
    syndrome 90
microsomal triglyceride transfer protein
    inhibitors (MTPi) 127, 230
    intestinal 232
    site of action 124
    systemic 230–1
mipomersen 232–4
MIRACL (Myocardial Ischaemia Reduction
    with Aggressive Cholesterol Lowering)
    64, 65, 66, 67
MISTRAL study (implitapide) 230
MK0524A (laropiprant) 25, 122, 125, 130
MK0859 (anacetrapib) 126, 130, 239
mortality
    effect of intensive statin therapy 67
    relationship to blood pressure and total
        cholesterol 109
Multiple Risk Factor Intervention Trial
    (MRFIT) 7, 108, 109, 112–13, 157
muscle pain, statin therapy see myopathy
    risk, statins
myeloperoxidase 215
    in ACS 218, 219
myocardial infarction see acute coronary
    syndromes
myoglobin, ACS 218
myopathy risk, statins 20–1, 69, 227, 228, 256

n3-PUFA, GISSI-HF trial 149, 151
natriuretic peptides 217–18
neglected groups 251–2
neural network techniques, use in risk
    prediction 171
neuroprotection, statins 82
New Zealand, guidelines for statin therapy
    168–70
NHANES 48, 50
NHFA/CSANZ, guidelines for statin therapy
    168–9
niacin (nicotinic acid) 24–5, 96–7, 237–8

clinical trials 36, 197
    effect on cIMT 198–9
evidence base 245
use in FH 125
Niaspan 24, 97
NIPPON DATA80 risk chart 161, 163
nitric oxidase production, effect of statins 82,
    188
nitric oxide (NO) 214
    effect of ADMA 216
nitrosating agents 214
nitrotyrosines 215
non-adherence to therapy 246, 250
    detection and improvement 254
non-fasting blood samples 257
non-HDL-C
    correlation with apoB 50–2
    as measure of cardiovascular risk 48–50,
        52–4
Northwick Park Heart Study 48
novel agents
    apolipoprotein B antisense 127, 130,
        232–4
    cholesterol absorption inhibitors (CAi)
        234
    direct HDL therapy 36, 239–40
    endothelial lipase inhibitors 240
    microsomal triglyceride transfer protein
        inhibitors (MTPi) 124, 127, 230–2
    niacin formulations 237–8
    nuclear receptors and transcription factors
        240
    plasma delipidation 239
    requirement for 227
    squalene synthase inhibitors 228–30
    see also cholesteryl ester transfer protein
        (CETP) inhibitors
NPC1L1 (Niemann-Pick C1-like 1) protein
    119, 124
NT-proBNP (N-terminal prohormone brain
    natriuretic peptide) 217–18
number needed to treat 158
Nurses' Health Study 48, 157, 257

obesity/ overweight 8–9
    in definition of metabolic syndrome 89,
        90
    increasing prevalence 4, 246
optical coherence tomography (OCT) 204
ORION (Outcome of Rosuvastatin Treatment
    on Carotid Artery Atheroma: a Magnetic
    Resonance Imaging Observation) 204

oxidative stress, biomarkers
    in ACS 219
    in primary prevention 214–16

pactimibe 126
    IVUS study 202
    trial in FH 123
Pathobiological Determinants of
    Atherosclerosis in Youth study 161
PCSK9 (proprotein convertase
    subtilisin/kexin type 9) 118, 234, 235
    inhibition 127, 236–7
peritoneal dialysis, cholesterol levels 136
physical activity 257
    relationship to blood pressure 107
    secondary prevention programmes 252
    value in diabetes and metabolic syndrome
        100
physical inactivity 9
pioglitazone, effect on cIMT 199
pitavastatin
    effect on synoviocytes 186
    efficacy and safety 20
    see also statins
PLAC-1 (Pravastatin Limitation of
    Atherosclerosis in the Coronary Arteries)
    study 196
plant sterols and stanols 97, 124, 125
plaque compliance and strain assessment
    204
plaque regression
    angiographic studies 196–7
    cIMT studies 197–9
    computed tomography studies 203
    IVUS studies 199–203
    MRI studies 204
plaque stabilisation, statins 82
plasma delipidation 239
pleiotropic effects of statins 82, 145, 177–9,
    190
    in aortic valve stenosis and sclerosis
        180–3
    in arthritis 183–6
    bioprosthetic valve protection 179–80
    in sepsis 186–9
PLUTO trial 122
PO2579 trial 122
'polypills' 255–6
population-specific prediction functions 161,
    162–5
POSCH (Program on the Surgical Control of
    the Hyperlipidaemias) 178, 196

Post-CABG trial 98
PPAR (peroxisome proliferator-activated
    receptor) agonists 240
pravastatin
    clinical trials 35
        angiographic study 196
        LIPID trial 35, 48, 50, 63, 98, 111, 139,
            158, 252, 256
        PPP 138–40
        PROSPER 158, 256
        PROVE-IT TIMI 22 62, 64, 65–6, 67, 68,
            69, 71, 80, 143, 200
        serial IVUS study 200
    effect on cIMT 198
    efficacy and safety 20
    risk of muscular symptoms 228
    use in children with FH 128
    use in hypertension (ALLHAT) 109
    see also statins
pre-alpha-HDLs 34
pre-beta-HDLs 34
pregnancy, management of FH 129–30
PREMIER (Prospective Registry Evaluating
    Myocardial Infarction: Events and
    Recovery) registry 252
prevention
    cost-effectiveness 250–1, 252
    see also primary prevention; secondary
        prevention
primary care 253–4
primary prevention
    biomarkers
        of inflammation 213–14
        multiple marker assessment 216
        of oxidative stress 214–16
    non-adherence 246
    risk stratification 212–13
    of stroke, role of statins 77–8
PRIMO (Prediction of Muscular Risk in
    Observational Conditions) study 228
PROCAM risk score 163
procoagulant state, sepsis, effect of statins
    188
PROGRESS (Perindopril Protection against
    Recurrent Stroke Study) 108
Prospective Pravastatin Pooling (PPP) project
    139
Prospective Studies Collaboration (PSC) 5, 6
PROSPER (PROspective Study of Pravastatin
    in the Elderly at Risk) 158, 256
protein isoprenylation, effect of statins 177,
    178

proteinuria, association with rosuvastatin 21
PROVE-IT TIMI 22 (Pravastatin or
    Atorvastatin Evaluation and Infection
    Therapy) 62, 64, 65–6, 67, 68, 69, 71, 80,
    143, 200
provider factors in undertreatment 250

QRISK2 score 164, 167
Quality and Outcomes Framework, UK 253
Quebec Cardiovascular Study 48

RAAVE (Rosuvastatin Affecting Aortic Valve
    Endothelium) study 182
Rac1, effect of statins 178
RADIANCE (Rating Atherosclerotic Disease
    change by Imaging with A New CETP
    Inhibitor) trial 36–7, 122, 126, 199
RANTES, effect of statins 188
Ras activation, effect of statins 178
REACH (Reduction of Atherosclerosis for
    Continued Health) Registry 245, 247
reactive oxygen species (ROS) 214
recombinant human lipoprotein AI$_{Milano}$ 239,
    240
    plaque regression 201, 202
REGRESS (Regression Growth Evaluation
    Statin Substudy) 198
relative risk 157
relative risk reduction 158
resins see bile acid sequestrants
REVERSAL (Reversal of Atherosclerosis with
    Aggressive Lipid Lowering) study 200
reverse cholesterol transport 47
Reynolds risk scores 164
rhabdomyolysis risk, statins 20–1, 69, 227,
    228, 256
rHDL (reconstituted HDL) infusions 36
rheumatoid arthritis, effect of statins 184–6
RhoA, effect of statins 178
rimonabant 240
risk
    concept of 157–8
    rational for absolute risk assessment
        156–7
risk assessment
    Framingham risk equations, validity in
        other populations 159–60
    future developments 170–1
    as guideline to therapy 167, 170
    inclusion of new markers 166–7
    in people with diabetes 165, 166
    population-specific tools 162–5

tools derived from Framingham Heart
        Study 159
    tools from populations other than FHS
        participants 160–1
    in women 161, 166
    in younger adults 161
    see also biomarkers
risk communication 255
risk factors 9–10
    associations with cardiovascular diseases,
        global differences 5–6
    attributable risks 6–9
    clustering 108
    global trends 3–5
risk stratification
    primary prevention 212–13
        biomarkers 213–16
    secondary prevention 217
        biomarkers 217–19
Riskard risk software 164
rosuvastatin
    association with proteinuria 21
    ASTEROID trial 145
    CORONA study 68–9, 146–9
    effect in aortic valve stenosis 182, 183
    effect on cIMT 198
    efficacy and safety 20
    GISSI-HF trial 149
    JUPITER study 246–9
    MRI study 204
    serial IVUS study 200
    trial in FH patients 122
    see also statins
RXRα agonists 240

SALTIRE (Scottish Aortic Stenosis Lipid
    Lowering Trial, Impact on Regression)
    182
Scandinavian Simvastatin Survival Study (4S)
    35, 48, 98, 143, 150, 158, 256
scavenger receptor B1 (SR-B1) 30, 31, 32
SCORE (Systematic COronary Risk
    Evaluation) risk charts 157, 160, 164
SEARCH (Study of the Effectiveness of
    Additional Reductions in Cholesterol and
    Homocysteine) 21, 68
SEAS (Simvastatin and Ezetimibe in Aortic
    Stenosis) study 182
secondary prevention 217
    biomarkers
        multiple markers strategy 219
        natriuretic peptides 217–18

secondary prevention (continued)
    oxidative stress 219
    troponins 217
    of stroke, role of statins 78
        SPARCL study 78–80, 82–4
secondary prevention programmes 252
selenocystein-tRNA, effect of statins 146
SENDCAP (St Mary's, Ealing, Northwick
    Park Diabetes Cardiovascular Disease
    Prevention) study 99
sepsis, effect of statins 186–9
SHARP (Study of Heart and Renal
    Protection) 23, 24, 140
side-effects
    of bile acid sequestrants 24
    of ezetimibe 23
    of mipomersen 233–4
    of MTPis 230, 231
    of niacin 24, 96–7
    of statins 20–1, 69, 227, 228, 256
simvastatin
    4S 35, 48, 98, 143, 150, 158, 256
    angiographic studies 196, 197
    combination with ezetimibe 73, 198
    combination with niacin 237
    comparison with atorvastatin in FH 119,
        121
    cost 70
    effect in aortic valve stenosis 182
    effect in sepsis 187
    efficacy and safety 20, 21
    MRI studies 204
    risk of muscular symptoms 228
    use in children with FH 128
    see also statins
SLx-4090 232
small dense LDLs 15, 45, 93
    formation 46
small vessel disease, stroke risk 80
smoking 8
    prevalence in developing countries 4
    prevalence in US 3
socioeconomic factors
    in CVD 2–3
    in undertreatment 249
socioeconomic status, inclusion in risk
    prediction tools 167
SPARCL (Stroke Prevention by Aggressive
    Reduction in Cholesterol Levels) study
    78–80, 82, 83–4, 179
    target LDL-C 80–2
spherical HDLs 31, 32, 34

squalene synthase 120
squalene synthase inhibitors 126, 228–30
stanols 97, 125
STARS (St Thomas' Atherosclerosis
    Regression Study) 196
statins 29, 156–7
    clinical trials 21–2, 35
        angiographic studies 196, 197
        in ACS 63–5
        effect on cIMT 198–9
        in ESKD, 4D study 136–7
        in heart failure 146–51
        after kidney transplantation, ALERT
            137–8
        MRI studies 204
        serial IVUS studies 199–201
    combination with ezetimibe 23, 24, 97, 121
    combination with niacin 24–5, 237
    contraindications 21
    CRP reduction 214
    effect on coronary calcification 203
    effect on kidney function 140
    effect on LDL particle composition 55
    efficacy 19–20
    evidence base 245
        JUPITER study 246–9
    guidelines for use 168–70
    and heart failure 143, 151–2
        clinical trials 146–51
        possible harmful effects 145–6
        potential beneficial effects 144–5
        relationship to mortality 147
    intensive therapy
        in ACS 65–6
        costs 70
        meta-analyses 66–9
        safety and efficacy 69–70
        stable CHD patients 61–3
        stroke prevention 80–1, 83
    interaction with beta-blockers 146
    mechanism of action 119, 229
    mode of action 19
    pleiotropic effects 82, 145, 177–9, 190
        in aortic valve stenosis and sclerosis
            180–3
        in arthritis 183–6
        bioprosthetic valve protection 179–80
        in sepsis 186–9
    side effects 20–1, 69, 227, 228, 256
    stroke prevention 77–8, 79, 83–4
        mechanisms of benefit 82, 83
        SPARCL study 78–80

target LDL-C 80–2
treatment gap 54
use in chronic kidney disease 136, 138–40
use in diabetes 94–6, 98, 100
use by elderly people 251
use in FH 119
    children 128, 129
use in hypertension 109–11
use by women 251
sterols 97, 124, 125
Still's disease, effect of atorvastatin 184, 185
stroke 77
    geographical differences 2
stroke prevention
    future perspectives 82–3
    LDL-C target levels 80–2
    role of statins 77–8, 79, 83–4
        mechanisms of benefit 82, 83
        SPARCL study 78–80
stroke risk
    4D study 137
    relationship to cardiovascular risk factors
        5, 6, 18
    relationship to LDL-C reduction 79
surface lipid exchange, lipoprotein particles
    46
syndrome X 89
    see also metabolic syndrome
synoviocytes, effect of statins 186
systemic juvenile idiopathic arthritis, effect of
    atorvastatin 184, 185

T cells, effect of statins 188
TAK-475-061 trial 123
TARA (Trial of Atorvastatin in Rheumatoid
    Arthritis) 185
therapeutic lifestyle change, value in diabetes
    and metabolic syndrome 100
therapeutic targets 52–3
thiazide diuretics 111
    lipid and lipoprotein effects 112–13
THROMBO study 48
thrombosis inhibition, HDLs 33
TNT (Treatment to New Targets) trial 30, 61,
    62, 63, 68, 69, 71–2, 80, 98, 139–40
    stroke prevention 78
TOMHS (Treatment of Mild Hypertension
    Study) 113
torcetrapib 36–7, 122, 126, 199, 201–2, 203,
    238–9
total cholesterol
    effect of antihypertensive drugs 112, 113

relationship to CHD risk 5, 6, 7, 8, 17–18
relationship to stroke risk 6
trends 3, 4–5
transcription factors, as therapeutic targets
    240
transient ischaemic attacks (TIA)
    SPARCL study 78–80
    see also stroke; stroke prevention
treatment gap 54
triglycerides
    in chronic kidney disease 135
    in definition of metabolic syndrome 90
    effect of antihypertensive drugs 112, 113
    effect on Friedwald equation 16
    effect of statins 19
    importance as risk factor 5
    relationship to LDL particle size and
        composition 54–5
    and risk of recurrent CHD 70–1
    see also hypertriglyceridaemia
triparanol 228
TRIPLE study 122, 124
troponins 217
type III hyperlipoproteinaemia (familial
    dysbetalipoproteinaemia) 49–50, 52

ubiquinone (coenzyme Q10) 228
    effect of statins 146
UKPDS risk engine 165, 166
undertreatment 245–6, 248
    contributing factors 249–50
    neglected groups 251–2
United States Renal Data System (USRDS)
    136
US NCEP ATP III, guidelines for statin
    therapy 168–9

VA-HIT (Veterans Affairs High-Density
    Lipoprotein Intervention Trial) 35, 97,
    99
valve interstitial cells (VICs) 181, 183
vascular cell adhesion molecule-1 (VCAM-1)
    expression, effect of HDLs 32, 33
verapamil, interaction with statins 21
very low-density lipoproteins (VLDLs) 44
    in diabetes and metabolic syndrome 93
    effect of statins 19
    synthesis 120

waist circumference 90
warfarin control, effect of statins 21
WEL-410 trial 122

WHO (World Health Organisation),
    definition of metabolic syndrome 90
women
    benefits of statin therapy 251
    risk prediction 161, 164, 166
Women's Health Study 48
World Health Report 2002 8–9

WOSCOPS (West of Scotland Coronary
    Prevention Study) 35, 139, 158

younger adults, risk assessment 161

zaragozic acids 229